# The Ultimate Childproofing Home Guide

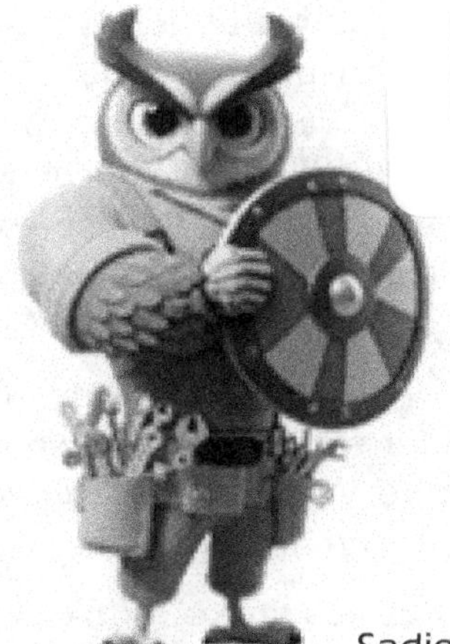

Sadie Hootenanny

**Infant/Non-mobile: (Birth - 6 months)**
**Infant Crawl/Roll: (5 months - 1 year)**
**Toddler/Pre-school: (1 year - 4 years)**
**School-age: (5 years - 6+ years)**

EVERPRESENT
North America Inc.
Copyright © 2026
ISBN: 979-8-9924367-3-0
AJ Baroody

Published by Everpresent North America Inc.
Second Edition: March 2026
UltimateChildproofingguide.com
Soft Cover:  ISBN: 979-8-9924367-3-0
AJ Baroody

---

## From the Author

**This book is packed with detailed information, and I'll admit it might sometimes feel overwhelming. But here's the thing: you don't need to implement every single tip or suggestion. Instead, think of it as a resource to heighten your awareness.** Use your best judgment and keep the key ideas in mind as you childproof your space. The goal is to help you spot potential hazards that might otherwise go unnoticed, not to make you worry about everything.

Childproofing is about taking reasonable precautions, not living in constant fear. The steps you take will give you peace of mind, knowing that you've created a safer environment for your kids. Minimizing regrets starts with being proactive. After all, your children are your top priority, and there's no need to cut corners when it comes to their safety.

That said, **it's essential to strike a balance.** You don't want to overprotect or shelter your kids from every little bump or bruise. These are natural parts of growing up and learning. Instead, take the necessary steps to protect them from severe dangers while allowing them to explore, grow, and experience life. Your role is to create a safe space where they can do that freely.

---

## Disclaimer

The information provided in this book is intended to serve as a general guide to childproofing and promoting safety in your home. While the author and publisher have made every effort to ensure the accuracy and completeness of the information contained herein, they make no guarantees, warranties, or representations, either express or implied, concerning the safety, efficacy, or appropriateness of any of the methods, products, or suggestions described in this book.

Childproofing is a complex and nuanced task; what may be appropriate and effective in one situation may not be in another. It is the reader's responsibility to assess the unique circumstances of their home and to exercise due diligence, caution, and common sense in implementing any childproofing measures. The reader is strongly encouraged to consult with a professional childproofing expert or other qualified professionals to ensure the safety of their home environment.

The author and publisher disclaim all liability for any injuries, losses, or damage that may result from the use or misuse of the information in this book, and they shall not be held responsible for any errors, omissions, or inaccuracies in the content. Remember, no book can replace the personalized advice and expertise of a certified professional in child safety. Your child's safety is of the utmost importance, and we urge you to prioritize it above all else.

---

### Acknowledgments

I am incredibly grateful to Lori. From the beginning, her role as a mother and a creative thinker has been at the heart of this project. Lori brought to the table her deep experience as a parent and an intuitive understanding of what truly matters when protecting children. Her insights, grounded in real-life challenges and triumphs, have shaped this book in ways that go beyond words.

Lori's creative spark and hands-on approach have enriched every chapter. She has an uncanny ability to see practical solutions where others see problems, and her suggestions are always thoughtful and actionable. Her contributions were not just helpful, they were transformation.

**Thank you, Lori, for your boundless creativity**, your wisdom, and, most of all, your unshakable support throughout this journey. You were more than a contributor; you were a partner in bringing this book to life. Your passion for child safety shines through every page, and this book is as much a reflection of your influence as it is of my work.

---

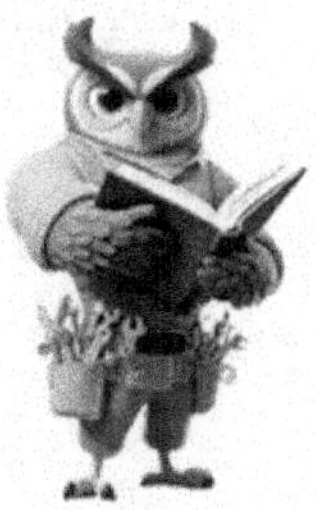

# Table of Contents

## Childproofing Chronicles

<u>**Book Introduction**</u>

The joy of watching a child explore, learn, and grow within the home is one of the most rewarding experiences for any parent. There's something magical about seeing your little one take their first wobbly steps, touch everything in sight with wide-eyed curiosity, and begin to understand the world around them. However, with this excitement comes an undeniable reality: with exploration comes risk.

According to the Centers for Disease Control and Prevention, a staggering 8.7 million children are treated in emergency departments for unintentional injuries every year, and many of these incidents happen right in the comfort of their own homes. That statistic is more than just a number; it's a reminder of how quickly a routine day can take a dangerous turn.

The home, with all its corners, edges, and seemingly innocent everyday objects, can present many hidden dangers for young children. Approximately 500,000 children under the age of 6 are treated in emergency rooms annually due to accidental poisoning, with medications and household cleaners being the top culprits.

This book is designed to be your trusted companion as you embark on the journey of childproofing. We know the challenges you face, and we're here to guide you every step of the way. Through expert insights, practical tips, and an easy-to-follow guide to common household dangers, we'll help you identify the areas that need attention and show you how to address them.

---

*"Within these walls, no harm shall reach the little feet that run free."*

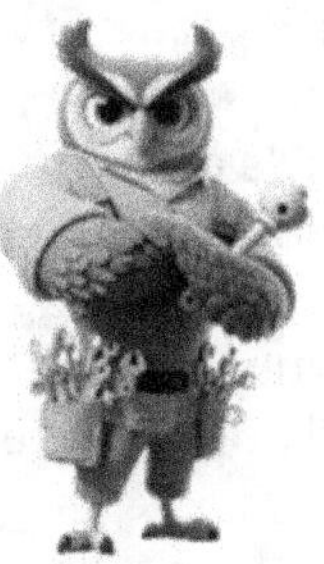

 # Foyer/Main Entrance

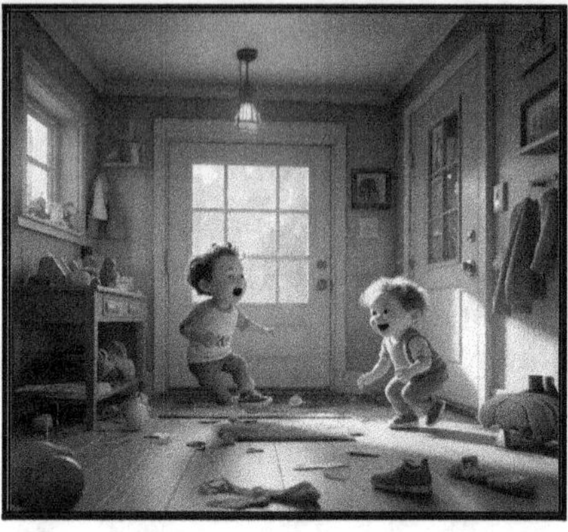

**Introduction:** Childproofing a foyer is a pivotal step in creating a safe home environment. The foyer, as the initial entry point into the home, often experiences high traffic and can sometimes become slippery, posing a significant risk for little ones prone to slips and falls. From utilizing anti-slip coatings and quality mats to establishing a safe footwear policy and ensuring adequate lighting, each aspect plays a crucial role in enhancing safety.

---

**Foyer/Main Entrance**
→ **Infant/Non-mobile: (Birth - 6 months)**
→ **Infant crawl/roll: (5 months - 1 year)**
→ **Toddler/Pre-school: (1 year - 4 years)**
→ **School-age: (5 years - 6+ years)**

# Clean Yourself Immediately

**Maintaining impeccable hygiene is paramount when caring for a child, especially newborns and infants.** Their developing immune systems make them particularly susceptible to germs and infections. Showering or washing up thoroughly before handling your child is a crucial preventative measure. **Routine tasks like diaper changing and feeding require meticulous attention to hygiene.** Washing your hands before and after these activities can significantly reduce the risk of contaminating the baby's area. Germs can easily irritate sensitive skin, making it essential to maintain a clean environment. To ensure a safe environment for your baby, encourage everyone to wash their hands before touching them. Regularly sanitizing commonly touched items, such as toys, pacifiers, and door handles, is also essential.

---

<u>**Foyer/Main Entrance**</u>
Infant/Non-mobile: (Birth - 6 months)
→ **Infant crawl/roll: (5 months - 1 year)**
→ **Toddler/Pre-school: (1 year - 4 years)**
→ **School-age: (5 years - 6+ years)**

# Tables and Stands

**Small tables, often used for keys or mail, can be dangerous for young children who might bump into them, leading to injuries. According to the CPS, each year in the U.S., around 2,400 young children (aged 0–6) are treated in emergency rooms for injuries caused by tables and stands tipping over.** It's essential to identify and pad surfaces that are at the right height to harm a child.

Various safety padding options are available, from corner guards to elasticized bumpers. Whichever you choose, ensure it's securely attached to prevent choking hazards. Coffee tables for infants or kitchen tables for older toddlers are particularly risky. By focusing on these details, you can create a safe, enjoyable environment for your child to explore.

---

<u>**Foyer/Main Entrance**</u>
Infant/Non-mobile: (Birth - 6 months)
Infant crawl/roll: (5 months - 1 year)
→ **Toddler/Pre-school: (1 year - 4 years)**
→ **School-age: (5 years - 6+ years)**

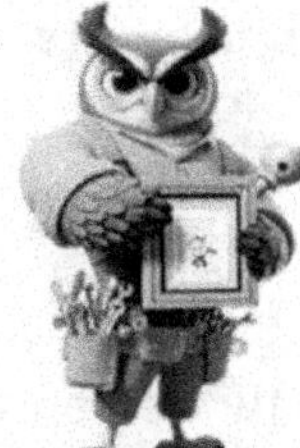

# Loose Picture Frames

**Picture frames, especially those loosely placed on tables, pose a hidden danger in homes with inquisitive toddlers.** Young children have a high risk of these frames being knocked over, and their sharp corners can cause injuries. Additionally, the glass in these frames can shatter if dropped, intensifying the hazard.

To ensure child safety, **consider wall-mounting frames or using adhesive methods like Velcro strips or Fun-Tak to secure free-standing frames on surfaces.** While displaying memories adds warmth to a home, prioritizing safety ensures a risk-free environment for children to explore.

---

# Slippery Floors

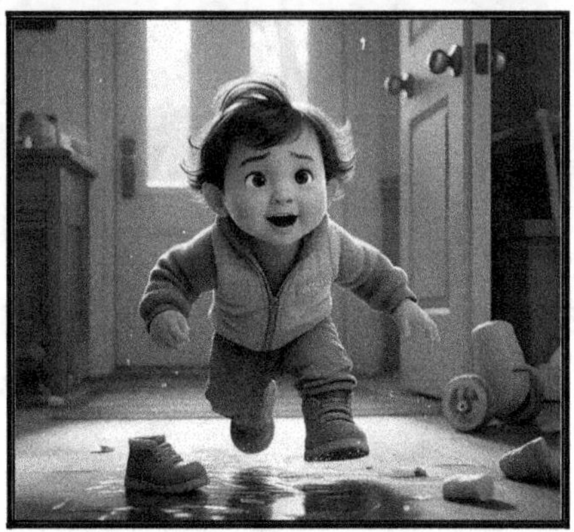

**Approximately 230,000 children ages 0-4 are treated in US emergency departments each year for fall-related injuries.** In our quest for childproofing and safety, it's essential to be mindful of our surroundings. Take a moment to check for any areas with sagging floors, as these can accumulate water over time, creating slip hazards, especially for little feet running around.

To further prevent slipping accidents, **ensure you have a doormat in place, especially during wet weather or when your pet comes indoors with muddy paws.** Standing water can quickly turn into a slipping hazard, and a doormat helps trap excess moisture and debris, keeping your floors safer for everyone.

While cleaning your home, **be cautious when using furniture polish on your console or other wooden surfaces.** Splatters of polish can inadvertently make the floor as smooth and slick as the table, increasing the risk of accidental slips. Take your time and clean mindfully, wiping away any excess polish that may have found its way to the floor.

---

**<u>Foyer/Main Entrance</u>**
Infant/Non-mobile: (Birth - 6 months)
Infant crawl/roll: (5 months - 1 year)
→ **Toddler/Pre-school: (1 year - 4 years)**
→ **School-age: (5 years - 6+ years)**

# Secure Throw Rugs

**Throw rugs and doormats, especially on hardwood or laminate floors, can be slip hazards if they move or bunch up.** While adults might navigate these with caution, children running around might not be as careful. To prevent accidents, it's vital to secure these mats with tape, especially near potentially dangerous areas like the top of stairs.

**Using the correct adhesive ensures mats stay put without damaging the floor.** According to a study published in the American Journal of Emergency Medicine, approximately 12,300 patients were treated in U.S. emergency departments for rug-related injuries. By securing your rugs and mats, you prioritize safety, making your home safer for everyone.

---

**<u>Foyer/Main Entrance</u>**
Infant/Non-mobile: (Birth - 6 months)
Infant crawl/roll: (5 months - 1 year)
→ **Toddler/Pre-school: (1 year - 4 years)**
→ **School-age: (5 years - 6+ years)**

# Coat Access

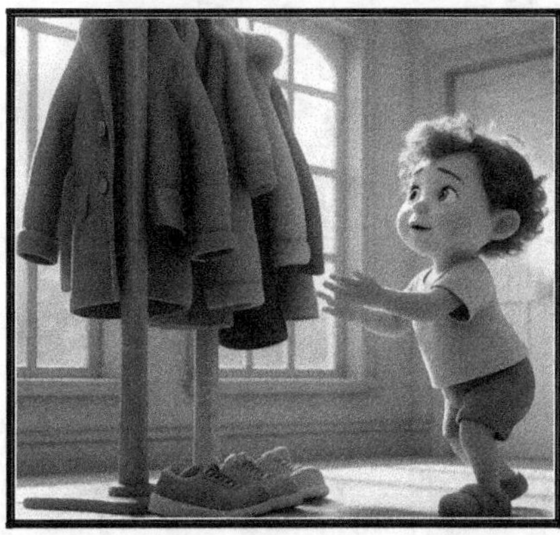

**Coat racks, although functional for hanging outerwear, can pose unexpected dangers that we shouldn't overlook.** These racks are often designed to be top-heavy, making them prone to tipping over with even a slight force applied. The sharp hooks they feature can also become hazardous, particularly for small children who may accidentally run into them or pull on their coats.

The risks don't stop there. **Coat pockets might contain items that are not safe for children**, and it's challenging to inspect every pocket thoroughly. Lighters, tobacco products, or unlabeled medicines might be lurking, presenting potential dangers to curious hands. To eliminate any potential hazards and prioritize everyone's safety, it's best to utilize the closet for coat storage instead. Using a coat storage closet creates a controlled and secure space where any potentially harmful items are kept out of reach of curious little ones.

---

**Foyer/Main Entrance**
Infant/Non-mobile: (Birth - 6 months)
Infant crawl/roll: (5 months - 1 year)
→ **Toddler/Pre-school: (1 year - 4 years)**
→ **School-age: (5 years - 6+ years)**

# TRIPPING HAZARDS

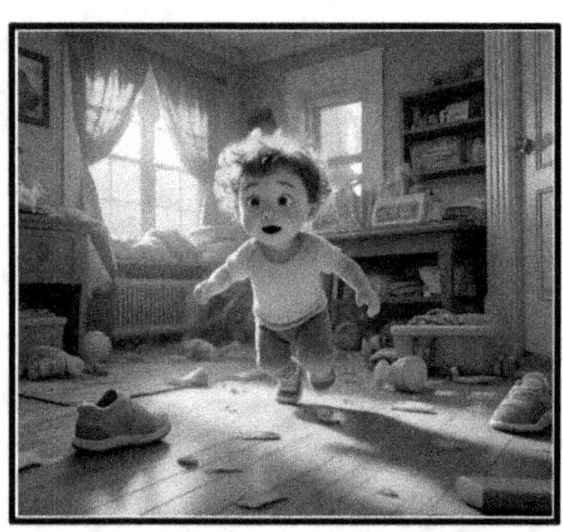

**Loose shoes and random items scattered at the doorway can be an unexpected tripping hazard, particularly when rushing into the house or carrying something bulky inside.** A simple misstep can lead to an unfortunate accident. To ensure a safe and clutter-free entrance, it's best to designate a specific spot for shoes.

**Consider keeping discarded shoes in a closet or storage bin near the doorway.** If you have the space, a bench with room underneath is an excellent solution. This way, both kids and adults can comfortably sit down to put on or take off their shoes. Once done, the shoes can be neatly tucked away out of sight and out of the way, ensuring a clear pathway for everyone.

---

🐛 According to a study published in the Journal of Injury & Violence Research, carpets and throw rugs were responsible for nearly 38,000 emergency room visits over a seven-year period. (Consumer Notice) And it gets worse.  Loose rugs and cluttered floors account for 25% of all home-based trips, and stairs without handrails increase the probability of a fall by 3 times. The foyer is the first place shoes, bags, and backpacks pile up. Making it one of the most overlooked danger zones in the home. (Sources: Journal of Injury & Violence Research *via ConsumerNotice.org; WifaTalents Slips, Trips & Falls Data Report 2026*)

---

**Foyer/Main Entrance**
Infant/Non-mobile: (Birth - 6 months)
→ **Infant crawl/roll: (5 months - 1 year)**
→ **Toddler/Pre-school: (1 year - 4 years)**
→ **School-age: (5 years - 6+ years)**

# Sneaker Odor/Bacteria

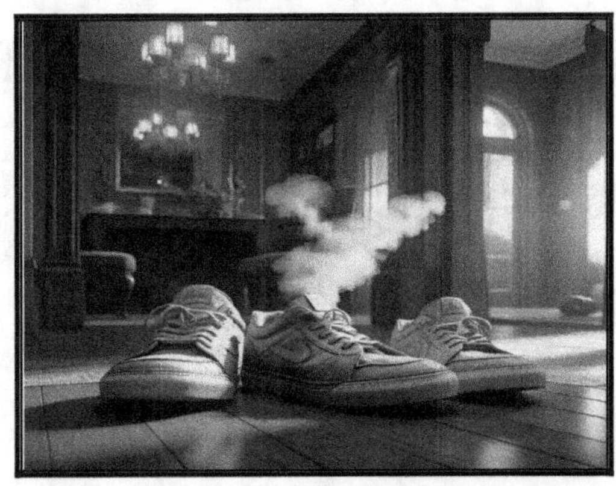

When it comes to taking care of your sneakers, **there are a few essential points to consider. One common issue is unpleasant odors, which are often caused by lingering bacteria in the soft, foamy insert**. To combat this, you can try spraying the inside with a good disinfectant or sprinkling some baking soda to absorb the moisture and odor. For more thorough cleaning, gently washing them can work wonders in refreshing your favorite pair. To ensure the longevity of your sneakers and maintain proper foot support, it's advisable to alternate the shoes you wear day after day. This practice helps prevent early arch breakdown. When purchasing new sneakers, it's vital to choose the right size. Shoes that are too big or too small can lead to discomfort, blisters, and potential foot issues, especially for growing kids. Children's feet grow rapidly, so it's essential to measure their feet regularly and get them properly fitted shoes.

<u>**Foyer/Main Entrance**</u>
Infant/Non-mobile: (Birth - 6 months)
Infant crawl/roll: (5 months - 1 year)
→ **Toddler/Pre-school: (1 year - 4 years)**
→ **School-age: (5 years - 6+ years)**

# Secure Doors

**Childproofing doorknobs in your home is crucial to prevent children from accessing dangerous areas or getting locked in rooms.** Different doorknobs require specific safety measures. For lever handles, install locks that require dual-action to open, use a Door Monkey, or create DIY solutions with rubber bands to restrict movement. For round doorknobs, use knob covers or Grip 'n Twist covers that are difficult for toddlers to operate. For oval or egg-shaped knobs, use custom covers or childproofing straps to prevent easy access. Additionally, pinch guards and door alarms should be installed, and children should be educated about the dangers of unsupervised access to certain rooms.

---

☙ Nearly half of all pediatric fingertip injuries are caused by door jams, and up to **91.6% of all traumatic amputations in children are specifically related to fingers being crushed in doors.** The Shock Factor: We often focus on the "latch side" (fingers getting pinched when the door shuts), but the hinge side is far more dangerous, exerting up to 40 tons of pressure per square inch. *American Journal of Pediatrics (2021) & The Journal of Trauma (CIRP).*

---

<u>**Foyer/Main Entrance**</u>
Infant/Non-mobile: (Birth - 6 months)
Infant crawl/roll: (5 months - 1 year)
→ **Toddler/Pre-school: (1 year - 4 years)**
→ **School-age: (5 years - 6+ years)**

# Screen Doors

Screen doors are a wonderful addition to many homes, allowing fresh air to circulate while keeping pests out. However, they can pose certain risks for households with young children. Upgrade to a more durable screen material that can withstand pushes and pulls from curious little hands. Consider materials like pet-resistant screens, which are tear and puncture-resistant.

Install a pneumatic or hydraulic door closer to ensure the door closes slowly, reducing the risk of it slamming on a child's fingers. Install a high latch or bolt out of the reach of children to prevent them from opening the door and wandering outside unsupervised. Sometimes, children may not recognize the screen and might walk or run into it. Place decals or stickers at their eye level to give them a clear visual indication that the screen door is closed.

---

**Foyer/Main Entrance**
Infant/Non-mobile: (Birth - 6 months)
Infant crawl/roll: (5 months - 1 year)
→ **Toddler/Pre-school: (1 year - 4 years)**
→ **School-age: (5 years - 6+ years)**

# FOYER CLOSET

**That innocent coat closet can be a treasure trove of hazards for curious explorers.** Heavy coats and bags topple easily when little hands start pulling. Keys, batteries, and small tools tucked in pockets or bags become choking hazards the moment children discover them.

**Start with a childproof door lock installed high enough that children cannot reach it.** This simple barrier prevents unsupervised closet adventures. Inside, organize strategically. Place small objects like keys and batteries on the highest shelves, preferably in labeled bins with secure lids. Install hooks high on the wall for bags and purses that might contain medications or sharp objects. Anchor these hooks securely so determined tugging cannot pull them down.

**Store heavy items like boots and bags at the bottom of the closet, pushed toward the back.** This lowers the center of gravity and reduces toppling risks when the door swings open. If cleaning supplies or chemicals have somehow ended up in the foyer closet, relocate them immediately to a higher, locked cabinet elsewhere. Always keep such items in original containers to prevent confusion and potential poisoning.

**Sharp objects need special consideration.** Umbrellas with pointed tips should be stored horizontally on high hooks with protective covers over the sharp ends. This keeps them both out of reach and less dangerous if somehow accessed.

**Minimize clutter by rotating seasonal items.** Keep only current season necessities in the foyer closet and store off-season gear in less accessible spaces. This reduces both hazards and temptation. As your child grows more adventurous, inspect the closet regularly, especially when rotating seasonal items. What worked six months ago might not suffice for your newly mobile explorer.

---

# INSTALL ENVIRONMENT DETECTORS

**Smoke detectors** belong on every floor, especially near sleeping areas. These lifesavers require regular maintenance to function when needed most. Test batteries monthly and replace them twice yearly. That chirping sound signals low battery power, so address it immediately rather than ignoring the annoyance.

**Keep detectors dust-free for optimal functionality**. If you have wired detectors, the periodic flashing light confirms they're working. For households with hearing-impaired members, choose detectors with visual and tactile alerts. A well-maintained smoke detector provides peace of mind and could save your family's life.

**Carbon monoxide detectors** are equally critical. The CDC reports over 20,000 children hospitalized annually from CO exposure. This colorless, odorless gas results from incomplete combustion in household appliances, making detection impossible without proper equipment.

**Install CO detectors near bedrooms and living spaces.** Test them regularly and ensure all fuel-burning appliances receive proper maintenance and ventilation. Watch for warning signs like orange flames in appliances, which indicate potential problems. Blue flames signal proper combustion.

**Inspect flues regularly for blockages that can cause CO buildup.** Ensure proper ventilation throughout your home and check appliances periodically for safety concerns. Never leave cars running in attached garages, even briefly. The CO can infiltrate your living spaces quickly and dangerously.

**If you rent, landlords must provide working detectors and maintain electrical and gas systems properly.** Don't hesitate to request maintenance or replacements. Your family's safety depends on these simple devices functioning correctly when needed. Regular attention to these often-forgotten items transforms your foyer from a potential danger zone into the safe, welcoming entrance your home deserves.

---

# KEY CONCERNS

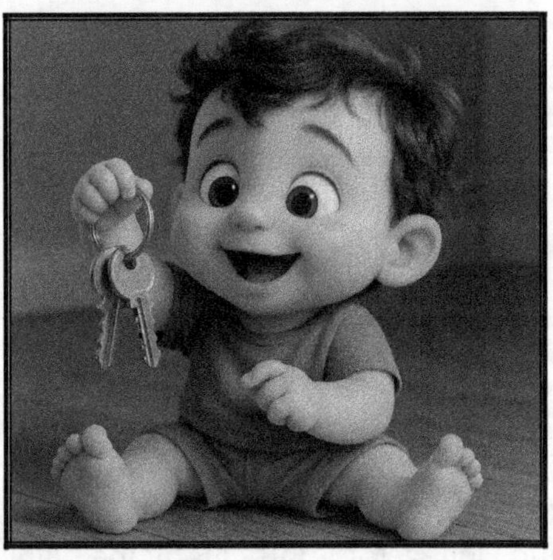

Keys serve a multitude of purposes, from unlocking doors and cabinets to accessing cars and gun safes. However, as versatile as they are, keys can pose significant risks to children if not handled cautiously. Keeping keys out of reach is essential to prevent children from accessing potentially dangerous items that could lead to accidents or injuries.

**Another important consideration is the presence of lead in both house and car keys, which is often mixed in with the brass.** Lead poisoning is a serious health concern, particularly for young children. Exposure to lead can lead to mental impairment, behavioral issues, hyperactivity, seizures, comas, and even death. To protect your children from lead exposure, it's essential to keep keys away from them. Babies and young children can absorb lead through their skin or accidentally ingest it by putting keys in their mouths. Always wash your hands thoroughly with soap and water after handling keys to minimize potential risks.

---

# BACKPACK WEIGHT

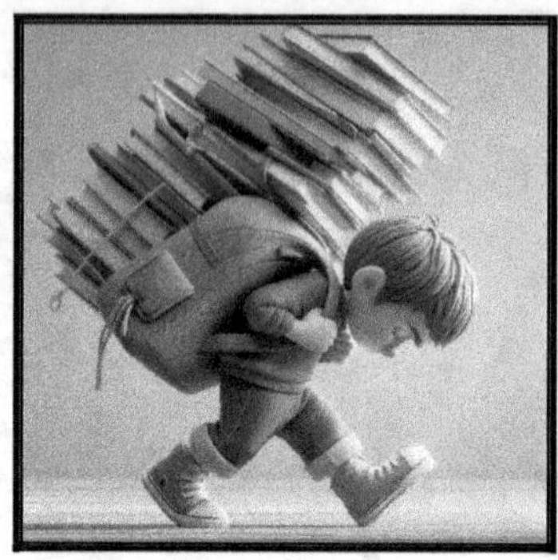

Attention to backpack weight and carrying method is essential to ensuring that children maintain good posture and avoid potential musculoskeletal issues. The American College of Sports Medicine highlights the impact of heavy backpacks on a child's posture, making it crucial to take appropriate preventive measures.

To prevent posture problems, the weight of a child's backpack should not exceed 10 percent of their body weight. You can calculate this by multiplying your child's weight in pounds by 0.10, which will give you the maximum recommended backpack weight in pounds. Consider using a rolling backpack as an effective solution to eliminate the weight burden. Encourage your child to vary how they carry their backpack each day to avoid placing excessive strain on the same muscles and joints.

---

🌰 That stuffed backpack your child lugs to school every day may be doing more damage than you think. **Every year, 5,000 children visit the emergency department for backpack-related injuries, and more than 14,000 children are treated annually for related problems.** With around 60% of orthopedic doctors reporting they are treating school-age children for back pain caused by backpack weight. Symmetryhealthchiropractic. The math is staggering: a child carrying a 12-pound backpack who sets it down just 10 times a day is lifting a cumulative total of 21,600 pounds. Roughly the weight of six mid-size cars. Symmetryhealthchiropractic. And most kids are carrying far more than they should. The American Academy of Pediatrics recommends a backpack weigh no more than 10% of a child's body weight. Yet studies show students on average carry 15% of their body weight. National Spine Health Foundation An MRI study published in the journal Spine made it even more concrete: imaging showed measurable compression of spinal discs and increased spinal curvature in children under_typical backpack_loads, with half of the children showing a significant spinal curve even at 18 pounds. And pain scores climbing sharply as weight increased. Wolters Kluwer *(Symmetry Health Chiropractic citing Children's Healthcare of Atlanta; National Spine Health Foundation / American Academy of Pediatrics; Wolters Kluwer / journal Spine MRI study)*

---

**<u>Foyer/Main Entrance</u>**
Infant/Non-mobile: (Birth - 6 months)
Infant crawl/roll: (5 months - 1 year)
→ **Toddler/Pre-school: (1 year - 4 years)**
→ **School-age: (5 years - 6+ years)**

# UMBRELLAS: AN OFTEN OVERLOOKED SAFETY MEASURE

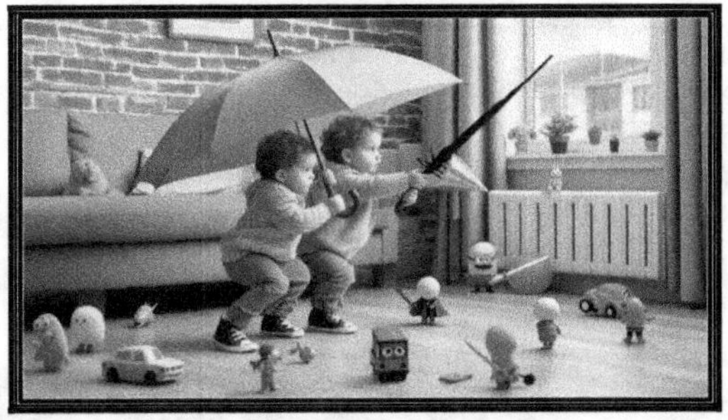

**Annually, approximately 1,000 children are injured by umbrellas and canes, including pokes and entanglements**. Umbrellas, often considered mundane household items, can pose a significant safety risk to young children. Their pointed ends and intricate mechanisms can cause accidental injuries. To create a safe home environment, it is essential to have childproof umbrellas. One effective way to minimize the risk is to store umbrellas in a secure, out-of-reach location. High shelves, locked closets, or designated umbrella holders are ideal options. This prevents children from accessing umbrellas unsupervised and potentially injuring themselves. Additionally, choosing umbrellas with rounded tips and child-friendly designs can further reduce the likelihood of accidents.

# |Ch 2| Living/Family Room

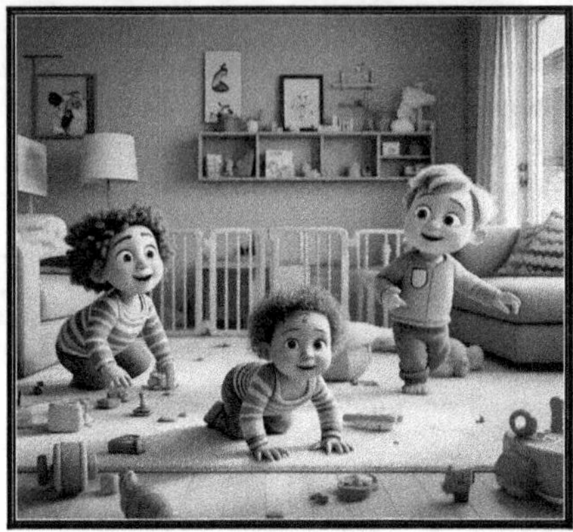

**Introduction:** The living room, often the heart of a home, is a hub of family activity. While it's a space for relaxation and bonding, it also presents numerous hazards for young explorers. This chapter delves into the essential steps to transform your living room into a safe haven for children. We cover everything from securing heavy furniture and electronics to ensuring cords and small decorative items are out of reach.

---

<u>Living Room/Family Room</u>
→ Infant/Non-mobile: (Birth - 6 months)
→ Infant crawl/roll: (5 months - 1 year)
→ Toddler/Pre-school: (1 year - 4 years)
→ School-age: (5 years - 6+ years)

# FIREPLACE

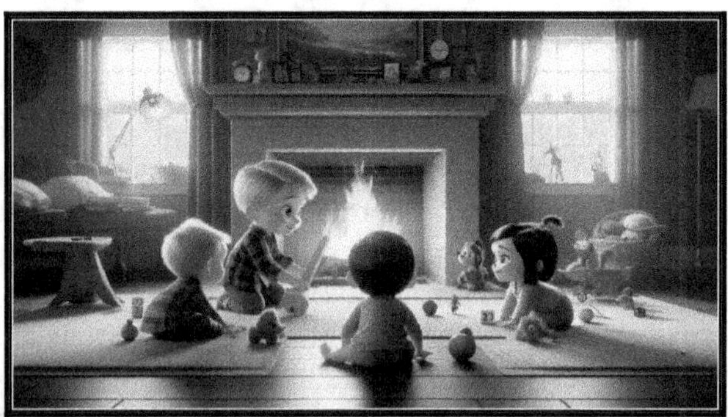

Over 1,000 children are injured each year from accidents involving fireplaces, candles, and other open flames in the U.S. Installing a

**baby safety fence around the fireplace effectively keeps curious toddlers at bay.** Ensure it is sturdy and tall enough to deter climbing attempts. Opt for heat-resistant glass doors that can function as a barrier to open flames.

**Creosote, a byproduct of burning wood, accumulates in chimneys and can ignite, causing dangerous chimney fires.** An annual sweep by a professional ensures this build-up is removed. Install carbon monoxide detectors in proximity to the fireplace and key areas throughout your home. This gas is undetectable by human senses, making these alarms vital.

The hearth, especially if made of stone or brick, can be a hazard for falls. Use specialized hearth padding or soft cushions to mitigate injury risks. Fireplace tools, while essential for maintaining a fire, can be hazardous in a child's hands. Store them securely, preferably in a locked cabinet or hung high out of reach.

---

<u>Living Room/Family Room</u>
Infant/Non-mobile: (Birth - 6 months)
→ **Infant crawl/roll: (5 months - 1 year)**
→ **Toddler/Pre-school: (1 year - 4 years)**
→ **School-age: (5 years - 6+ years)**

# FLOOD LAMP

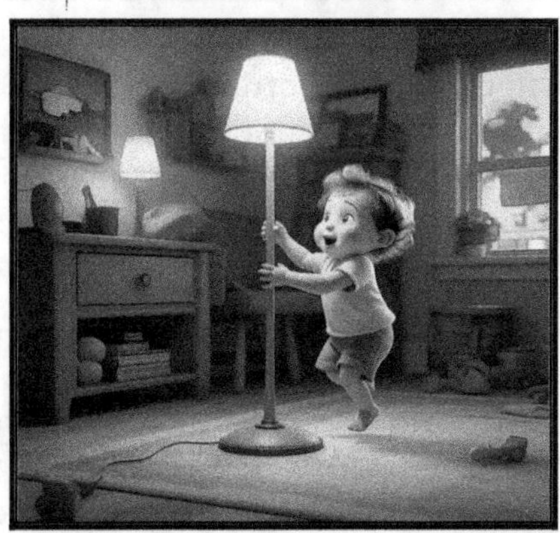

Though practical and stylish, floor lamps can present safety hazards, particularly the torchiere style that directs light upwards. These lamps have earned their torch-like name due to their potential to cause fires when knocked over. The combination of an unstable base and the presence of electricity makes them a significant risk in any home. **A common cause of accidents with torchiere floor lamps is their top-heavy design.** A slight bump or collision with furniture, pets, or even energetic children can cause the lamp to tip over. Once on the ground, the hot bulb or other electrical components can encounter flammable materials, leading to a potentially devastating fire. Choose lamps with a stable and sturdy base, ideally with a broad footprint to prevent tipping.

---



# Standing Fans

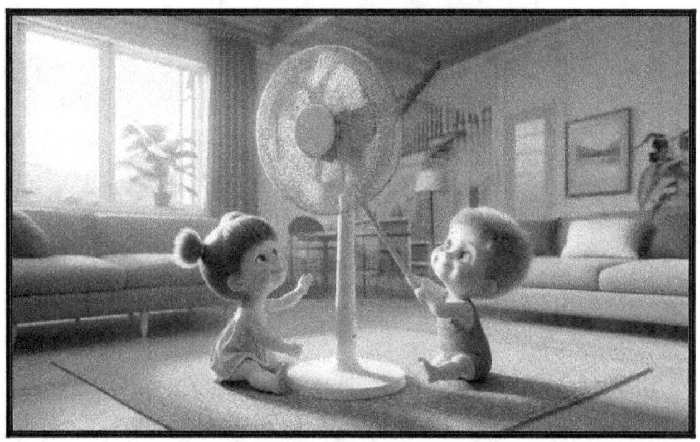

**Annually, approximately 2,500 children are injured by electric fans, including cuts from blades and electrical hazards.** Standing fans, while essential for comfort, especially during warmer months, can pose potential hazards to young children. Their curiosity and natural inclination to explore can lead them to these fans, making it crucial for parents and guardians to ensure their safety.

**Position the fan on a tall piece of furniture or a dedicated fan stand that is out of the reach of children.** Invest in high-quality fan guards with smaller gaps, which ensure tiny  fingers can't slip through. Ensure the fan's base is sturdy to prevent it from being easily tipped over. Some fans come with broader bases or weighted bottoms for added stability. Use cord organizers or covers to keep the fan's electrical cord out of sight and reach, preventing tripping or tugging hazards.

---

# Table edges

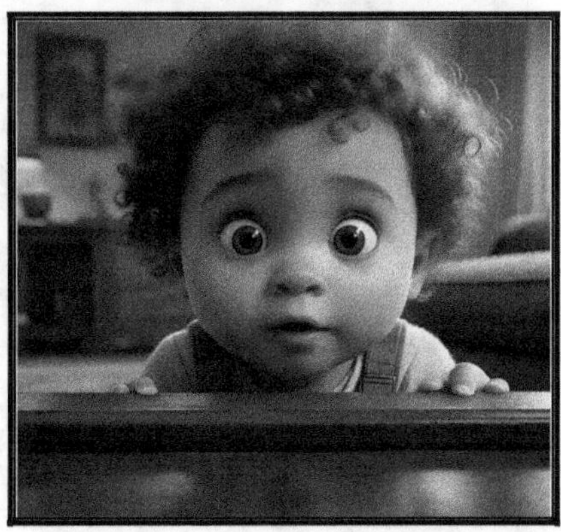

**Tables at a child's head height pose the greatest injury risk. If your table stands less than 36 inches tall, childproofing becomes essential. Children bump heads while climbing or playing nearby, often with surprising force.**

Safety padding comes in various forms: corner guards for sharp angles, long padded strips for edges, and elasticized bumpers for curved surfaces. Choose based on your table's design and your child's typical play patterns. Install the padding securely and inspect it regularly to ensure it remains firmly attached. Damaged or loose padding becomes a choking hazard itself.

Secure tables to walls using anchors or safety straps to prevent tipping when climbed. Remove small objects like figurines, coins, and beads that present choking risks. Keep table surfaces clear of clutter to reduce tripping hazards and improve visibility. As your child grows and becomes more mobile, reassess your approach. What works for a crawler may need adjustment once that same child starts climbing furniture like a miniature mountaineer.

---

# Record Player and Records

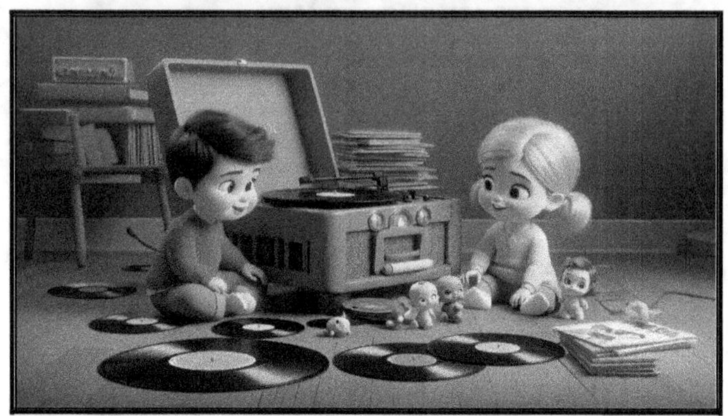

Record players fascinate toddlers who see them as spinning rides waiting to happen. Keep players on high, stable surfaces out of reach. Use the dust cover religiously to protect both the equipment and curious fingers from the needle. Store vinyl records vertically on high shelves or in locked cabinets.

---

🍃 Vinyl records are made of Polyvinyl Chloride (PVC), and until recently, many were stabilized with lead or softened with phosphates, which can make up to 40% of the weight of a soft plastic product. If a teething toddler chews on the edge of a vintage record, they aren't just damaging your music; they are directly ingesting **"the most hazardous plastic for children's health."** PVC is known to off-gas VOCs and, when chewed, can leach endocrine-disrupting chemicals. *Center for Health, Environment & Justice (CHEJ) and The Ecology Center.*

Vintage records (pre-2008) are particularly suspect as they were produced before modern regulations on lead and phthalates in consumer goods.

---

# CANDLES

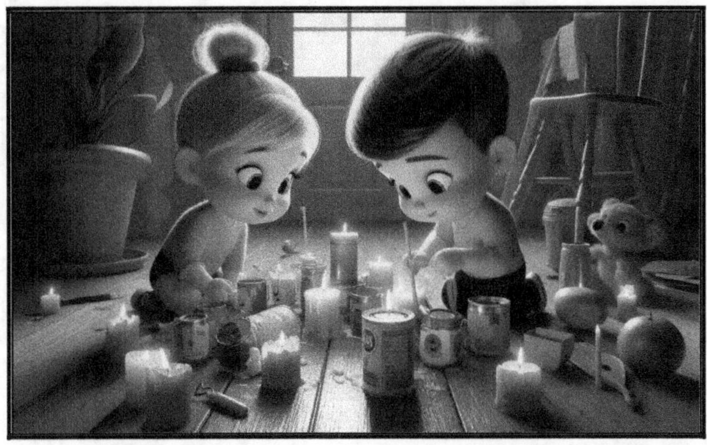

Candles create ambiance but pose serious fire risks around children. **Place them on high shelves completely out of reach.** Better yet, switch to flameless LED candles that provide the same warm glow without flames, wax drips, or potential disasters. If you insist on real candles, never leave them lit unattended around children, and use hurricane glass covers to protect flames from curious hands.

---

🌿 Children under the age of **five** are at the highest risk for death or injury from candle fires, and they are the victims in roughly **20% of all home candle fire incidents** where unsupervised children are involved. **The Shock Factor:** A small, decorative flame can turn into a full-blown structure fire in less than **two minutes**, often before a child even realizes they should call for help. *American Red Cross & U.S. Fire Administration (FEMA).*

"Unsupervised" doesn't mean "left home alone" it means a parent stepped into the kitchen for 60 seconds while a candle was burning in the living room.

---

# Fish Tanks

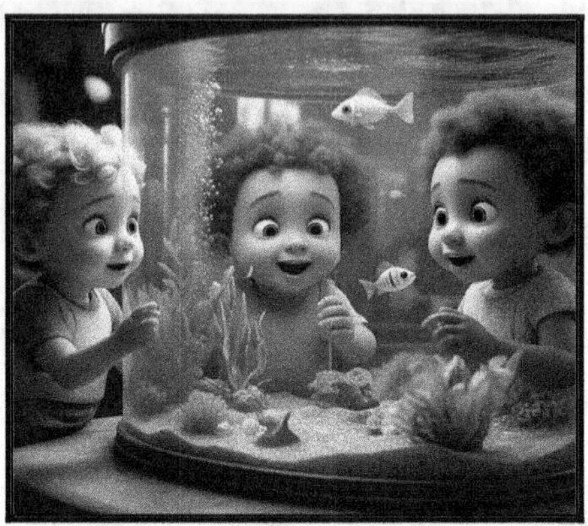

**Fish tanks require extensive childproofing beyond simply keeping children from touching the water.** Choose a sturdy surface designed specifically for aquariums, placed away from high-traffic areas and active play spaces. Use a secure lid designed for your tank size to prevent curious hands from reaching inside.

**Anchor both the tank and stand to the wall using heavy-duty furniture straps or wall anchors.** Locate wall studs with a stud finder for maximum security. Install straps on the tank stand's back and follow manufacturer instructions carefully. Test gently after installation to confirm the tank cannot tip.

**Manage electrical cords with organizers, keeping them out of reach along the tank's back.** Install childproof outlet covers nearby. Choose tank decorations that secure firmly and avoid sharp or small objects that could become choking hazards. Select child-friendly fish species known for peaceful temperaments.

**Teach children about respecting the fish tank** and explain why touching the water or glass disturbs the fish. When cleaning, use child-safe products and rinse thoroughly before reintroducing fish. Keep emergency supplies accessible for quick response to tank issues.

---

# UNFINISHED FURNITURE

Unfinished furniture brings rustic charm but also serious hazards. Rough surfaces cause splinters, and unstable construction creates tipping risks. According to the CPS, unfinished wooden furniture contributes to the 250,000 annual furniture-related injuries affecting children. Splinters can cause infections or inflammation, while falls from low tables and stands account for over a quarter of fractures in children under two.

**Begin by sanding every surface thoroughly, paying special attention to edges and corners.** Use fine-grit sandpaper for a smooth finish that eliminates wood fibers. Apply water-based, non-toxic sealants, varnishes, or paints designed for use around children. This protective layer prevents splinters and moisture damage that could create new hazards over time.

**Secure all exposed nails, screws, and bolts firmly**. Add padding or corner protectors to sharp edges. Unfinished furniture often lacks the stability of mass-produced pieces, especially handmade or older items. Anchor taller pieces like bookshelves and dressers to walls using anti-tip straps. This prevents catastrophic tipping when children climb.

**Inspect regularly for new rough spots, loose hardware, or developing hazards.** Furniture condition changes over time, and vigilance keeps children safe as they grow and explore more adventurously.

---

❦ That unfinished dresser or bookcase sitting against the wall is far more dangerous than it looks. According to a 30-year study published in Injury Epidemiology, 560,203 children under 18 were treated in U.S. emergency departments for furniture tip-over injuries, averaging one child every 46 minutes. And the danger is concentrated in the very youngest: over 75% of tip-over fatalities involve children under six years old, and 91% happen right in the child's own home. The culprit is often an unanchored dresser with open drawers — children between ages 2 and 5 are at the highest risk, using drawers like rungs on a ladder to climb and reach something higher up. (Sources: Injury Epidemiology Journal *via TuckerLawyers.com; CPSC Anchor It! campaign via TerryBryant.com; Kids In Danger, kidsindanger.org*)

---

# SECURE THROW RUGS

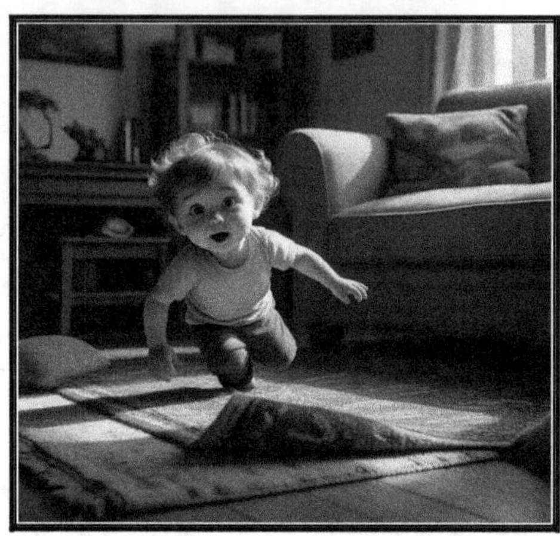

**Over 20,000 children slip and fall annually due to loose rugs and mats, suffering fractures, sprains, and head injuries.** Homes with hardwood or laminate flooring face particular challenges. Throw rugs shift and bunch under active feet, and wet mats near entrances become dangerously slippery.

**Use strong, double-sided tape to secure mats firmly in place.** Apply tape across the entire underside, especially edges, to prevent corners from flipping up. Prioritize high-traffic areas like entrances, hallways, and bathrooms. Pay special attention to rugs near cellar stairs or elevated surfaces where a misstep could have severe consequences.

**Choose adhesives recommended by manufacturers that won't leave sticky residue on your floors.** Follow application instructions carefully for optimal results. Regularly check that tape remains effective and replace when adhesion weakens.

# ANTIQUE FURNITURE

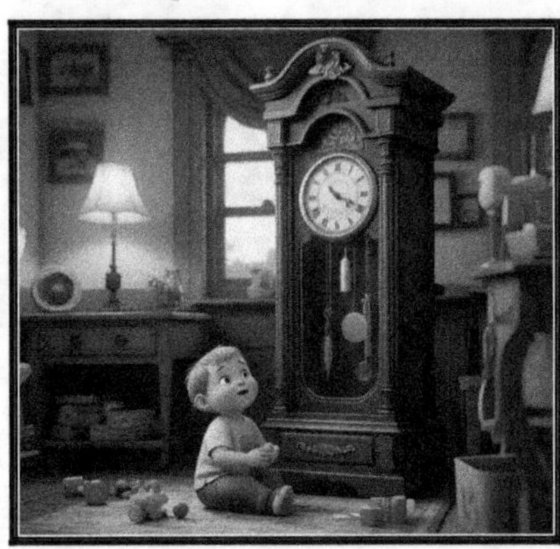

**Antique furniture holds sentimental value but wasn't designed with child safety in mind.** Vintage cribs feature slat spacing that can trap heads. Old trunks slam down on fingers. Antique sewing machines start with simple pedal presses, creating pinch points and operational hazards.

**Consider placing valuable antiques in rooms children cannot access or storing them until kids are older.** Use baby gates to create child-free zones protecting both furniture and children. If you must keep antiques in shared spaces, implement extra supervision and clear safety rules.

**Lead-based paint poses significant health risks on older furniture.** Never attempt to strip such paint yourself, as this releases harmful particles. Instead, seal existing paint or cover with non-toxic alternatives. Consult antique dealers or appraisers for specialized guidance on preserving pieces while ensuring safety.

**You can enjoy the beauty and history of cherished furniture while protecting your family.** Create a harmonious home where antiques and children coexist safely through thoughtful placement, honest assessment of risks, and appropriate protective measures. The memories you create matter more than any object, no matter how beautiful or historically significant.

---

# Anchor Taller Furniture!

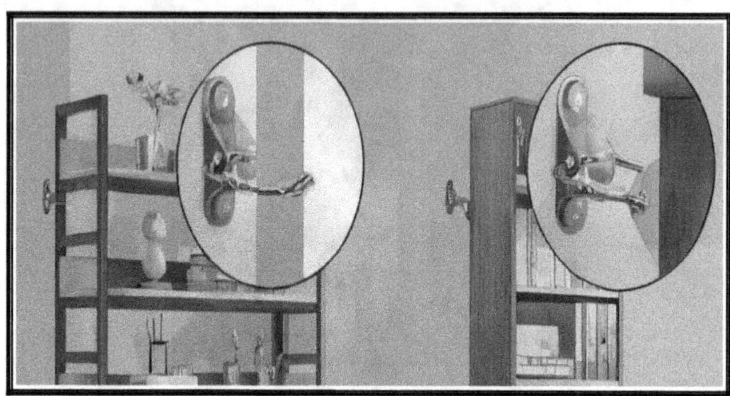

**Approximately 300 children die each year in the U.S. from furniture tip-overs, such as bookshelves and dressers, emphasizing the need for anchoring heavy furniture to walls.** Anchoring tall furniture is not just a recommendation; it's an absolute must when childproofing your home. Children are naturally curious and love to climb, pull, and explore every corner of the house. While wonderful to watch, this sense of adventure can quickly become dangerous if heavy furniture is not properly secured.

**According to the U.S. Consumer Product Safety Commission, a child is sent to the emergency room every 30 minutes due to a furniture or TV tip-over.** This is not just a rare occurrence; it's an alarmingly common problem affecting families nationwide. Proper anchoring can drastically reduce the risk of your child being hurt by toppling furniture.

**It's not just tall or oversized furniture that needs to be anchored.** Any piece that a child might climb or pull on can pose a hazard if it's not secured. Bookshelves can look like the perfect climbing structure to a child. Use heavy-duty metal straps to anchor dressers to the wall. Ensure the straps can support not only the weight of the furniture but also the weight of whatever's inside the drawers. Entertainment centers should be anchored securely to prevent tipping, and you should also anchor the TV separately for added safety.

❦ *According to the American Academy of Pediatrics,* **a child is rushed to the emergency department at least once every single hour of every single day with injuries from furniture or TV tip-overs. Specifically,** 77% of all tip-over deaths from 2000 to 2019 involved kids under the age of six.

<u>**Living Room/Family Room**</u>
Infant/Non-mobile: (Birth - 6 months)
Infant crawl/roll: (5 months - 1 year)
→ **Toddler/Pre-school: (1 year - 4 years)**
→ **School-age: (5 years - 6+ years)**

# PLAYPENS

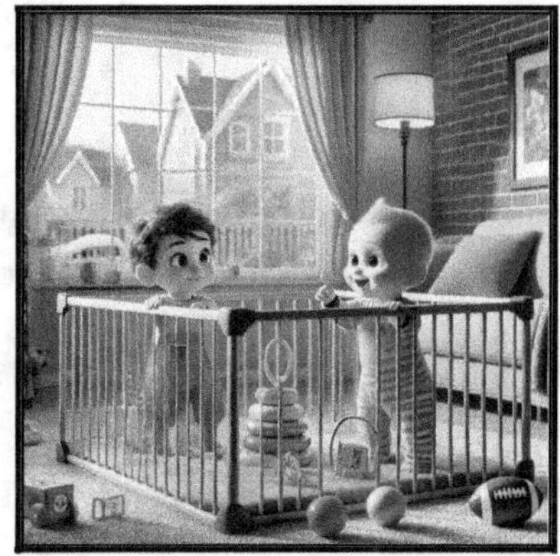

**Playpens offer parents peace of mind by providing a contained safe space for babies and toddlers. However, safety requires attention to important details.** The playpen's base should be firm and flat. Never add extra mattresses or thick blankets, as these create suffocation risks. If using a sheet, ensure it fits snugly over the existing mattress or pad.

**Inspect the playpen regularly for wear and tear.** Check mesh sides carefully for holes or loose threads that could cause entanglement or strangulation. These hazards develop gradually, so weekly inspections catch problems before they become dangerous.

**Choose playpen toys carefully.** Avoid anything with small parts that could be swallowed or long cords that pose strangulation risks. As your child grows more active and mobile, remove large toys that could serve as stepping stones for adventurous escape attempts. Even the safest playpen never replaces adult supervision. Always keep your child within sight, remembering that playpens provide a contained play environment but not a substitute for watchful care giving.

# LEAD PAINT

**Lead paint presents serious health risks,** particularly in homes built before 1978 when lead-based paint was common. Approximately 500,000 children aged one to five in the United States have elevated blood lead levels, with many cases linked to lead-based paint and contaminated dust in older homes.

**Children under six are especially vulnerable** because their developing bodies absorb lead more readily than adults. The consequences can be severe and long-lasting: brain damage, seizures, delayed growth, learning disabilities, behavioral problems, and hearing loss. In extreme cases, lead poisoning causes coma, convulsions, or death.

**Early identification is crucial** for prevention and treatment. If a sibling or playmate has been diagnosed with high blood lead levels, have your child tested immediately. They may have been exposed to the same environmental hazards. Any suspicion of lead exposure warrants immediate medical consultation. Healthcare professionals can conduct blood lead level testing and provide appropriate guidance and treatment.

**Protect your family by regularly inspecting your home for lead-based paint**, particularly if you live in an older house. Take necessary precautions when renovating or disturbing painted surfaces. Lead dust created during home improvement projects spreads easily and poses significant risks. Stay informed about potential hazards in your environment, from old playground equipment to imported toys that may contain lead.

Being proactive and informed helps you prevent lead exposure and create a healthy environment for your family. Together, we can work toward a safer, lead-free future for our children, one careful inspection and informed decision at a time.

---

🏵 **Approximately 500,000 children aged 1–5 in the U.S. have elevated blood lead levels (≥5 µg/dL),** with many cases linked to lead-based paint and contaminated dust in older homes. *(Childrenshospital.org)*

---

# Electrical Outlet Safety

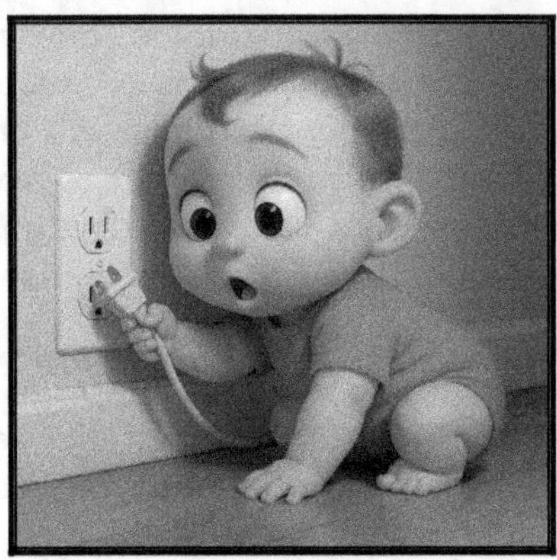

**Each year, more than 15,000 children are injured by inserting objects into open electrical outlets**, resulting in shocks and burns. Install outlet covers or safety caps on all electrical outlets within the reach of children. These covers are designed to fit securely over the outlets, making it difficult for little fingers to access the electrical openings.

**Consider replacing standard outlets with tamper-resistant ones, also known as childproof outlets.** These outlets have built-in safety shutters that automatically close the electrical openings when not in use. To insert a plug, equal pressure must be applied to both sides of the outlet, preventing children from inserting objects into the slots and reducing the risk of electric shock.

**Research shows that 100% of 2-4 year olds were able to remove some types of plastic outlet caps in under 10 seconds,** making tamper-resistant outlets a more reliable solution. When using any electrical devices, ensure proper ventilation by opening windows and allowing fresh air to circulate.

---

# CANNABIS VAPES AND WEED

When it comes to childproofing your home, one area that often gets overlooked is the safe storage of cannabis products. Whether you use cannabis for medical or recreational purposes, it's critical to ensure that these items are stored securely and kept out of reach of children. The potential dangers of accidental exposure to cannabis, especially for young children, are genuine, ranging from mild disorientation to severe poisoning.

**Store all cannabis products in a locked, childproof container.** Whether it's cannabis flowers, edibles, oils, or vapes, the key is to ensure that children cannot access these items. Store the locked container in a high place, well out of reach of curious little hands. A high-up locked cabinet provides double protection, ensuring that even the most determined child can't get into something they shouldn't.

**Cannabis products, much like medications, should be stored in child-resistant packaging.** Many cannabis products today are required by law to be sold in childproof containers, but the responsibility doesn't end there. After each use, ensure you properly seal the containers. Use bold, visible labels that identify the product as cannabis, so there's no room for confusion. Never leave vapes, edibles, or cannabis products where children can mistake them for everyday snacks.

---



# LOOSE PICTURE FRAMES

**Loose picture frames on tables pose hidden dangers for toddlers in their grabbing phase.** One enthusiastic swipe can send frames crashing down, with sharp corners causing head injuries and shattering glass creating even more hazards. Wall-mounted frames eliminate this risk entirely. Use sturdy picture hooks or screws to anchor frames securely out of reach. For freestanding frames you want to keep on tables or shelves, adhesive Velcro strips or museum putty work wonders keeping them firmly attached. This simple solution ensures frames stay put even when curious hands explore. While showcasing cherished memories adds warmth to your home, safety must always come first.

---



# Recliner/Rocking Chairs

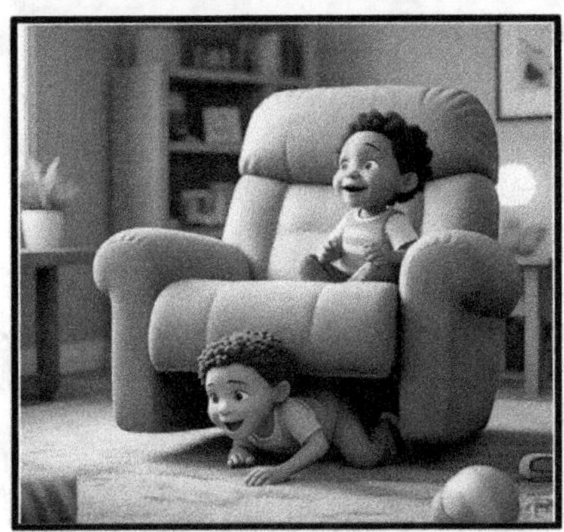

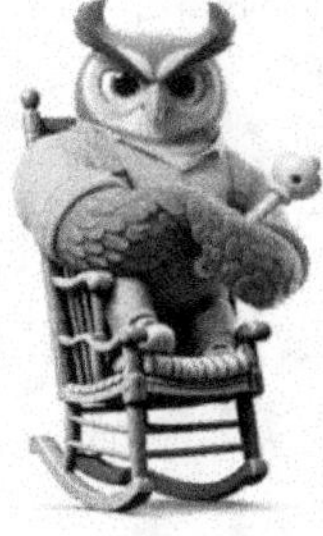

**Recliners pose unexpected dangers with their numerous moving parts.** The speed at which they open and close creates entrapment risks for heads, hands, and arms. Test the crushing force by placing a pencil in the mechanism; if it snaps under pressure, fingers face the same risk. Some recliners have spaces underneath where children can crawl and become stuck. Fasten fabric or barriers behind footrests to block access.

Since 1980, the CPS has recorded at least eight fatalities and several serious injuries to children under five caused by recliner entrapment. One

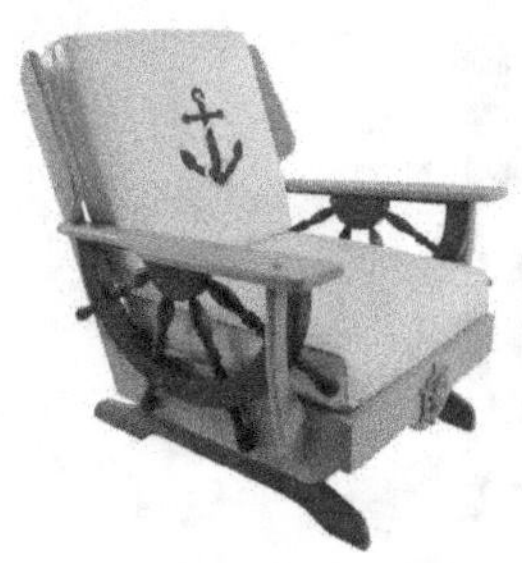

investigation from 1980 to 1985 alone confirmed three deaths and two brain injuries in toddlers aged twelve to thirty months who became caught under footrests. Never allow young children to operate recliners, and keep controls out of reach to prevent unintended adjustments.

**Traditional rocking chairs** bring cozy comfort but also present hazards. Curved edges threaten toes and fingers, especially for children unaware of risks. Gaps between spindles on arms and backrests can trap limbs or heads. Choose rockers with narrow gaps or add safety cushions to reduce entrapment risks. Educate children that rockers are for sitting only, never climbing or playing.

**Platform rockers** eliminate tipping risks but still pose dangers. The gliding motion creates gaps between seat and base where arms or fingers can become caught and crushed. Use cushions or fabric covers to shield these gaps. Teach children never to place hands near moving parts.

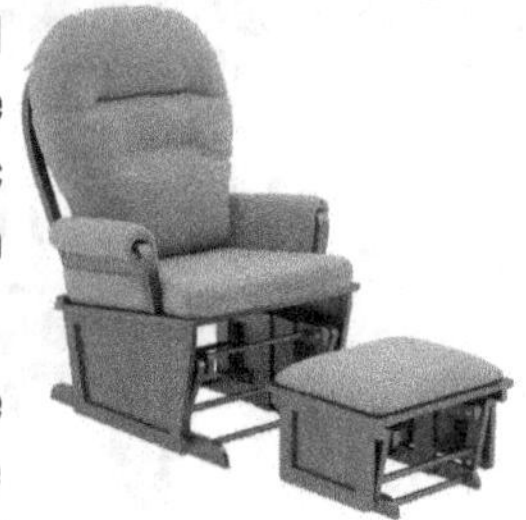

**Platform rockers** with side panels offer the safest option, providing enclosed, secure seating with protective barriers reducing injury risks.

---

🐛 Since 1980, the *U.S. Consumer Product Safety Commission* has recorded **at least 8 fatalities** and several serious injuries to children under five caused by entrapment in recliner mechanisms One investigation from 1980–1985 alone confirmed **3 deaths and 2 brain injuries** in toddlers aged 12–30 months who became caught under footrests

---

**Living Room/Family Room**
Infant/Non-mobile: (Birth - 6 months)
→ **Infant crawl/roll: (5 months - 1 year)**
→ **Toddler/Pre-school (1 year - 4 years)**
→ **School-age: (5 years - 6+ years)**

# Couch Slipcover

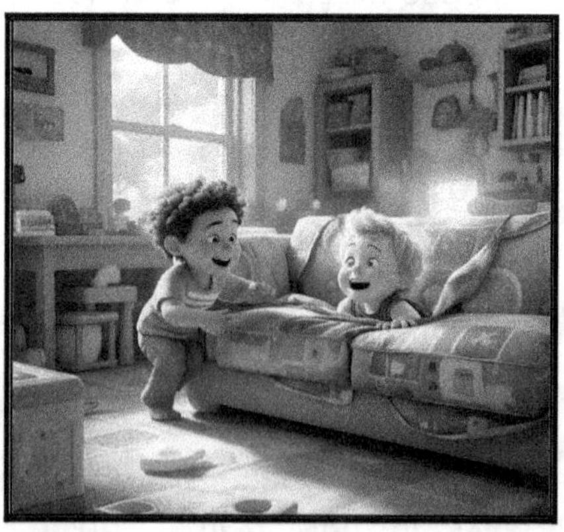

**Slipcovers require thoughtful selection for homes with children.**

Choose hypoallergenic, durable fabrics that withstand active play without fraying or tearing. Custom-fitted slipcovers prevent loose fabric from creating tripping hazards. Look for anti-slip features preventing covers from sliding off and causing accidents.

Avoid slipcovers with dangling accessories like tassels or fringe that present choking hazards. Ensure stitching is secure and robust to prevent small parts from loosening. Select easy-to-clean, stain-resistant fabrics maintaining hygiene and preventing bacterial growth from food spills.

---

**Living room**
Infant/Non-mobile: (Birth - 6 months)
Infant crawl/roll: (5 months - 1 year)
→ **Toddler/Pre-school: (1 year - 4 years)**
→ **School-age: (5 years - 6+ years)**

## CHECK FURNITURE CUSHIONS FOR SMALL CHOKING HAZARDS

**Check furniture cushions regularly for hidden dangers.** Children exploring cushions may find medications, small batteries from remotes, sharp objects like pins, or heavy items that could cause furniture to tip if pulled. The CPS has recorded fatalities when loose foam beads or cushion fillings escaped through tears and caused choking or airway blockage. Any small piece fitting through a 1.25-inch cylinder poses serious choking hazards for toddlers.

---

**Living Room/Family Room**
Infant/Non-mobile: (Birth - 6 months)
Infant crawl/roll: (5 months - 1 year)
→ **Toddler/Pre-school: (1 year - 4 years)**
→ **School-age: (5 years - 6+ years)**

## TRAVEL TRUNKS

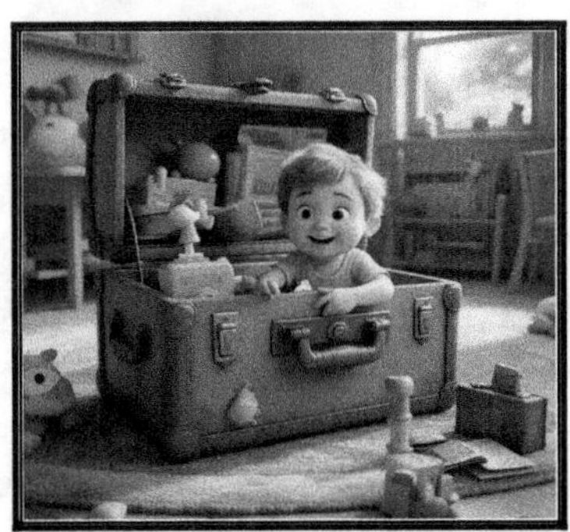

**Old-style travel trunks bring vintage charm but present unique childproofing challenges.** Heavy lids can slam shut, injuring fingers.

Install soft-close hinges or lid support hinges preventing sudden closures. Remove or secure old-fashioned locks and latches to prevent pinching or trapping.

**Clean interiors thoroughly and deodorize with baking soda to eliminate must and mold.** Sand rough patches and line with soft fabric protecting against scratches. Attach corner protectors to sharp metal corners. Ensure metal clasps, handles, and decorative elements are securely attached or remove them to prevent choking hazards.

**Anchor tall trunks to walls using furniture straps. Place non-slip pads underneath preventing unexpected sliding, especially on smooth floors.** Consider transforming trunks into cushioned seating areas, reducing how often the lid opens. If using for storage, store only child-safe items inside.

---

**Living Room/Family Room**
→ Infant/Non-mobile: (Birth - 6 months)
→ Infant crawl/roll: (5 months - 1 year)
→ Toddler/Pre-school: (1 year - 4 years)
→ School-age: (5 years - 6+ years)

# Vacuuming Importance and Carpet concerns

**Regular vacuuming plays a pivotal role in child safety beyond mere cleanliness.** Children spending significant time on floors exploring face hazards from small objects like coins, toy parts, and food crumbs. Prompt removal of these items reduces choking risks. Over 7,000 children are injured annually by vacuum cleaners themselves through cord entanglement and suction hazards, so store vacuums carefully.

**Carpets trap allergens including dust, pet dander, and pollen.** For infants and toddlers with sensitive respiratory systems, these allergens trigger reactions or exacerbate asthma. HEPA-filtered vacuums capture 99.97% of particles as small as 0.3 microns, including dust mites, mold spores, bacteria, and viruses. This prevents recirculation and provides thorough cleaning essential for allergen-prone environments.

**Carpet selection impacts health significantly.** Certain carpets emit volatile organic compounds containing ethyl benzene, formaldehyde, styrene, and acetone. Prolonged exposure causes headaches, nausea, respiratory irritation, and severe health problems. One chemical, p-dichlorobenzene, has been linked to fetal abnormalities in animal testing and causes nerve damage and respiratory issues in humans.

**Choose low VOC carpets or natural fiber options like wool or sisal with lower emissions**. Ensure backing and adhesives are also low VOC. Maintain proper ventilation during and after installation to disperse lingering chemicals. Look for Green Label Plus certification indicating strict low VOC emission standards.

---

<u>**Living Room/Family Room**</u>
Infant/Non-mobile: (Birth - 6 months)
Infant crawl/roll: (5 months - 1 year)
→ **Toddler/Pre-school: (1 year - 4 years)**
→ **School-age: (5 years - 6+ years)**

# SPACE HEATER SAFETY

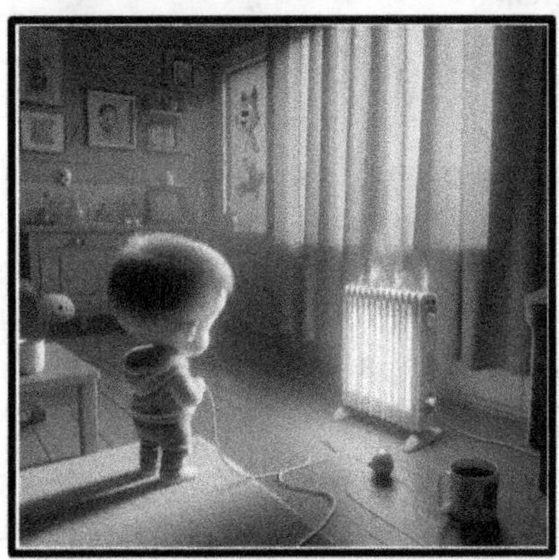

**More than 1,800 children suffer burns or fires annually from portable heaters.** Space heaters require careful placement and supervision. Position on flat, stable surfaces away from traffic where they won't be bumped. Maintain at least three feet clearance from flammable materials including curtains, furniture, and bedding.

**Choose heaters with tip-over protection providing automatic shut-off** and overheat protection preventing fires. Cool-to-touch exteriors prevent burns if accidentally touched. Never leave space heaters unattended with children present. If leaving the room even briefly, turn off the heater.

**Set up safety barriers or gates around heaters** providing extra protection for toddlers. Regular maintenance prevents dust buildup creating fire hazards. University of Chicago Medicine reports portable heaters reach temperatures exceeding 392°F and cause an estimated 2,300 burn injuries annually in preschoolers, along with nearly 1,700 heater-related fires leading to 160 injuries and 80 deaths.

❦ Portable space heaters aren't just cozy. They're risky. Hotter than 392°F and able to tip easily, these heaters cause an **estimated 2,300 burn injuries annually in preschoolers (ages 0–6)**. Combined with nearly 1,700 annual heater-related fires. **Leading to 160 injuries and 80 deaths.** They pose a hidden hazard in everyday comfort zones. *-University of Chicago Medicine*

**Living Room/Family Room**
Infant/Non-mobile: (Birth - 6 months)
→ **Infant crawl/roll: (5 months - 1 year)**
→ **Toddler/Pre-school: (1 year - 4 years)**
→ **School-age: (5 years - 6+ years)**

# EXTENSION CORD CONCERNS

**Extension cords pose tripping, electrocution, and fire risks.** Replace frayed cords immediately. Use extension cords temporarily only, never as permanent solutions. Avoid overloading cords and match polarized appliances with polarized cords ensuring proper grounding. Cover unused outlets with safety caps. Insert plugs fully and unplug by pulling the plug itself, not the cord.

**Never remove the third prong from three-wire cords,** as it prevents shock and electrocution. Check regularly for overheating; warm plugs or softening plastic indicate immediate replacement needs. Never run cords under carpets, rugs, or radiators, and don't staple or nail them, as this damages protective covering.

**Living Room/Family Room**
Infant/Non-mobile: (Birth - 6 months)
Infant crawl/roll: (5 months - 1 year)
→ **Toddler/Pre-school: (1 year - 4 years)**
→ **School-age: (5 years - 6+ years)**

# ELECTRICAL OUTLET SAFETY

**More than 15,000 children annually insert objects into electrical outlets,** resulting in shocks and burns. Install tamper-resistant outlets with built-in safety shutters requiring equal pressure on both sides to insert plugs. Research shows 100% of 2-4 year olds removed certain plastic outlet caps in under ten seconds, making tamper-resistant outlets far superior.

<u>**Living Room/Family Room**</u>
Infant/Non-mobile: (Birth - 6 months)
→ **Infant crawl/roll: (5 months - 1 year)**
→ **Toddler/Pre-school: (1 year - 4 years)**
→ **School-age: (5 years - 6+ years)**

# Use a Cord Concealment Device

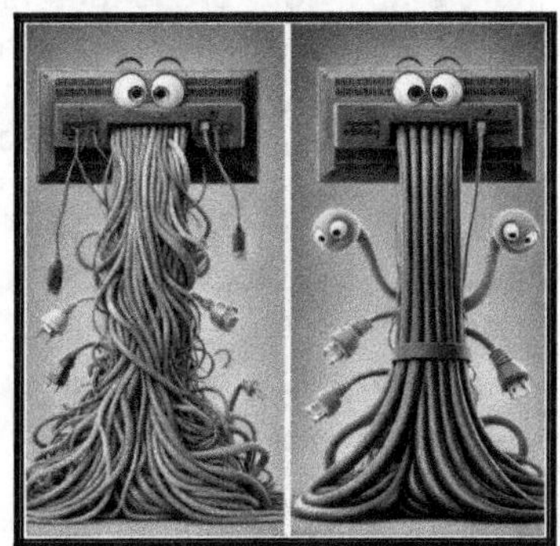

Use cord concealment systems in entertainment centers and home offices organizing multiple cables. These prevent tripping, entanglement, and make cord identification easier. Choose durable, flame-retardant materials with adequate capacity for all cords.

<u>**Living Room/Family Room**</u>
Infant/Non-mobile: (Birth - 6 months)
Infant crawl/roll: (5 months - 1 year)
→ **Toddler/Pre-school: (1 year - 4 years)**
→ **School-age: (5 years - 6+ years)**

# Install Power Strip Covers

**More than 10,000 children are injured annually by power strips and surge protectors.** Secure power strips to walls or furniture using adhesive strips or mounting brackets. Choose surge protectors adding automatic shut-off during electrical faults. Use cord management accessories keeping cords bundled and organized. Inspect regularly for damage and educate children about electrical safety.

__Living Room/Family Room__
Infant/Non-mobile: (Birth - 6 months)
Infant crawl/roll: (5 months - 1 year)
→ **Toddler/Pre-school: (1 year - 4 years)**
→ **School-age: (5 years - 6+ years)**

# Secure Empty Lamp Light Sockets

Empty lamp sockets present serious hazards. **Over 21,000 preschoolers annually are treated for inserting fingers or objects into empty sockets.** After unplugging lamps, insert socket safety caps fitting securely and preventing access to inner components. Inspect caps periodically and replace if worn. Position lamps stably away from edges and high-traffic areas.

---

🌰 **Every year, more than 21,000 preschoolers (under age 6) in the U.S. are treated in emergency rooms after inserting fingers or objects into empty lamp sockets or outlets.** Over 80% are in the toddler-to-preschool range, and many snacks, playtime, and kitchen moments involve curious hands meeting live terminals, often leading to painful burns and shocks. *(ESFI, Elictrical Safety Foundation International)*

---

__Living Room/Family Room__
Infant/Non-mobile: (Birth - 6 months)
→ **Infant crawl/roll: (5 months - 1 year)**
→ **Toddler/Pre-school: (1 year - 4 years)**
→ **School-age: (5 years - 6+ years)**

# Small and Button Batteries

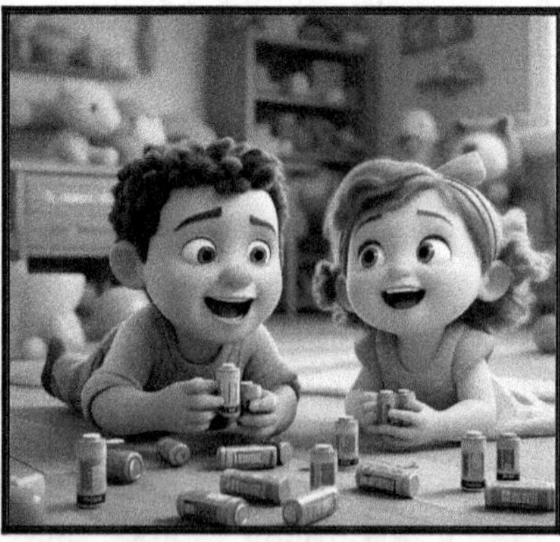

**Button batteries pose life-threatening risks when swallowed.** Johns Hopkins Medicine reports an average of 3,500 button battery ingestions annually, with incidence increasing over the last decade. Store batteries in containers with childproof latches, completely out of reach and sight. Ensure battery compartments on devices are screw-secured or taped closed.

**Clean battery leaks immediately wearing gloves in well-ventilated areas.** Dispose of damaged batteries properly and promptly. If you suspect a child swallowed a battery, seek emergency medical attention immediately, even without symptoms. Symptoms might include coughing, drooling, discomfort, or appetite decline. Over 10,000 children are injured annually mishandling remote controls through electrical shocks and swallowing small parts.

---

<u>**Living Room/Family Room**</u>
→ **Infant/Non-mobile: (Birth - 6 months)**
→ **Infant crawl/roll: (5 months - 1 year)**
→ **Toddler/Pre-school: (1 year - 4 years)**
→ **School-age: (5 years - 6+ years)**

# Loud Noise Concerns

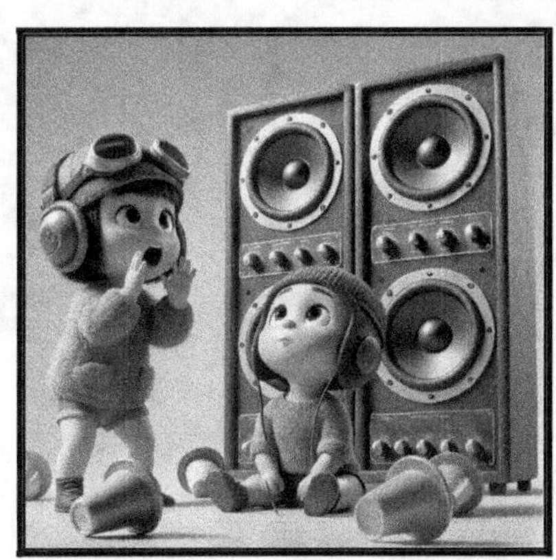

**Protecting children's hearing requires awareness of volume levels and noise exposure.** The CDC emphasizes that children's ears are more sensitive than adults', and prolonged loud sound exposure causes hearing damage. Monitor volumes on all electronic devices. Limit time in unavoidable loud environments and use noise-canceling headphones or earmuffs when necessary.

**Check toy volumes regularly and reduce them or dampen speakers with tape.** Teach older children safe listening practices with headphones, encouraging lower volumes and regular breaks. Schedule regular hearing check-ups for early detection of any issues.

**Beyond physical safety, monitor content children consume on TV,**

**radio, and social media.** Use parental controls restricting inappropriate content by age ratings. Engage children in discussions about what they watch, helping them distinguish fiction from reality. Co-view programs when possible, set viewing limits, and preview new content before allowing access. Choose trusted platforms offering child-friendly profiles displaying only age-appropriate material. Education and guidance help children develop healthy relationships with technology and media.

---

<u>**Living Room/Family Room**</u>
Infant/Non-mobile: (Birth - 6 months)
Infant crawl/roll: (5 months - 1 year)
→ **Toddler/Pre-school: (1 year - 4 years)**
→ **School-age: (5 years - 6+ years)**

# KNOW WHAT YOUR CHILD IS WATCHING

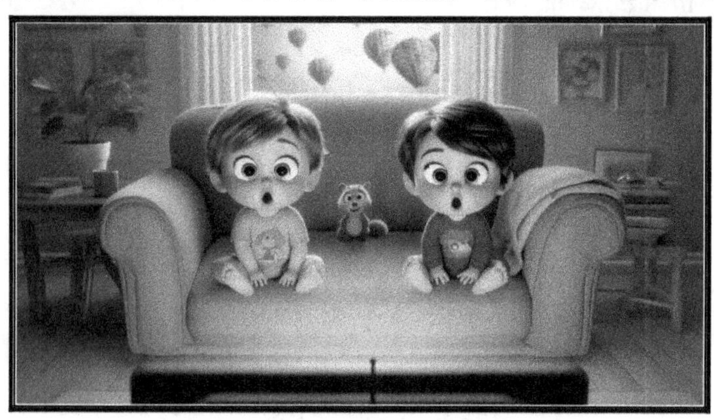

### Media and Content Safety

Childproofing extends beyond physical safety to encompass the content children consume visually and audibly. In today's digital age, children face vast exposure to TV, radio, and social media, making parental vigilance crucial.

**Parental Controls:** Modern televisions and streaming platforms offer parental control settings. Use these features to restrict access to inappropriate content based on age ratings or specific themes.

**Educate and Discuss:** Engage children about what they watch and listen to. Open discussions help them understand the difference between fiction and reality and provide context for confusing or mature themes.

**Co-Viewing and Co-Listening:** Whenever possible, watch TV shows or listen to radio programs with your children. This allows you to gauge content appropriateness while offering bonding and discussion opportunities.

**Set Viewing Limits:** Limit screen time and radio listening. Encourage other activities like reading, outdoor play, or family games to ensure a balanced routine.

**Review Content:** Before allowing children to watch new shows or listen to new stations, preview the content yourself. This gives clear insight into suitability for your child's age and maturity level.

**Use Trusted Platforms:** Opt for platforms and channels known for producing child-friendly content. Many streaming services offer kids' profiles displaying only age-appropriate content.

Media safety isn't just about restricting access but educating and guiding children to make informed choices as they grow. Creating a safe media environment allows children to learn, be entertained, and develop a healthy relationship with technology.

---

**Living Room/Family Room**
→ **Infant/Non-mobile: (Birth - 6 months)**
→ **Infant crawl/roll: (5 months - 1 year)**
→ **Toddler/Pre-school: (1 year - 4 years)**
→ **School-age: (5 years - 6+ years)**

# INSECTS AND PESTS

**There are over 200,000 cases of insect and animal bites among children annually in the U.S., with allergic reactions posing serious health risks.** Understanding how to protect your children from various household pests is crucial for maintaining a safe home environment. (Source: Centers for Disease Control and Prevention (CDC) - Venomous Bites and Stings)

---

## Mosquitoes

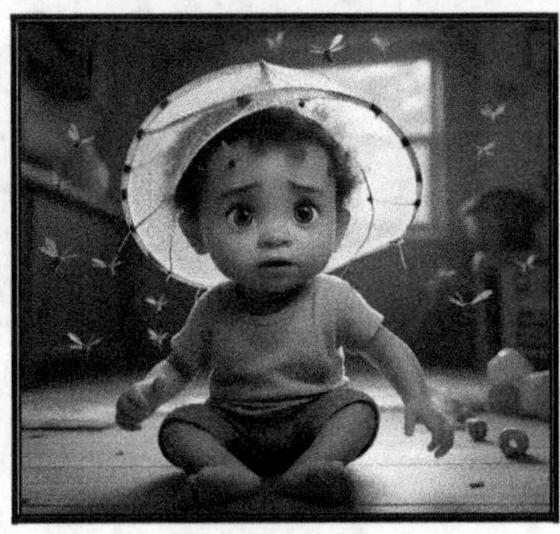

Mosquitoes can transmit various diseases, with malaria alone affecting hundreds of millions of people worldwide. When outdoors, use insect repellents containing DEET, picaridin, or lemon eucalyptus oil. Wear long-sleeved shirts, long pants, socks, and closed-toe shoes during mosquito-prone hours. Eliminate standing water around your home, as mosquitoes lay their eggs in stagnant water.

---

## Houseflies

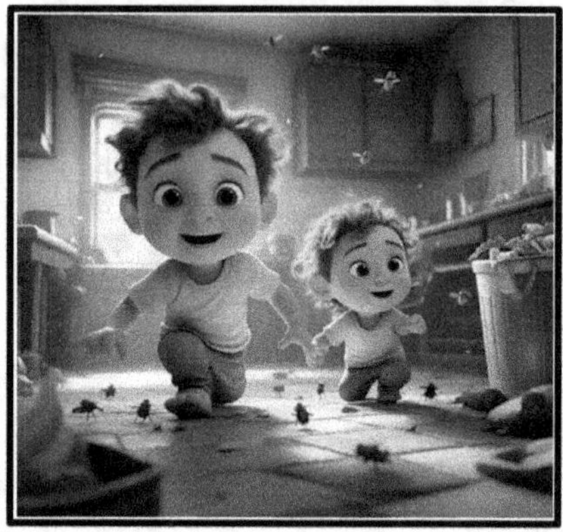

**Flies can carry harmful bacteria and diseases.** Maintain good hygiene by regularly cleaning your living spaces and disposing of garbage promptly. Store food in airtight containers and install fly screens on doors and windows.

---

## Bedbugs

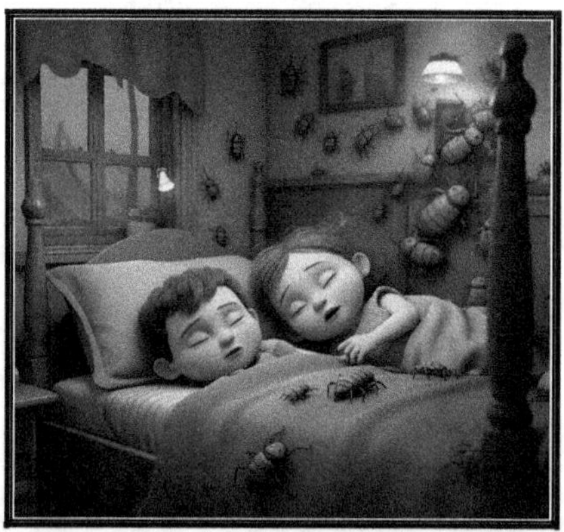

For bedbugs, inspect furniture regularly and use mattress encasements designed to prevent bedbugs from entering or escaping.

---

# Fleas

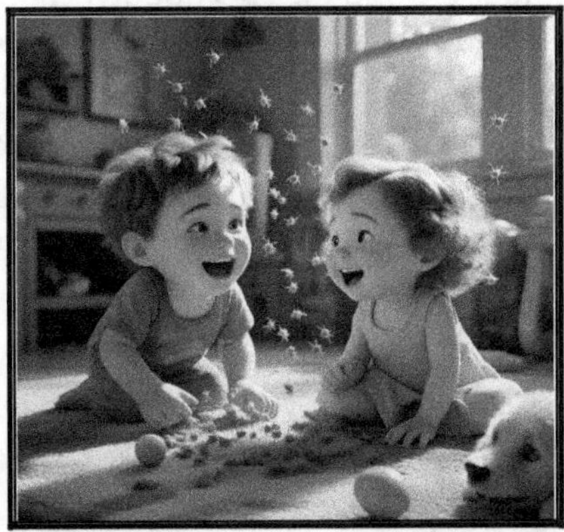

**Fleas can infest homes even without pets, attracted to warmth and movement.** They hitch rides on humans from outdoors and thrive in humid areas. Inspect regularly for dark specks, bites, or flea dirt on pets. Vacuum floors, carpets, and furniture frequently, disposing of bags outside immediately. Wash bedding and linens in hot water to kill all life stages. Treat pets and home simultaneously to break the flea cycle. Consult professionals for severe infestations and exercise caution in outdoor areas when traveling.

---

# Bees and Wasps

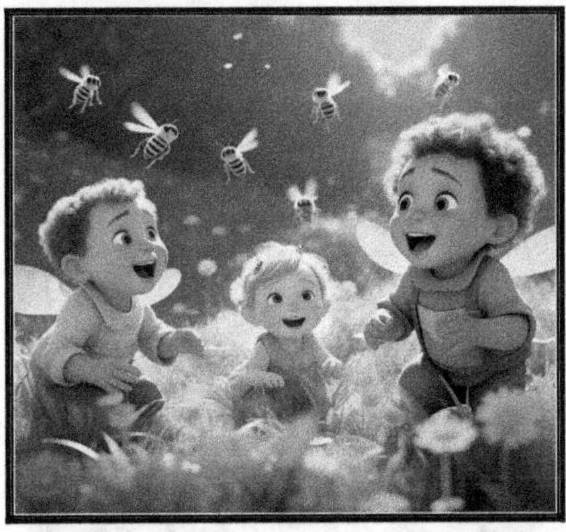

These insects are most active in warmer months. While ecologically important, their stings can be painful or trigger severe allergic reactions in children. Check outdoor areas regularly for nests in trees, shrubs, gutters, eaves, or underground. Cover food and drinks outdoors and clean up immediately after meals. Dress children in neutral or light colors rather than bright, floral patterns. Teach kids to stay calm and move away slowly rather than swatting. Keep outdoor trash bins tightly sealed. Plant natural deterrents like marigolds, citronella, and eucalyptus. Monitor for allergic reactions after stings and seek immediate medical help if needed.

## Brown Recluse and Black Widow

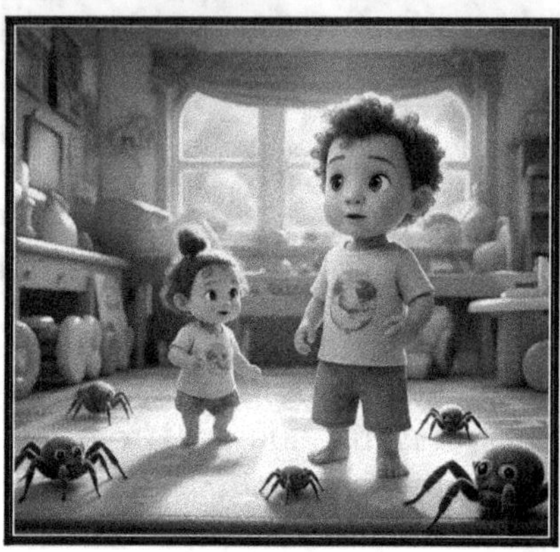

**For more dangerous pests like brown recluse and black widow spiders, regular cleaning and reducing clutter in basements, garages, and attics is essential.** Seal entry points by checking for cracks in the foundation and gaps in windows or doors. Fire ants require immediate treatment when mounds are spotted, and children should be taught to recognize and avoid fire ant mounds.

## Cockroaches

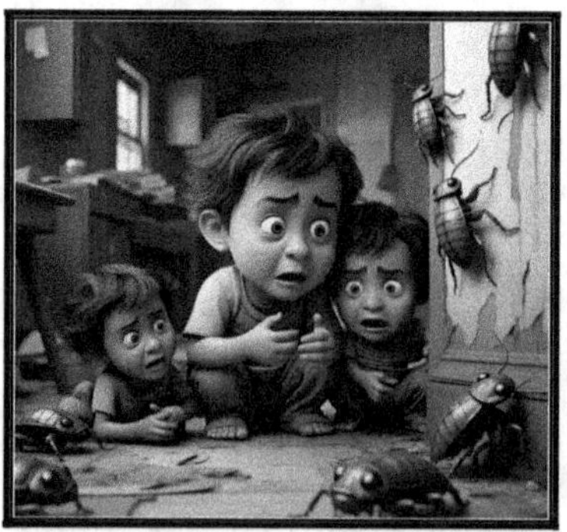

**Cockroaches carry diseases and trigger allergies and asthma in children.** Their droppings, shed skins, and bodies contaminate food and play areas. Seal cracks, holes, and gaps in kitchens and bathrooms to prevent entry. Clean up food crumbs and spills immediately, vacuum and sweep regularly. Store all food, including pet food, in airtight containers and avoid leaving food out overnight. Empty trash bins regularly, keep them sealed, and store away from entry points. For infestations, hire professional pest control. Use natural repellents like bay leaves or cucumber slices. If using pesticides, keep them away from children and pets, follow label instructions, and consider gel-based baits in inaccessible areas.

---

## Ticks

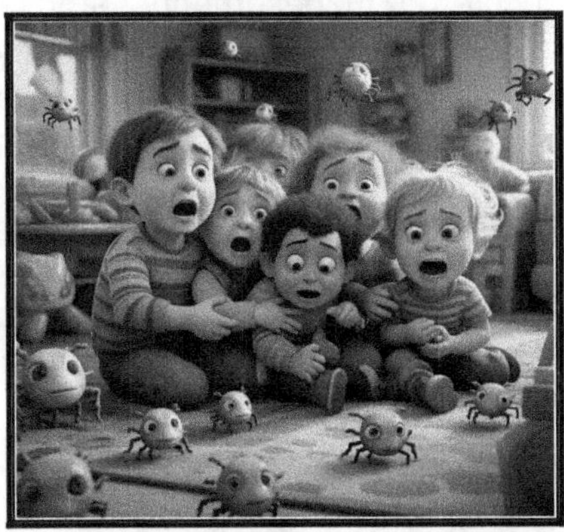

**Ticks transmit various diseases, so careful removal is essential.** Stay calm and use fine-tipped tweezers to grasp the tick close to the skin without squeezing or crushing it. Pull gently upward with steady motion without twisting or jerking. Clean the bite area and hands with rubbing alcohol, iodine, or soap and water. Save the tick in a sealed container for identification if concerned. Monitor the bite site for rashes or unusual symptoms over the following weeks. To prevent tick exposure outdoors, wear long-sleeved shirts and long pants, use insect repellents containing DEET or picaridin, treat clothing with permethrin, and perform regular tick checks on yourself, children, and pets after outdoor activities.

---

## Mice and Rats

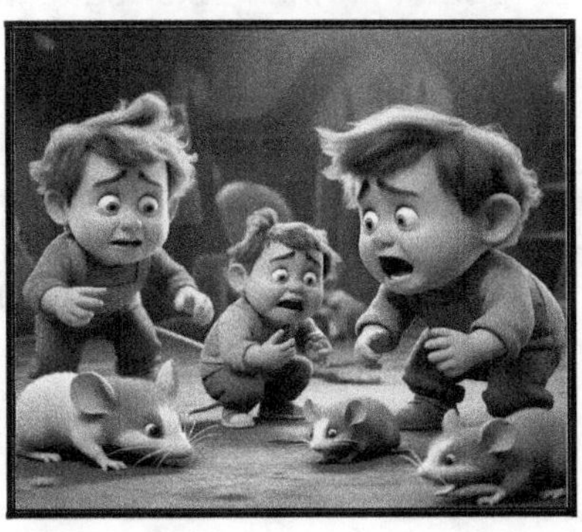

**Mice and rats contaminate food, chew wires creating fire hazards, and spread diseases.** Children may try to touch them, risking bites or pathogen exposure. Inspect your home regularly for cracks, holes, and gaps, sealing them with caulk or steel wool. Ensure doors and windows close tightly, install door sweeps, and repair torn screens. Store food in airtight containers, especially grains and cereals, and promptly clean up spills and crumbs. Use garbage cans with tight-fitting lids, empty regularly, and reduce clutter in basements, attics, and garages. Use enclosed bait stations or child-safe electric traps in areas inaccessible to children. Avoid rodenticides as they're harmful if ingested; if necessary, use child-resistant bait stations. Consider professional pest control for significant infestations. Teach children never to touch or approach rodents and watch for signs like droppings, gnaw marks, or nests.

---

<u>**Living Room/Family Room**</u>
→ **Infant/Non-mobile: (Birth – 6 months)**
→ **Infant crawl/roll: (5 months – 1 year)**
→ **Toddler/Pre-school: (1 year – 4 years)**
→ **School-age: (5 years – 6+ years)**

# House Plants

**Approximately 33,000 annual calls to U.S. poison control centers involve children ingesting plant parts, mostly toddlers exploring by mouthing objects.** Houseplants account for around 102,000 poison control calls yearly involving children under six, resulting in approximately 11,700 doctor or ER visits and about 150 severe cases requiring hospitalization.

Dieffenbachia contains calcium oxalate crystals causing intense burning in the mouth, difficulty swallowing, swelling, oral irritation, drooling, and vomiting. Philodendron shares the same defense mechanism, causing swelling of lips, tongue, and throat, accompanied by vomiting and diarrhea. Pothos also contains insoluble calcium oxalates causing intense burning and irritation in the mouth, lips, and tongue. Oleander is highly toxic in all parts, even small amounts causing vomiting, diarrhea, plummeting heart rate, and potentially death. ZZ Plant harbors calcium oxalate crystals in thick leaves causing oral irritation, pain, drooling, and sometimes vomiting. Peace Lily contains calcium oxalate crystals causing painful irritation of the mouth, lips, and tongue.

Keep poison control contact information readily available and seek medical attention immediately if ingestion occurs. Educate children about plant safety and create awareness in your home.

---

# Artificial Plants

**Choose high-quality, non-toxic artificial plants made without harmful chemicals like BPA and PVC.** Select plants with securely attached leaves and stems to avoid choking hazards from small, detachable parts. Use heavy pots or planters and add weight with rocks or sand to prevent tipping when pulled or tugged. Place plants on high shelves, use hanging or wall-mounted planters to keep them out of reach during the mouthing phase. Avoid plants with small fake fruits or berries that resemble real food and pose choking risks.

Secure larger plants to floors or furniture with adhesive strips or museum putty. Use wall brackets for tall plants to prevent them from falling. Teach children that artificial plants are for looking, not touching, and create simple rules about designated play areas. Regularly inspect plants for wear and tear, tighten or replace loose pieces with strong adhesive, and wipe down plants with a damp cloth to prevent dust buildup that can irritate children with allergies.

---

**Living Room/Family Room**
Infant/Non-mobile: (Birth - 6 months)
→ **Infant crawl/roll: (5 months - 1 year)**
→ **Toddler/Pre-school: (1 year - 4 years)**
→ **School-age: (5 years - 6+ years)**

# Air Fresheners and Ozone Generators

**Many air fresheners contain chemicals that may cause respiratory irritation and exacerbate asthma or allergies.** Children may ingest these products out of curiosity, causing harmful reactions. Choose products labeled non-toxic or natural with fewer synthetic chemicals and avoid those containing phthalates and formaldehyde. Ensure proper ventilation by opening windows when using air fresheners. Keep products out of reach of children and pets and use them sparingly, only when necessary. **Ozone generators produce ozone gas that can irritate the respiratory system, causing coughing, throat irritation, and shortness of breath, especially for those with asthma.** High levels can lead to ozone poisoning and severe respiratory distress. Use ozone generators only in unoccupied spaces and turn them off before entering. Follow manufacturer recommendations for safe ozone levels and ensure adequate ventilation to disperse ozone. Consider hiring trained professionals for odor removal or purification using ozone generators.

<u>**Living Room/Family Room**</u>
Infant/Non-mobile: (Birth - 6 months)
→ **Infant crawl/roll: (5 months - 1 year)**
→ **Toddler/Pre-school: (1 year - 4 years)**
→ **School-age: (5 years - 6+ years)**

# POTPOURRI CONCERNS

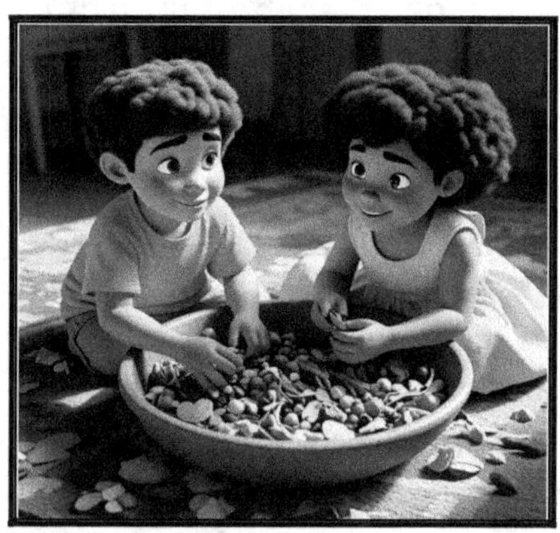

Potpourri might look beautiful and smell wonderful, but **it presents real dangers to young children**. Those colorful beads, stones, and shells that make potpourri so decorative are exactly what attracts little hands and mouths. For infants and toddlers who explore the world by putting things in their mouths, these small pieces become serious choking hazards.

The dangers go beyond choking. Larger **pieces can cause gastrointestinal blockages** if swallowed, leading to painful complications that require medical intervention. The oils and liquid refreshers used to maintain potpourri's scent contain harmful chemicals that can cause irritation or poisoning when ingested. Even the fumes from burning potpourri or oil warmers can irritate young respiratory systems, particularly affecting children with asthma or breathing sensitivities.

**Keep potpourri stored in secure containers** completely out of reach, and avoid displaying it where curious hands can grab it. If you love pleasant scents in your home, consider safer alternatives like essential oil diffusers or scented candles placed well above child level. Talk with your children about why potpourri isn't safe to touch or taste, encouraging them to come to you if they find any around the house. Check your potpourri containers regularly for broken pieces that could pose choking risks, and discard damaged items immediately.

---

**<u>Living Room/Family Room</u>**
Infant/Non-mobile: (Birth - 6 months)
Infant crawl/roll: (5 months - 1 year)
→ **Toddler/Pre-school: (1 year - 4 years)**
→ **School-age: (5 years - 6+ years)**

# SLIDING GLASS DOOR

Sliding glass doors create a beautiful connection between indoor and outdoor spaces, but they need careful attention when you have young children. According to the American Academy of Pediatrics and Centers for Disease Control, o**ver 58,000 door-related injuries happen annually to children ages zero to four in the United States, with around 20,000 kids under 18 treated each year for glass door or window injuries.** These familiar home features cause impacts, cuts, fractures, and even partial amputations among preschoolers every year.

**Start by installing door finger guards** to prevent those inevitable pinched fingers when little hands get caught in the sliding mechanism. Apply safety film to the glass so that if it breaks, the pieces stay together rather than scattering dangerous shards everywhere. If your door leads to a balcony, deck, or patio, install sturdy barriers or railings to prevent falls, making sure vertical bars are close enough together that children cannot squeeze through.

**Install childproof locks high enough to stay out of reach of small hands.** Apply colorful stickers or decals at your child's eye level to make the glass more visible and prevent collisions. Consider door alarms that alert you when the door opens, and add anti-lift devices to prevent unauthorized access from outside. Regular maintenance ensures everything continues working safely as your children grow and test boundaries.

---

🌿 *According to the American Academy of Pediatrics or the Centers for Disease Control and Prevention.* In the U.S., over **58,000 door-related injuries** occur annually in children ages 0–4, and around **20,000 kids under 18** are treated each year for glass door or window injuries. This means that **thousands of preschoolers,** even in familiar home spaces, suffer from sliding glass door impacts, cuts, fractures, and even partial amputations every year.

---

<u>**Living Room/Family Room**</u>
Infant/Non-mobile: (Birth - 6 months)
Infant crawl/roll: (5 months - 1 year)
→ **Toddler/Pre-school: (1 year - 4 years)**
→ **School-age: (5 years - 6+ years)**

# WINDOW BLIND STRING CONCERNS

**More than 1,000 children suffer strangulation or entanglement injuries from window blind cords each year in the United States, according to Safe Kids Worldwide.** Approximately 3,000 children are injured annually by window treatments including drapes and curtains. These numbers make cordless window treatments essential for homes with young children.

**The safest approach is installing cordless blinds or curtains throughout your home.** These options are increasingly available and eliminate strangulation risks entirely. If cordless blinds aren't feasible right now, shorten existing cords and secure them to walls using cord cleats or tie-down devices, keeping them taut to prevent loops or dangling sections. Retrofit older blinds with safety devices like cord cleats, tensioners, or wraps that keep cords securely positioned.

**Arrange furniture away from windows and blinds so children cannot climb up and reach cords.** Keep cribs, beds, and play areas completely separate from window areas. Supervise children in rooms with window blinds and explain why they should never play with cords. Use safety kits designed specifically for blind cords, which often include multiple devices to secure and manage cords safely.

**Inspect your blinds regularly for wear, fraying, or damage, replacing or repairing damaged cords immediately.** When moving into a new home or apartment with older blinds lacking safety features, prioritize updating them or using temporary solutions until safer blinds can be installed. Window blind cord safety requires ongoing attention, especially as children grow and explore new areas. Regularly reassess your safety measures to protect your child's well-being and prevent accidents.

---

# CONSIDER INSTALLING
# SHATTER PROOF WINDOWS

**Choosing Plexiglass or shatterproof glass over regular glass significantly enhances safety throughout your home.** These materials are engineered for much greater impact resistance, making windows highly resistant to accidental bumps and knocks from active children, pets, or everyday household activity. They're less likely to crack or break under considerable pressure, providing crucial protection in homes with young children.

**In play areas and children's rooms, Plexiglass and shatterproof glass provide an added safety layer.** During rough play or accidental collisions, these materials are far less likely to break and cause harm. Unlike regular glass, they don't shatter into sharp, dangerous pieces when broken, significantly reducing injury risk. For commercial settings, these materials improve security by making it more difficult for intruders to break in through windows and doors. In regions experiencing severe weather like hurricanes or tornadoes, impact-resistant windows and doors help protect homes and buildings from flying debris and other hazards.

**Plexiglass and shatterproof glass work well in numerous applications including windows, doors, skylights, displays, signage, protective barriers, and even eye-wear.** Their versatility makes them suitable for both residential and commercial settings. They're easy to clean and maintain, practical for busy environments like restaurants and retail stores. Plexiglass, a form of acrylic plastic, is more environmentally friendly than traditional glass manufacturing processes.

---

# French Door Concerns

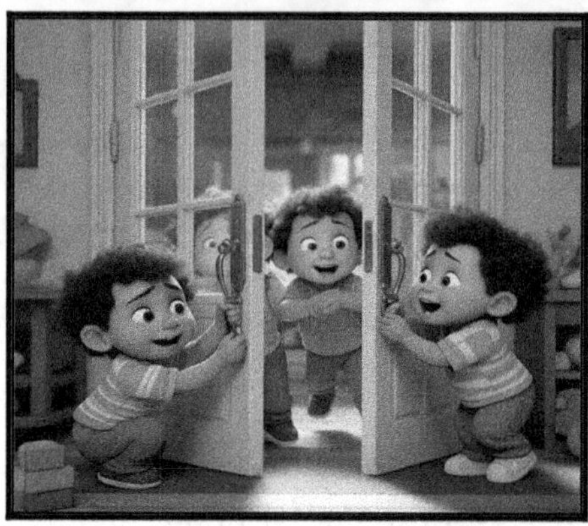

**Each year in the United States, tens of thousands of toddlers and preschoolers under age four are injured by glass-panel doors like French or patio doors.** A study published in Injury Prevention found that 41% of all door-related injuries occurred in children aged four or younger. Hospital reviews note that glass doors can cause deep lacerations damaging nerves or arteries. Simple moments like running into an unmarked door have led to emergency room visits and surgery.

**Install child safety locks on French doors** to prevent your child from opening them without your knowledge. These locks can be placed at the top or bottom of doors and typically require a key or specific action to unlock, ensuring only adults can operate them. Doorknob covers are affordable, easy to install, and prevent children from turning knobs to open doors.

**For families with very young children, install safety gates at French door entrances to restrict access, especially useful in areas where close supervision might be challenging.** Add shatter-resistant window film to glass panels to reduce injury risk from impacts. The film holds glass together, minimizing dangerous shard scattering in accidents.

If your French doors have key locks, **keep keys completely out of children's reach, using a key chain or high shelf for storage.** Nothing replaces supervision and education. Teach your child about hazards associated with opening doors without adults present and encourage them to seek assistance when needed.

**Regularly inspect French doors** to ensure they function correctly, fixing loose hinges, handles, or locks promptly to maintain childproofing effectiveness. Be cautious positioning furniture near doors, as children might use it as climbing aids to reach doorknobs or locks. Keep furniture away from doors to eliminate this risk. If doors have blinds or curtains with cords, secure them out of reach using cord cleats or tie-down devices.

---

🐝 Each year in the U.S., the equivalent of **tens of thousands of toddlers and preschoolers, many under age 4, are injured by glass-panel doors like French or patio doors.** A 1999–2008 study published in the journal Injury Prevention found that 41% of all door-related injuries occurred in children aged 4 or younger. Hospital reviews note that glass doors can cause deep lacerations damaging nerves or arteries. In real-world incidents, simple moments like running into an unmarked door have led to emergency room visits and even surgery. *Consumer Product Safety Commission*

---

<u>**Living Room/Family Room**</u>
Infant/Non-mobile: (Birth - 6 months)
Infant crawl/roll: (5 months - 1 year)
→ **Toddler/Pre-school: (1 year - 4 years)**
→ **School-age: (5 years - 6+ years)**

# WINDOW AIR CONDITIONER CONCERNS

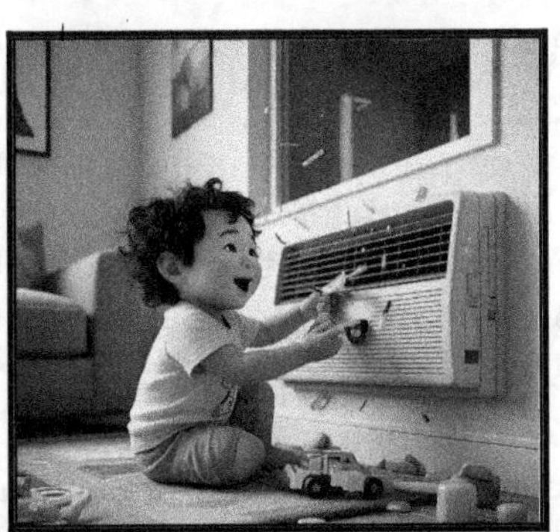

**More than 2,500 children are injured annually by window air conditioners, including falls and electrical hazards,** according to the Centers for Disease Control and Prevention. Regular maintenance is crucial. Inspect and maintain AC units to ensure they function correctly and safely, checking for loose or damaged parts and repairing or replacing them promptly.

**Install a window lock in addition to using window guards to secure windows in closed positions when AC units are in use, preventing children from accidentally opening windows and accessing units.** Use window air conditioner brackets that attach units to window frames for added stability, helping prevent tipping or falling from accidental pushes or bumps.

**If window blinds or curtains are near AC units, ensure cords are safely secured and out of children's reach, as loose cords pose strangulation risks.** Install window stops or wedges to limit window opening to safe levels, preventing children from accidentally opening windows wide enough to reach AC units. Keep remote controls out of children's reach, storing them in designated places when not in use.

**Always supervise children near window AC units, educating them about potential dangers and reminding them not to touch or play with units.** If AC units are located near blinds or curtains, properly secure them to avoid tangling or entanglement hazards. Install childproof window locks or guards requiring adults to unlock or release windows for safe operation. Teach older children how to safely operate AC units and what to do in emergencies like overheating or unusual noises.

---

**Living Room/Family Room**
Infant/Non-mobile: (Birth - 6 months)
→ **Infant crawl/roll: (5 months - 1 year)**
Toddler/Pre-school: (1 year - 4 years)
School-age: (5 years - 6+ years)

# <u>NO</u> BABY WALKERS

Baby walkers may appear convenient for helping infants learn to walk, but they pose significant dangers to children. Contrary to popular belief, baby walkers actually delay development of essential motor skills by preventing infants from learning proper balance and weight distribution needed for independent walking.

**The mobility of baby walkers leads to falls down stairwells or over ledges, resulting in severe injuries.** Their speed and unpredictability make it difficult for parents to react quickly enough to prevent accidents. Even with attentive parents, constantly monitoring a child in a baby walker proves challenging. This lack of supervision can lead to dangerous situations.

**Baby walkers grant access to hazards typically out of reach for crawling infants.** Children in walkers may reach sharp objects, toxic cleaning products, or electrical outlets, increasing injury or poisoning risks. They allow babies to access hot surfaces or liquids they normally couldn't reach, leading to burns or scalds. The devices place stress on infants' legs and hips, potentially causing discomfort or developmental issues. Using baby walkers on uneven surfaces like patios or driveways is especially dangerous, as they may tip over or become unstable.

**Due to safety concerns, some countries have banned or strictly regulated baby walker sales and use.** According to Consumer Report, from 2021 to 2023, an estimated 2,467 injuries per year involving baby walkers, jumpers, or exercisers were treated in U.S. emergency departments for children under five. In 2023, over 3,000 injuries were reported from these products combined. From 2014 to 2023, baby walkers or jumpers accounted for 34,558 nursery equipment injuries, ranking ninth among nursery products.

Instead of baby walkers, consider safer alternatives that promote safe exploration and development, such as stationary activity centers, playpens, or simply allowing your child to learn walking at their own pace without aids. Always consult with pediatricians and child safety experts for guidance on appropriate aids and childproofing measures.

---

**Living Room/Family Room**
Infant/Non-mobile: (Birth - 6 months)
→ **Infant crawl/roll: (5 months - 1 year)**
→ **Toddler/Pre-school: (1 year - 4 years)**
→ **School-age: (5 years - 6+ years)**

# MONEY CONCERNS

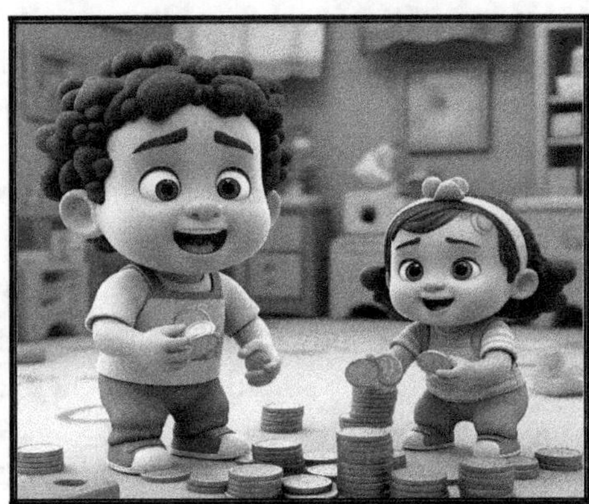

**While money is essential in our daily lives, it poses unexpected hazards to young children.** Coins are especially dangerous for curious toddlers still exploring the world through their mouths.

**The most immediate risk is choking.** Coins are just the right size to become lodged in a child's airway. Their shiny appearance and easy-to-grasp size make them particularly attractive to little ones, increasing ingestion risk. Some coins contain metals that can be toxic if ingested. Prolonged contact with or swallowing certain coins can lead to metal poisoning with serious health implications.

**Money changes hands frequently and carries a multitude of germs.** Children who handle money and then touch their mouths or eyes can be exposed to various bacteria and viruses. While less common, paper money or damaged coins can have sharp edges that might cut or scratch skin.

---

**Living Room/Family Room**
Infant/Non-mobile: (Birth - 6 months)
Infant crawl/roll: (5 months - 1 year)
→ **Toddler/Pre-school: (1 year - 4 years)**
→ **School-age: (5 years - 6+ years)**

# HIDDEN DANGERS OF KNICKKNACKS

Knickknacks, with their intriguing designs and colors, often captivate attention, especially from young children. However, beneath their decorative charm lie potential risks that parents and caregivers should recognize. Due to their small size, children might mistake knickknacks for toys and place them in their mouths, posing significant choking risks, especially for toddlers. Some knickknacks have sharp edges or parts that can break off, leading to cuts or other injuries.

**From 1995 to 2015, over 750,000 U.S. children under age six were treated in emergency rooms after swallowing small household items like figurines, coins, or beads. An average of 100 incidents per day.** Research shows these objects, especially spherical ones, are among the most likely to dangerously block toddlers' airways.

Keep decorative items on higher shelves or surfaces well out of your child's reach. If stored in cabinets, equip them with childproof locks to prevent curious hands from accessing them. Periodically check areas where children play or spend time to ensure no small items have been left within grasp. Talk to children about differences between toys and decorative items, emphasizing the importance of not putting unfamiliar objects in their mouths. While knickknacks add aesthetic appeal to homes, recognizing and mitigating risks they pose to young children is essential.

---

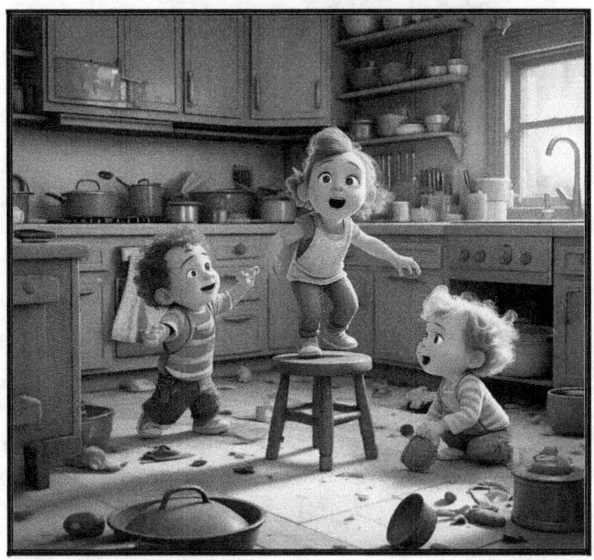

**Introduction:** The kitchen, often referred to as the heart of the home, is a bustling hub of activity, filled with enticing aromas, intriguing gadgets, and the promise of delicious meals. Yet, for all its warmth and allure, it also presents a myriad of potential hazards, especially to curious little ones. From sharp utensils to hot surfaces and from toxic cleaning agents to easily accessible cabinets, the kitchen can be a veritable minefield for children. As we delve into this chapter, we will explore comprehensive strategies and practical tips to transform your kitchen into a safe haven, ensuring that your child's exploratory adventures don't turn into dangerous misadventures. Let's embark on this essential journey of safeguarding the space where family memories are often made, ensuring it remains a place of joy, bonding, and safety.

---

**Kitchen**
Infant/Non-mobile: (Birth - 6 months)
Infant crawl/roll: (5 months - 1 year)
→ **Toddler/Pre-school: (1 year - 4 years)**
→ **School-age: (5 years - 6+ years)**

# SLIDING GLASS DOORS

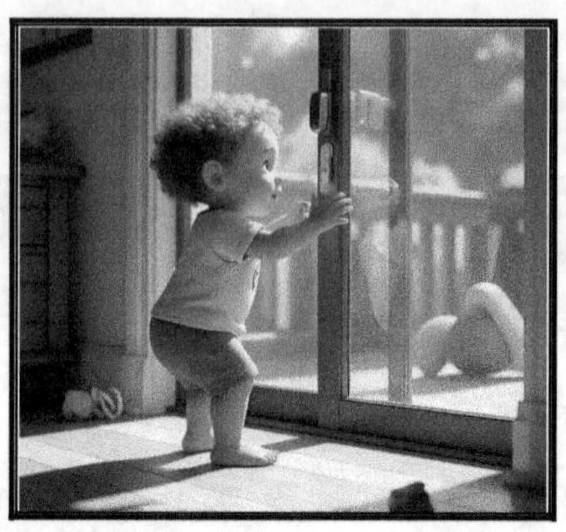

**Install door finger guards or stoppers to prevent children's fingers from getting caught in the sliding mechanism.** Replace standard glass with safety glass or add safety film that holds pieces together upon impact to reduce injury from broken glass. If the door leads to a balcony, deck, or patio, install sturdy barriers or railings with vertical bars close enough together to prevent children from squeezing through. Use childproof locks positioned high enough to be out of children's reach and apply colorful stickers or decals at a child's eye level to increase visibility and prevent collisions. Always supervise young children around sliding glass doors and educate them about potential dangers. Consider installing door alarms that sound when the door is opened and use anti-lift devices on the track to prevent unauthorized lifting from outside.

---

❦ A sliding glass door looks harmless. It's just a door. But to a toddler, it's practically invisible. A study published in PubMed analyzing data from the National Electronic Injury Surveillance System found that children sustained an estimated 1,392,451 door-related emergency room visits over just a 10-year period. That's roughly one child injury every 4 minutes. And the danger isn't just impact. According to the U.S. Consumer Product Safety Commission, over 15,000 children are treated annually for injuries related to glass doors. And in one tragic documented case, a toddler wandered outside through an unlocked sliding door and drowned in a backyard pool.

Even sticker warnings don't fully solve the problem. Researchers found that 22 glass door injuries occurred even when a design, decal, or separation bar was already visible on the glass. Meaning children (and adults) simply don't register the barrier in time. *PubMed / National Electronic Injury Surveillance System; U.S. CPSC via RyanSlidingDoorRepair.com; California State Department of Public Health study*

# KITCHEN ISLAND

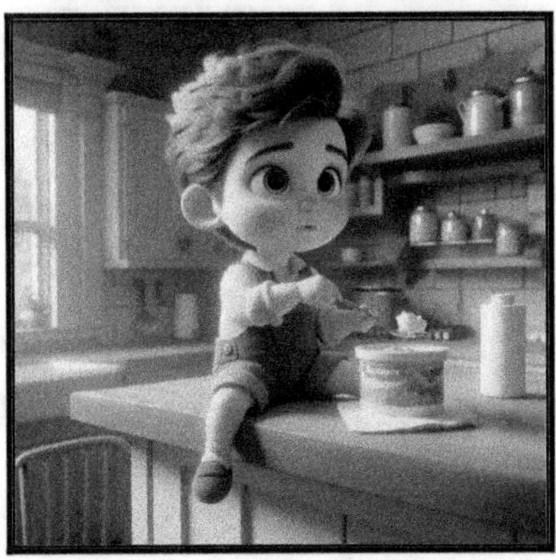

**Kitchen islands provide 360-degree access, making sharp knives and hot surfaces easily reachable for children.** Drawers can become stepping stools for climbing, and mobile islands on wheels risk trapping fingers or toes. Approximately 150,000 children are treated annually for burns and scalds from hot foods and beverages, often during meal preparation. Falls from islands contribute significantly to the 2.5 million annual fall-related ER visits in children under five, and children are evaluated every 46 minutes for tip-over injuries involving furniture. Use rear burners when cooking to keep hot surfaces away from edges. Install childproof locks on drawers, especially those containing knives. Maintain a clutter-free zone to reduce tripping hazards. Always ensure an adult is present and vigilant when children are in the kitchen, and educate them about potential dangers while establishing clear safety rules.

---

🍎 Kitchen islands, central to family life, double as hidden hazards for little ones. Falls from islands contribute **significantly to the 2.5 million annual fall related ER visits in children under 5,** while the kitchen remains the top site for burns. 20–30% are caused by contact with hot objects like pots and pans. In fact, children are evaluated every 46 minutes for tip-over injuries involving furniture; kitchen islands are often just tall pieces of furniture waiting for climbing hands. *The American Academy of Pediatrics (AAP)*

---

# Hydro Garden

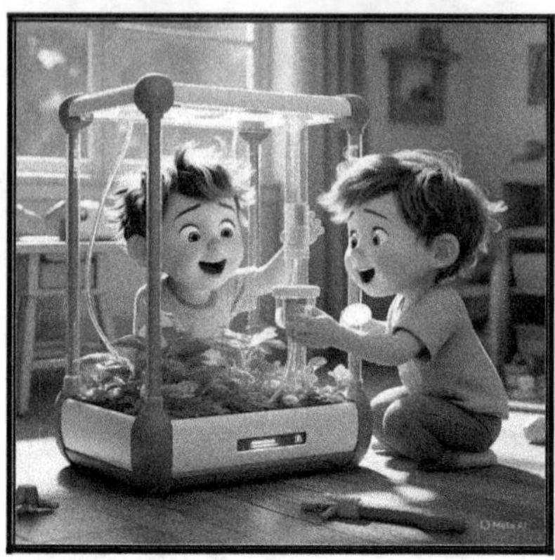

**Secure all electric components like lights and water pumps by tucking cords away with organizers or clips, or use cord covers to prevent curious fingers from yanking anything.** Place the hydro garden on an out-of-reach counter or use a small, clear guard to shield plants and equipment from little hands. Consider a mesh or fabric barrier that allows light through but prevents access. Choose non-toxic plants so if your child reaches a leaf or two, they won't be harmed. Stick to familiar kitchen herbs that are safe if ingested.

---



# Tablecloths Vs. Placemats

**Scald burns result in over 2,500 hospitalizations of children annually in the United States.** Young children may pull on tablecloth edges, causing dishes, hot beverages, or other items to tip over, posing burn or injury risks. Tablecloths hanging too low can become tripping hazards. Use tablecloth clips or weights to secure the cloth and opt for shorter lengths to minimize tripping. Placemats present fewer risks but can be chewed on by teething children or slide off tables, potentially taking dishes with them. Choose placemats made of non-toxic, BPA-free materials and select ones with anti-slip backing to prevent movement.

Experts estimate tens of thousands of related injuries yearly, including about 10,000 high-chair falls involving kids yanking items like placemats, and over 560,000 tip-over injuries affecting children under six. Place mats are generally the safer choice from a childproofing perspective.

---

🐞 Though no national registry logs 'tablecloth pull' injuries, experts estimate tens of thousands of related injuries each year: about **10,000 high-chair falls** alone involve kids yanking items like placemats or hot plates, and over **560,000 tip-over injuries.** Including those from pulling cloths, affect children under six. Even a simple placemat slipping underfoot has led to broken bones in toddlers. *Nationwide Children's Hospital*

---

**Kitchen**
Infant/Non-mobile: (Birth - 6 months)
Infant crawl/roll: (5 months - 1 year)
→ **Toddler/Pre-school: (1 year - 4 years)**
→ **School-age: (5 years - 6+ years)**

# Garbage/Recycling Cans

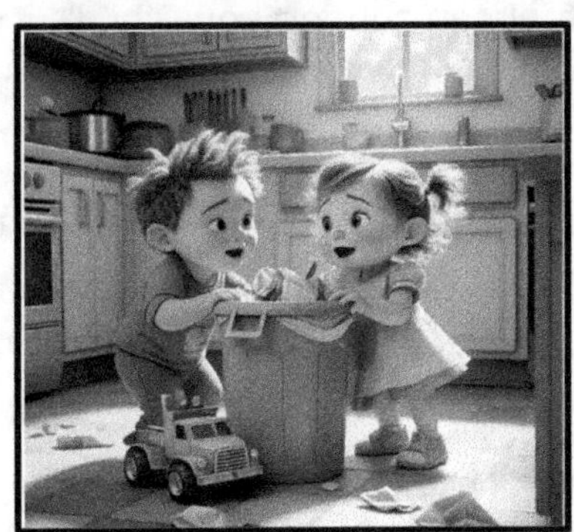

**Choose childproof lids with locking mechanisms or lids requiring force to open, preventing children from accessing harmful or sharp objects.** Store cans in locations not easily accessible, such as locked cabinets or off-limit rooms. Explain to children that these containers are not toys and should never be touched without an adult present. Dispose of hazardous materials like cleaning products, batteries, and electronics properly, keeping them out of children's reach and following local regulations. Always supervise children's interactions with garbage and recycling cans. If children are old enough to help, create a designated, secure recycling area with child-friendly bins placed away from hazardous materials.
**Kitchen**

Infant/Non-mobile: (Birth - 6 months)
Infant crawl/roll: (5 months - 1 year)
→ **Toddler/Pre-school: (1 year - 4 years)**
→ **School-age: (5 years - 6+ years)**

# FOOTSTOOL CONCERNS

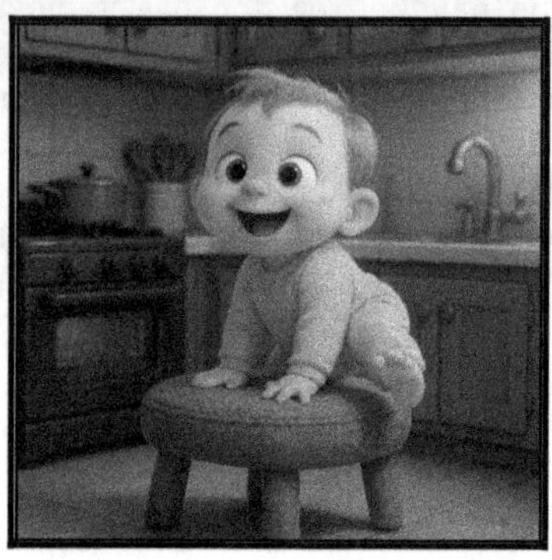

**Choose footstools with sturdy, wide, stable bases to prevent tipping.** Select heights appropriate for your child's age and size so they can comfortably and safely use them. Check the manufacturer's weight limit and ensure the footstool can support your child's weight plus any items they might carry. Always supervise children when using footstools and teach them to use them only for their intended purpose, not as toys. Consider footstools with non-slip surfaces for better traction and add padding or covers to sharp edges or corners to make them safer.

---

<u>Kitchen</u>
→ Infant/Non-mobile: (Birth - 6 months)
→ Infant crawl/roll: (5 months - 1 year)
→ Toddler/Pre-school: (1 year - 4 years)
→ School-age: (5 years - 6+ years)

# IMPORTANCE OF UNPLUGGING APPLIANCES

**Over 75,000 children sustain injuries from household appliances like blenders, mixers, and toasters annually in the U.S. Unplugging appliances when not in use prevents electrical shocks or burns from children fiddling with cords or buttons.** It also prevents accidental operations, particularly concerning with devices like toasters or blenders. Unplugging reduces overheating and fire hazards from electrical faults and minimizes exposure to residual fumes from ovens after cleaning or cooking. This habit also provides an opportunity to educate children about responsibility and awareness, equipping them with knowledge for the future.
<u>Kitchen</u>

Infant/Non-mobile: (Birth - 6 months)
Infant crawl/roll: (5 months - 1 year)
→ **Toddler/Pre-school: (1 year - 4 years)**
→ **School-age: (5 years - 6+ years)**

# CHARGING AREA (PHONES, TABLETS, ETC...)

**Place charging stations on high shelves or counter tops out of reach.** Secure cords against walls or furniture with cord covers or cable clips to prevent tripping. Install outlet covers to prevent children from inserting objects into sockets and use surge protectors to limit electrical shock risks. Always supervise children around electrical outlets and cords, and teach them about the dangers of electricity. **Consider wireless charging pads for a cleaner, safer solution or invest in dedicated charging stations with built-in cord management and safety features.** Regularly inspect the area for damaged cords or outlets. Keep counter tops clear of clutter to prevent children from climbing, and be mindful of hot appliances like stoves and ovens when placing charging stations.

---

**Kitchen**
Infant/Non-mobile: (Birth - 6 months)
→ **Infant crawl/roll: (5 months - 1 year)**
→ **Toddler/Pre-school: (1 year - 4 years)**
→ **School-age: (5 years - 6+ years)**

# KITCHEN FLOOR SAFETY

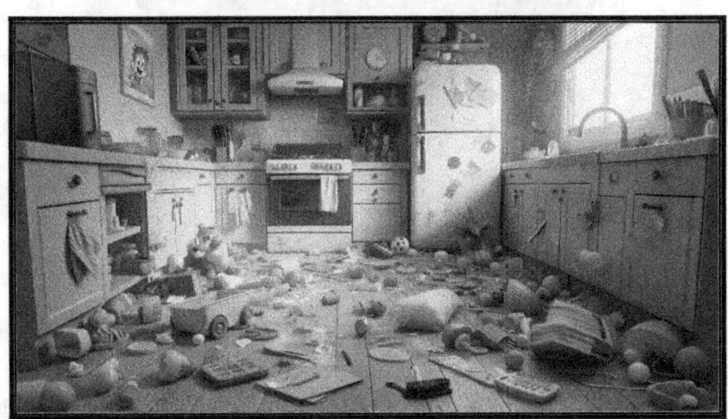

Approximately 2,000 children under age five die annually in the U.S. from choking on food or small objects. Regularly sweep or vacuum floors to keep them clear of small objects like coins, beads, or pet food that pose choking hazards. Teach children about the dangers of putting objects in their mouths. Use area rugs with non-slip backing in high-traffic areas or play zones and place non-slip mats near sinks or bathtubs. Provide slip-resistant footwear for children. Regularly inspect floors for sharp objects like broken glass, promptly cleaning up or repairing hazards. Keep tools and sharp objects in locked cabinets or drawers. Organize electrical cords and keep them out of the way using cord covers or hiding them behind furniture. Secure cords with clips or ties to keep them safely out of reach.

---

🍎 To childproof your kitchen floor to the extreme, install hospital-grade, flash coved linoleum that curves up the wall to eliminate 90-degree corners where bacteria and allergens accumulate. Pair this with a high-density, closed-cell foam underlayment to provide medical-grade impact attenuation, effectively turning the entire room into a "soft-fall" zone. *According to the American Academy of Pediatrics (AAP) standards for child-care facilities.*

---

**Kitchen**
Infant/Non-mobile: (Birth - 6 months)
Infant crawl/roll: (5 months - 1 year)
→ **Toddler/Pre-school: (1 year - 4 years)**
→ **School-age: (5 years - 6+ years)**

# REFRIGERATOR SAFETY

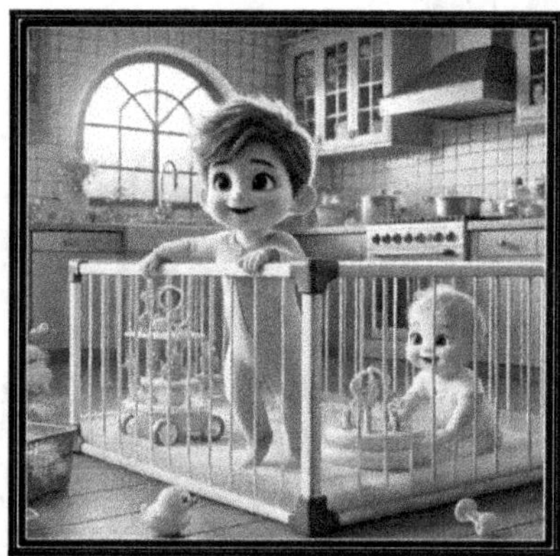

**Install childproof magnetic locks on fridge doors that unlock with a special magnetic key, invisible until needed.** Add adjustable strap locks for extra security. Use handle covers requiring a two-handed twist to open, ensuring only adults can access contents.

**Decorate with stickers placed strategically over handles to distract children.** Keep tempting snackable items on top shelves out of reach and place less desirable foods on bottom shelves. Put treats in containers labeled with boring names like "Mom's Kale Smoothies." Use non-slip fridge mats that are easy to clean and install a fridge door alarm that sounds if left open too long. If your fridge has an ice or water dispenser, install a childproof lock or temporarily turn off the water supply.

**Install shelf guards to prevent items from being pulled out and use sliding trays that lock in place when not in use.** Add a magnetic chalkboard or whiteboard to the front for children to draw on, and place cute fridge magnets shaped like animals as "guardians" to keep food safe from mischievous hands.

---

**Kitchen**
Infant/Non-mobile: (Birth - 6 months)
Infant crawl/roll: (5 months - 1 year)
→ **Toddler/Pre-school: (1 year - 4 years)**
→ **School-age: (5 years - 6+ years)**

# BREAST MILK SAFETY

**Always wash hands thoroughly with soap and water before expressing or handling breast milk.** Store in clean, BPA-free bottles or bags, labeling each with the date and time.

**Refrigerate for up to four days at 32-39°F or freeze for up to six months in a regular freezer or 12 months in a deep freezer.**

**Never microwave breast milk** as it causes hot spots and destroys nutrients. Thaw frozen milk by placing the container in warm water or using a bottle warmer. Gently swirl to mix separated layers without vigorously shaking. Avoid adding fresh milk to frozen milk. Check temperature before feeding; it should feel lukewarm, not hot.

**Use freshly expressed or thawed milk within two hours at room temperature.** Follow manufacturer's instructions for cleaning and sterilizing breast pumps.

**Be mindful of alcohol consumption and medications as they can pass into breast milk.** If you have an infectious illness, consult a healthcare professional before continuing breastfeeding, though it can usually continue with precautions.

---

Kitchen
→ Infant/Non-mobile: (Birth - 6 months)
→ Infant crawl/roll: (5 months - 1 year)
Toddler/Pre-school: (1 year - 4 years)
School-age: (5 years - 6+ years)

# Baby Formula

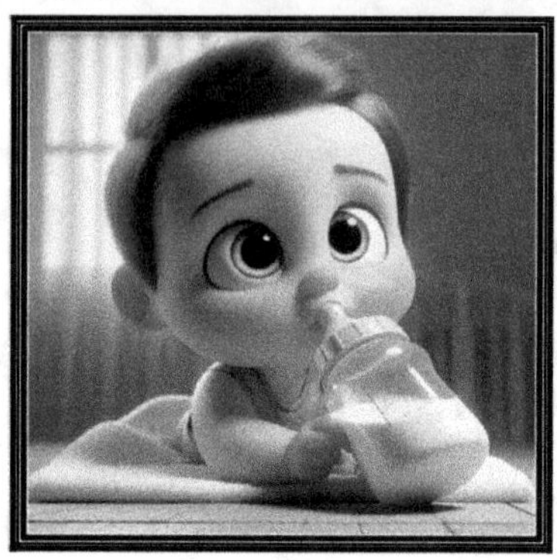

**Store formula in airtight containers on high shelves inside locked cabinets or pantries, creating a fortified vault.** Use containers with double lids for extra security. Hide formula in plain containers labeled with boring names like "Mom's Protein Powder" or use false bottom containers with uncooked pasta or rice on top. Use lockable measuring spoons or prepare pre-portioned formula packs in advance, sealed and stored in childproof containers. Place automatic formula makers on high counter tops and unplug when not in use. **Consider childproof locks on power cords or outlets.** Store manual mixing tools in high, secure cabinets or lockable drawers. Install smart locks controlled via app or use magnetic locks hidden inside cabinets that only open with a special magnetic key. Place a fun, interactive toy on top of the formula container as a "guard." Establish a regular feeding routine and set up a distraction station with favorite toys or books nearby.

---

Kitchen
Infant/Non-mobile: (Birth - 6 months)
→ Infant crawl/roll: (5 months - 1 year)
→ Toddler/Pre-school: (1 year - 4 years)
→ School-age: (5 years - 6+ years)

# Salmonella

**Salmonella causes approximately 1.35 million cases annually in the U.S., resulting in 26,500 hospitalizations and 420 deaths. Children under five are particularly vulnerable, with 43% of infected individuals**

**in a 2024 outbreak being under age five.**

Encourage frequent hand washing with soap and warm water, especially before handling food, after using the bathroom, and after playing outside. Cook all food thoroughly, especially meat, poultry, and eggs, using a meat thermometer to check safe internal temperatures.

**Promptly store cooked food in the refrigerator or freezer and avoid leaving perishable items at room temperature for more than two hours.** Clean all kitchen surfaces and utensils with hot, soapy water, especially after handling raw meat, poultry, or eggs.

Use separate cutting boards and utensils for raw meat and other foods to prevent cross-contamination. Teach children about food safety and hygiene practices, explaining why these guidelines are essential for preventing illness.

---

**Kitchen**
Infant/Non-mobile: (Birth - 6 months)
Infant crawl/roll: (5 months - 1 year)
→ **Toddler/Pre-school: (1 year - 4 years)**
→ **School-age: (5 years - 6+ years)**

# STOVE SAFETY

**Install stove guards to prevent children from reaching pots and pans, choosing heat-resistant materials. Use knob covers to prevent children from turning stove knobs, opting for transparent covers for easy visibility.** Create a "no-go" safety zone around the stove using visual cues like floor mats or tape.

**Always supervise children in the kitchen, especially during cooking.** Use back burners whenever possible and turn pot and pan handles toward the back of the stove. Use stable cookware to prevent tipping. Teach children about fire dangers and what to do in emergencies. Keep a fire extinguisher nearby and ensure all adults know how to use it.

**Have emergency numbers readily available and teach older children how to call for help.** Never use an oven to heat your home. Gas ovens can produce carbon monoxide when left open for extended periods, leading to poisoning. Ovens running continuously can overheat and cause fire risks. Open oven doors are accessible to children who might touch them or try to climb, causing severe burns or creating tripping hazards. Teach older children about oven dangers and the importance of not playing near or with them.

---

# HIGHCHAIR SAFETY

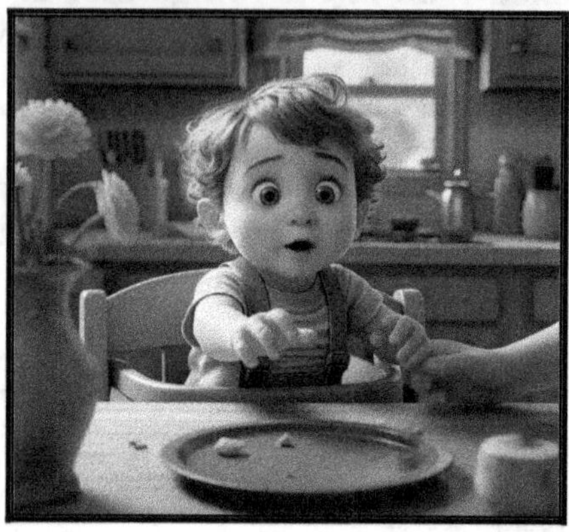

**Over 200,000 children are injured annually by furniture and fixtures, including falls from highchairs. In 2023, U.S. emergency departments treated 14,484 highchair-related injuries, a 47.8% increase from 9,803 in 2014. Children aged 7 to 23 months are most frequently injured, with approximately 94% of injuries resulting from falls due to climbing or standing.** Securely strap children into highchairs before each use to prevent falls, slipping, and difficulty feeding. Without proper strapping, children can wiggle, move, slip down, or access hazardous items like hot drinks or sharp utensils, leading to burns, cuts, or choking. Closely supervise children while seated and regularly inspect highchairs for wear or damage. Follow manufacturer guidelines for maintenance and usage.

---

**Kitchen**
Infant/Non-mobile: (Birth - 6 months)
Infant crawl/roll: (5 months - 1 year)
→ **Toddler/Pre-school: (1 year - 4 years)**
→ **School-age: (5 years - 6+ years)**

# KITCHEN COUNTERS

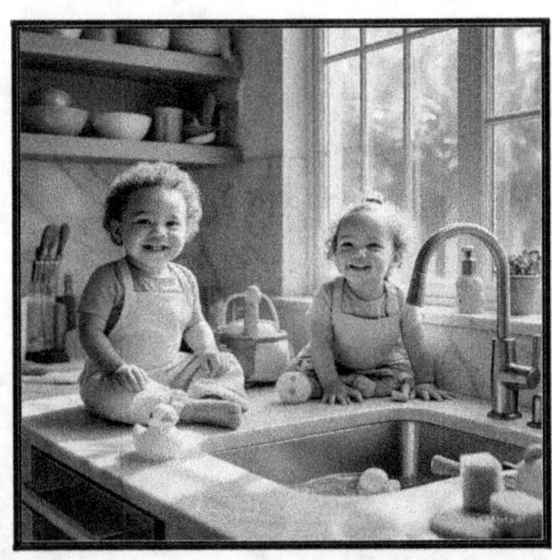

**Discourage children from sitting on counters as they can easily lose balance and fall from the height, potentially hitting their heads or suffering other injuries.** They may reach dangerous objects like knives, scissors, or hot pots and pans, risking burns or cuts. Counters may have contact with food, cleaning products, or harmful substances that could lead to contamination if children touch these surfaces and put their hands in their mouths. Sitting or standing on counter tops can cause damage over time, and allowing this behavior encourages children to climb onto other high surfaces like tables or shelves, increasing accident risks. **Provide children with safe, comfortable places to sit and play, such as child-sized tables or chairs.** Teach them about potential risks and the importance of using appropriate furniture. Always supervise children, especially in areas with potential hazards.

---

**Kitchen**
Infant/Non-mobile: (Birth - 6 months)
Infant crawl/roll: (5 months - 1 year)
→ **Toddler/Pre-school: (1 year - 4 years)**
→ **School-age: (5 years - 6+ years)**

# DISHWASHER

**Keep detergent pods and cleaning supplies out of reach in secure cabinets or drawers with childproof latches, as colorful pods can be enticing but hazardous if ingested.** Install a latch or lock on the dishwasher door to prevent younger children from opening it and accessing dangerous items like sharp knives or glassware. Use childproofing straps to secure the door. Promptly unload the dishwasher once it completes its cycle, ensuring sharp utensils are out of reach. Supervise children around kitchen appliances to ensure safety and teach proper kitchen etiquette.

---

# Cabinet Locks

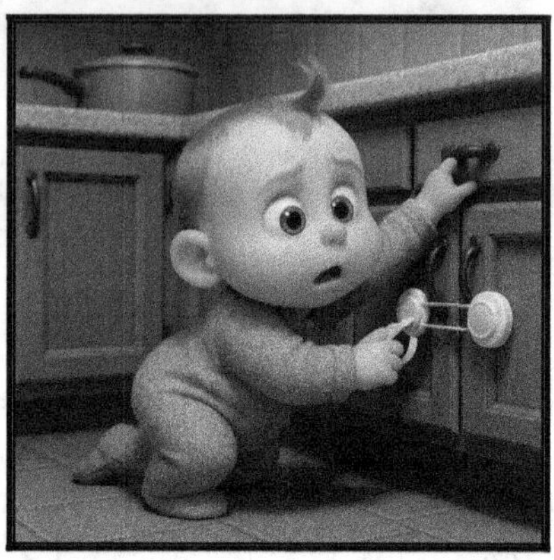

**More than 15,000 children are injured annually by sharp edges or entrapment in kitchen cabinets and drawers. Each year, over 100,000 children are exposed to dangerous household chemicals, leading to numerous ER visits for irritation, burns, or poisoning.** Install childproof locks or latches on cabinets containing hazardous items like cleaning supplies, sharp objects, or medications. Choose from adhesive locks, sliding locks, or magnetic locks. Consider locks for cabinets with messy items like flour or sugar to avoid choking hazards and unnecessary cleanups. Always keep hazardous cabinets locked, even when in the room, as accidents happen quickly. Store frequently needed items in lower cabinets so children won't be tempted to climb or reach for locked cabinets. Explain to children why certain cabinets are off-limits using simple, age-appropriate language. Regularly check locks and latches to ensure they function correctly and adjust as needed as your child grows.

---

**Kitchen**
Infant/Non-mobile: (Birth - 6 months)
Infant crawl/roll: (5 months - 1 year)
→ **Toddler/Pre-school: (1 year - 4 years)**
→ **School-age: (5 years - 6+ years)**

# Chairs with Wheels

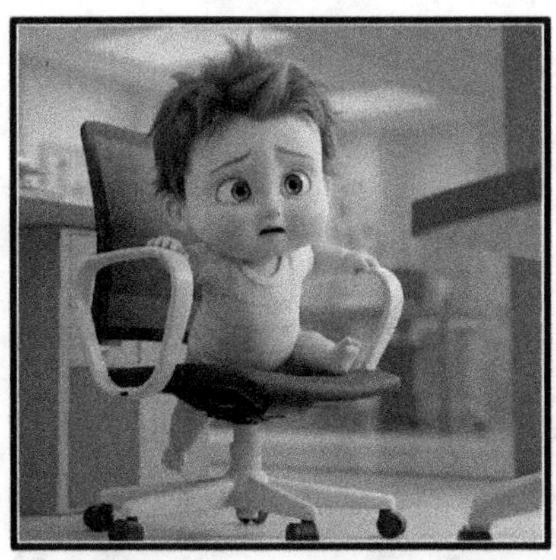

Opt for child-friendly furniture with stable bases, rounded edges, and no moving parts. Designate specific areas as safe play zones free from rolling chairs. Actively supervise playtime and intervene if you notice unsafe behavior. Use chair stops or locking mechanisms to prevent chairs from moving freely when not in use. Teach children about safe chair use, encouraging them to sit properly without rocking or tilting. Keep areas around rolling chairs clear from obstacles or hazards to prevent collisions and tripping.

---

**Kitchen**
Infant/Non-mobile: (Birth - 6 months)
Infant crawl/roll: (5 months - 1 year)
→ **Toddler/Pre-school: (1 year - 4 years)**
→ **School-age: (5 years - 6+ years)**

# Install Ground Faults

GFCIs protect households from electrical shocks. Receptacle type GFCIs integrate into homes instead of conventional outlets, offering protection against ground faults and extending protection to other outlets along the circuit. Circuit breaker type GFCIs can be incorporated into panel boxes to shield selected circuits, responding to short circuits or overloads. Portable type GFCIs are ideal when permanent installation isn't practical, offering temporary protection. The National Electrical Code mandates GFCI protection in specific zones including exterior outlets, bathroom circuits, garage outlets, kitchen sockets, and all outlets in crawl spaces and unfinished basements. For comprehensive safety, integrate GFCIs even where not required. GFCI circuit breakers can replace regular circuit breakers in older home panels. If homes use fuses, receptacle or portable GFCIs can be incorporated in key areas.

---

# Garbage Disposal

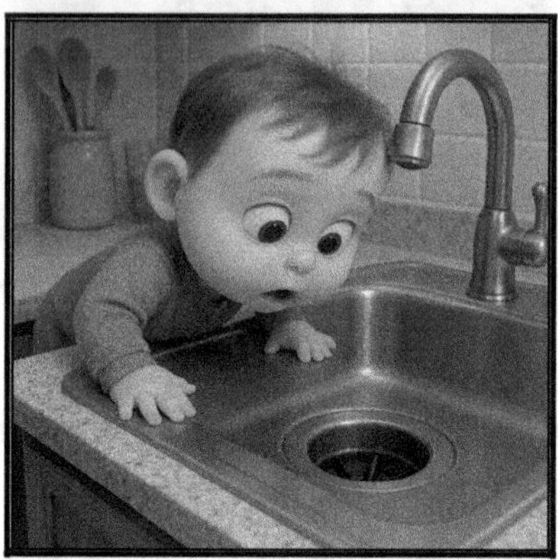

**Cover the switch with a clear plastic guard to prevent accidental activations while allowing visibility.** Consider installing a safety switch requiring a key or special code to operate. Teach children that garbage disposals are not toys and should only be used by adults. Insert a rubber stopper when not in use to prevent anything from accidentally falling in. Never leave children unsupervised in the kitchen, always keeping a watchful eye near the garbage disposal area.

---



# Trash Compactor Safety

**Install a childproof lock on the trash compactor to prevent children from accessing it.** Position it out of reach whenever possible by mounting higher on the wall or placing in a locked cabinet. Keep the key out of children's reach in a safe location. Constantly supervise children around the trash compactor. Educate children about the hazards, explaining it's not a toy and should only be used by adults.

---

# TEST WATER

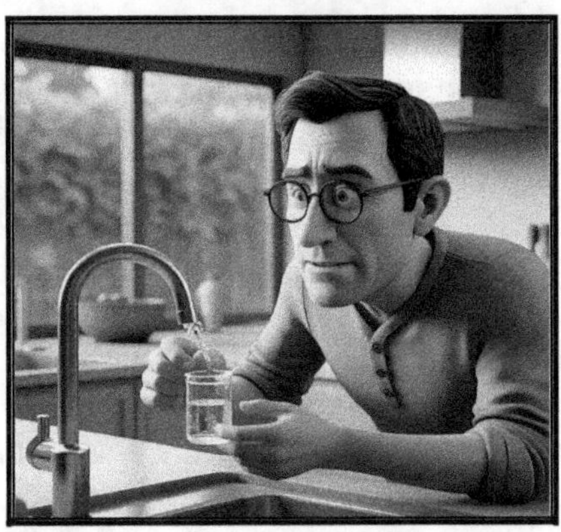

**Children, especially infants, have sensitive systems susceptible to waterborne pathogens and contaminants. Lead can have detrimental effects on cognitive development.** Water purity is crucial for baby formula preparation, as contaminated water can introduce harmful bacteria or chemicals and interfere with nutrient absorption. Identify potential contamination sources like older plumbing with lead-based pipes or proximity to industries or farms. Purchase home water testing kits targeting bacteria, lead, and harmful chemicals. Use frequently used taps for samples.

**Consider laboratory analysis for in-depth testing, especially in areas with known water issues.** Install suitable water filters like faucet attachments for removing lead or whole-house systems for comprehensive treatment. Regularly maintain your water system by cleaning and flushing heaters and tanks. Educate your family about which taps have treated water and are safe for drinking. Ensure anyone preparing baby formula uses only safe, treated water.

---

# Ice Maker Safety

**Check your refrigerator's user manual to activate the child lock function on the ice dispenser, preventing children from accessing ice and potentially spilling it or getting injured.** Ensure the freezer door has a childproof lock or latch if your ice maker is inside the freezer compartment. Explain to children the dangers of playing with the ice maker and that it's not a toy. Store ice scoops in high cabinets or drawers where children cannot reach them to prevent choking on ice cubes. Periodically check the ice maker and surrounding area for loose or broken parts, repairing or replacing them promptly. Always supervise young children in the kitchen, especially when using appliances like the refrigerator and ice maker. them repaired or replaced promptly.

> **Supervise Children in the Kitchen:** Always supervise young children when they are in the kitchen, especially when using appliances like the refrigerator and ice maker. This will help prevent accidents and ensure their safety.

---



# Educating Older Siblings

**Establish clear safety rules and protocols for everyone to follow, including activating safety devices, locking doors and cabinets after use, unplugging electronics when not in use, and always supervising younger siblings.** Assign age-appropriate safety responsibilities to older siblings who can help younger ones understand and follow rules, keep hazardous items out of reach, and be aware of dangers. Older siblings should lead by example, consistently following safety rules and demonstrating responsible behavior. **Encourage open communication about safety concerns and help younger siblings understand why measures are essential.** Conduct regular safety drills like fire drills or emergency evacuation plans. Foster a supportive environment where siblings look out for each other's safety, encouraging older siblings to be protective and nurturing. Provide age-appropriate supervision based on developmental needs and capabilities.

---



---

<u>**Kitchen**</u>
Infant/Non-mobile: (Birth - 6 months)
→ **Infant crawl/roll: (5 months - 1 year)**
→ **Toddler/Pre-school: (1 year - 4 years)**
School-age: (5 years - 6+ years)

# PLAYPEN IN THE KITCHEN

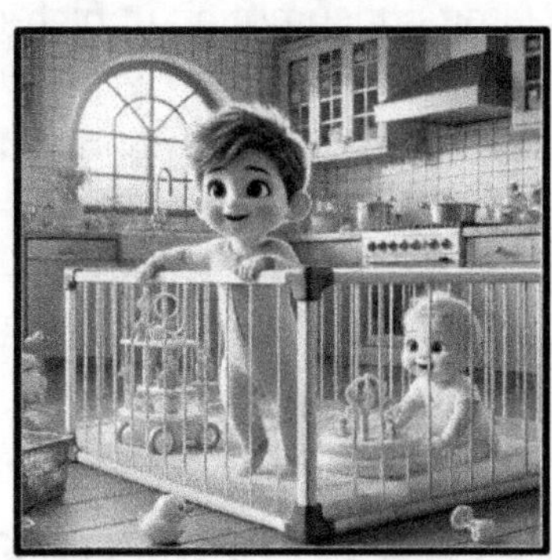

**A playpen creates a secure space for children to play while you focus on kitchen tasks, keeping them away from sharp objects, hot surfaces, and other hazards.** Use stove knob covers to prevent little hands from turning on burners and keep the playpen away from hot appliances. Maintain constant supervision and never leave children unattended in the playpen near the kitchen. Childproof the entire kitchen by securing cabinets and drawers with hazardous items and using safety locks on oven doors and refrigerators. Educate children about kitchen safety from an early age to help them understand dangers and develop good safety habits.

---

**Kitchen**
→ **Infant/Non-mobile: (Birth - 6 months)**
→ **Infant crawl/roll: (5 months - 1 year)**
→ **Toddler/Pre-school: (1 year - 4 years)**
→ **School-age: (5 years - 6+ years)**

# Mercury Concerns

**Mercury, particularly harmful to children with developing nervous systems, is found in older thermometers and barometers.** If broken, mercury vaporizes, creating inhalation risks. Fluorescent light bulbs contain small amounts requiring proper cleanup if broken. Some older batteries, especially button batteries, may contain mercury, and old paints from before the 1990s used mercury as a fungicide. Mercury accumulates in aquatic food chains with higher concentrations in predatory fish. Avoid or consume in moderation high-risk fish like shark, swordfish, king mackerel, and tilefish.

**Albacore or white tuna has higher mercury levels than light tuna.** Store mercury-containing items out of children's reach where they won't break. Dispose of old thermometers or fluorescent bulbs at designated hazardous waste sites. Limit consumption of high-mercury fish following recommended guidelines, especially for children and pregnant women.

**Teach older children about mercury dangers and the importance of not handling items that might contain it.**

---

**Kitchen**
Infant/Non-mobile: (Birth - 6 months)
Infant crawl/roll: (5 months - 1 year)
→ **Toddler/Pre-school: (1 year - 4 years)**
→ **School-age: (5 years - 6+ years)**

# Risks of Raw Sprouts

Raw sprouts can be contaminated with harmful bacteria like E. coli and salmonella from fertilizers used during growth. While rinsing decreases infection risk, it doesn't guarantee safety. Cooking sprouts effectively diminishes harmful bacteria, so ensure they reach the right temperature to neutralize pathogens. Raw diet enthusiasts must practice meticulous food handling and washing techniques. Stay updated with safety guidelines and consistently practice safe food preparation to enjoy nutritional benefits while ensuring safety.

---

# The Hidden Dangers in Candy: Lead Exposure

**Each year, U.S. poison centers receive about 102,000 calls for candy-related exposures in kids under six, with nearly 12,000 requiring medical treatment and over 140 involving serious symptoms. Imported candies,** especially those with chili, tamarind, or lead-ink wrappers, have tested above FDA's safe limit and are linked to elevated blood lead levels in young children. Lead is particularly harmful to young children, causing developmental lags, learning challenges, and behavioral disorders. Some imported candies contain more lead due to varying international standards, and lead may be present in wrapper inks or materials. Check where candies are imported from and lean toward trusted brands and sellers. Regularly check for product recalls or advisories related to lead content. Discourage children from chewing or playing with candy wrappers.

---

❦ Each year, U.S. poison centers receive about **102,000 calls** for candy-related exposures in kids under 6. Nearly **12,000** leading to medical treatment and **over 140 involving serious symptoms**. Imported candies, especially those with chili, tamarind, or lead-ink wrappers, have tested above FDA's safe limit (0.1 ppm), and linked to elevated blood lead levels in young children. *Washington State Dept of Health*

---



# Nut Concerns

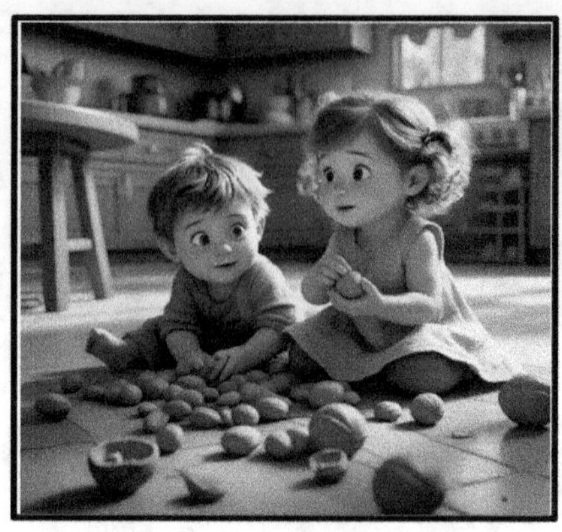

**Up to 6% of children under age three have food allergies, with peanut allergy being most concerning due to its potential to trigger anaphylaxis.** Initial indicators include itching, hives, or a runny nose, which can rapidly escalate to chest pain, swelling of throat and mouth, difficulty breathing, dizziness, and severe headaches. Seek medical attention immediately. Anaphylaxis can develop within minutes of exposure. Insect stings, medications, and latex can also trigger allergic reactions.

**Use separate counter tops, utensils, and storage areas for allergen-free foods to minimize cross-contamination.** Read labels carefully as allergens might be present in trace amounts or under different names. When dining out, communicate food allergies to staff. Train parents and caregivers to recognize when and how to administer an EpiPen correctly and always have emergency contacts readily available.

---

<u>Kitchen</u>
Infant/Non-mobile: (Birth - 6 months)
Infant crawl/roll: (5 months - 1 year)
→ **Toddler/Pre-school: (1 year - 4 years)**
→ **School-age: (5 years - 6+ years)**

# KNIFE SAFETY

**More than 200,000 children are treated annually for cuts and lacerations from sharp household objects.** Store knives in knife blocks or on magnetic strips mounted high on walls out of children's reach. Use lockable drawers or cabinets with childproof locks. Use knife guards or sheaths to cover blades when not in use. Educate older children about knife safety and responsible handling, emphasizing keeping knives away from younger siblings. Always supervise young children in the kitchen and keep them at a safe distance from cooking areas.

**Consider childproof gadgets like knife edge protectors or blade covers.** Use child-friendly utensils with rounded edges and blunted tips for younger children. Some knife sets come with locking mechanisms securing blades in handles when not in use. Knife locking straps can help secure blades to handles. Keep counter tops clear and clean, putting away knives immediately after use.

---

<u>Kitchen</u>
→ **Infant/Non-mobile: (Birth - 6 months)**
→ **Infant crawl/roll: (5 months - 1 year)**
→ **Toddler/Pre-school: (1 year - 4 years)**
→ **School-age: (5 years - 6+ years)**

# Bacteria Concerns

**Wash hands thoroughly with soap and water after handling raw meat, poultry, and eggs, cleaning all surfaces, utensils, and cutting boards that contacted them.** Avoid cross-contamination by using separate cutting boards and utensils for raw meats. Handle unpasteurized foods carefully and wash hands and surfaces after handling. Wash fruits and vegetables thoroughly under running water before consumption. Always wash hands after handling reptiles, amphibians, or their habitats as they can carry Salmonella.

**Ensure homemade pet food is properly cooked and wash hands and surfaces after handling.** Use hot, soapy water to clean surfaces, cutting boards, and utensils, sanitizing counter tops and equipment regularly. Store perishable foods at appropriate temperatures, keeping refrigerators at 40°F or below and freezers at 0°F or below. Be aware of food poisoning symptoms like stomach cramps, diarrhea, vomiting, and fever, seeking medical attention if they occur.

**Use color-coded cutting boards to differentiate between food groups.** If you have a child with allergies, designate specific cutting boards and utensils for allergen-free foods. Use separate utensils for different food groups and thoroughly wash with hot, soapy water after use.

---

<u>Kitchen</u>
Infant/Non-mobile: (Birth - 6 months)
Infant crawl/roll: (5 months - 1 year)
→ **Toddler/Pre-school: (1 year - 4 years)**
→ **School-age: (5 years - 6+ years)**

# Pots and Pans

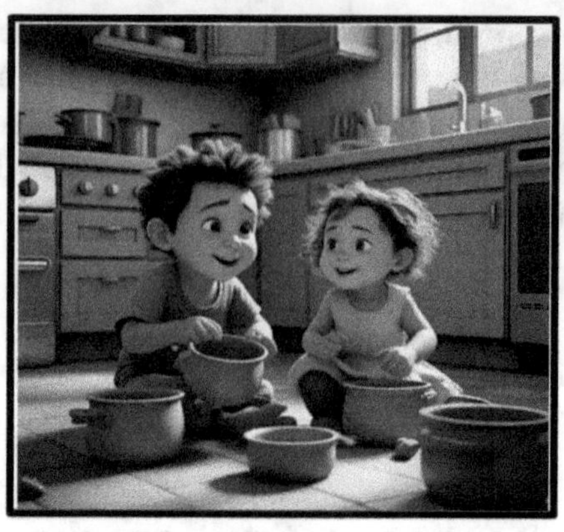

**More than 47,000 preschoolers ages 0-6 are treated annually in U.S. emergency rooms for burns or scalds from pots, pans, or hot liquids, often after pulling a pan off the stove.** Use rear burners when cooking to keep hot cookware away from the front. Turn pot and pan handles inward, away from the stove's front, to prevent children from grabbing them. Install childproof locks on all lower cabinets where pots and pans are stored. Store heavy items on lower shelves or in lower cabinets to avoid them falling. Use wall-mounted pot racks out of children's reach or ensure hanging racks are inaccessible. Educate children about kitchen safety, explaining that pots and pans can be hot and dangerous. Always supervise children in the kitchen and avoid leaving them alone near the stove or hot cookware. Let pots and pans cool down before moving or storing them. Consider using silicone handle covers providing heat-resistant barriers for safer handling.

---

🍏 According to the The *U.S. Consumer Product Safety Commission (CPS)* Every year, more than **47,000 preschoolers (ages 0–6) in the U.S. are treated in emergency rooms for burns or scalds from pots, pans, or hot liquids**. Often after simply pulling a pan off the stove. Toddlers are at highest risk: studies show they pull down pots or pans more than any other cause when reaching.

---

<u>**Kitchen**</u>
Infant/Non-mobile: (Birth - 6 months)
Infant crawl/roll: (5 months - 1 year)
→ **Toddler/Pre-school: (1 year - 4 years)**
→ **School-age: (5 years - 6+ years)**

# FRYING FOOD DANGERS

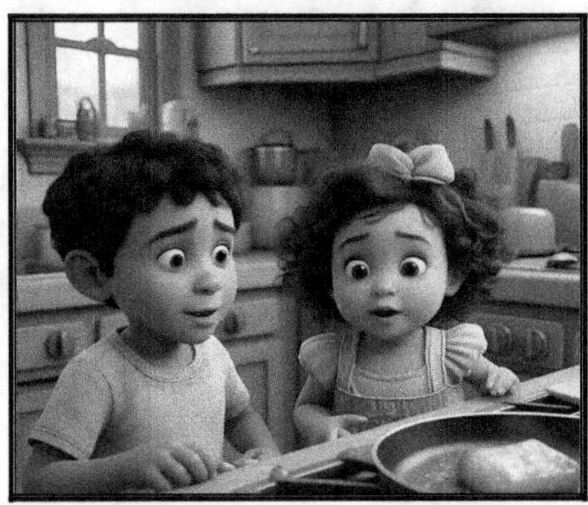

**Use splatter guards for frying pans to prevent hot oil and grease from splashing.** Designate a safe area in the kitchen away from the stove for your child to stay while cooking, setting up a play area or providing toys. Turn handles inward to prevent accidental spills and cook on back burners when possible. **Consider using lids to partially cover pans, containing splatters and reducing hot oil escape.** Educate children about hot surface dangers and why they should stay away from the stove. Always supervise children closely and never leave them unattended when cooking with hot oil. **Use long-handled utensils like tongs and spatulas to maintain a safe distance.** Wait for oil to cool before transferring to storage containers and keep containers out of reach. Be prepared for emergencies with a fire extinguisher or fire blanket accessible and know how to use them.

---

<u>**Kitchen**</u>
→ **Infant/Non-mobile: (Birth - 6 months)**
→ **Infant crawl/roll: (5 months - 1 year)**
→ **Toddler/Pre-school: (1 year - 4 years)**
→ **School-age: (5 years - 6+ years)**

# FLUORIDE IN DRINKING WATER

**Health Canada's expert panel found fluoride levels in Canadian drinking water may be associated with reduced IQ scores in children,** recommending considering cognitive effects when setting health-based values. Use child-safe or non-fluoridated toothpaste for young children who haven't mastered spitting it out. Always supervise children while brushing, ensuring they use only a pea-sized amount and spit it out. Store toothpaste out of children's reach. Many municipalities add fluoride to water supplies, and excessive consumption can lead to dental fluorosis in children. **Consider water filters designed to remove fluoride or use fluoride-free bottled water.** Check labels if wanting to limit intake. Mixing powdered or concentrated formula with fluoridated tap water can increase fluoride intake. Consider using fluoride-free bottled water or filtered water for formula preparation. **Discuss with your pediatrician about best water sources and whether fluoride supplements are necessary.** Some processed foods are made with fluoridated water, contributing to overall intake. Preparing meals at home with non-fluoridated water helps control consumption. Some children are prescribed fluoride supplements, so store these safely and give only in recommended doses. Regular dental checkups help monitor fluoride levels and adjust treatments as necessary.

---

🍏 Health Canada's expert panel reviewed evidence suggesting that fluoride levels commonly found in Canadian drinking water may be **associated with reduced IQ scores in children.** They recommended considering cognitive effects when setting health-based values for fluoride in drinking water.

---

<u>**Kitchen**</u>
→ **Infant/Non-mobile: (Birth - 6 months)**
→ **Infant crawl/roll: (5 months - 1 year)**
→ **Toddler/Pre-school: (1 year - 4 years)**
→ **School-age: (5 years - 6+ years)**

# Microwaved Food Hot Spots

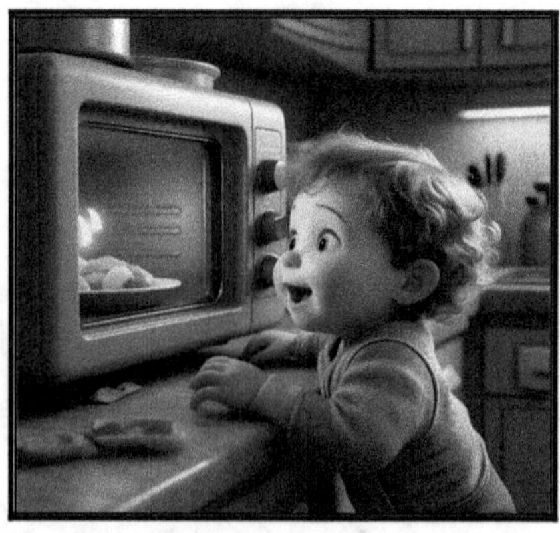

**Approximately 3,500 children suffer burns or scalds from microwave ovens annually, often from mishandling hot containers or steam.** Microwaves can cause uneven heating with dangerously hot areas while others remain lukewarm, posing burn risks to infants' sensitive mouths and throats. If microwaving, stir food or formula multiple times during heating to distribute heat evenly. Always test temperature on your wrist before feeding. Alternative methods include bottle warmers designed for heating to the right temperature, warm water baths for gradual, even heating, or stove top heating allowing more consistent temperature control.

---

**Kitchen**
Infant/Non-mobile: (Birth - 6 months)
→ **Infant crawl/roll: (5 months - 1 year)**
→ **Toddler/Pre-school: (1 year - 4 years)**
→ **School-age: (5 years - 6+ years)**

# THE DANGER OF KITCHEN SPICES

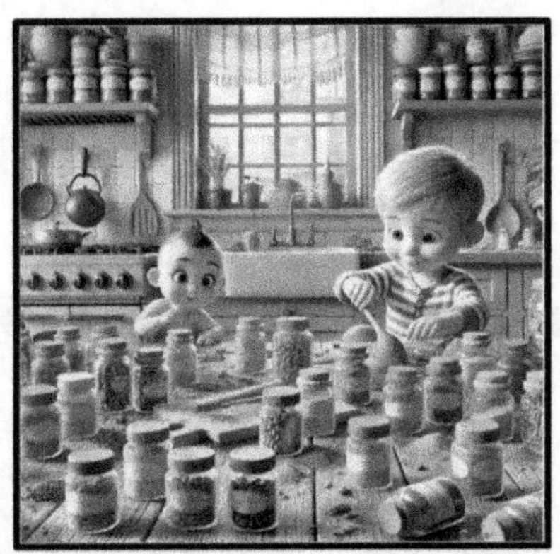

**Over a quarter of imported spices like chili powder and turmeric contain dangerous lead levels.** Studies show just a few bites can raise preschool children's blood lead by 25-30%, driving some toddlers above the 10 µg/dL danger level. Nearly 29% of spices in homes of lead-poisoned kids were contaminated. Nutmeg can cause hallucinations and seizures even in small amounts. Chili powder can cause severe discomfort if ingested, inhaled, or contacts skin. Cloves and bay leaves are choking hazards and can cause internal discomfort if swallowed whole. Toxic varieties of star anise can be harmful, and large amounts of fennel and anise seeds can cause difficulty breathing. Black and white pepper can irritate eyes, nose, and throat. Store all spices, especially dangerous ones, on high shelves or upper cabinets. Install childproof locks on drawers storing spices.

**Clearly label every container so you can quickly identify what children might have consumed.** As children grow, teach them about spice dangers and let them safely explore scents and flavors under supervision. Avoid open displays or easily accessible storage. Ensure no spices are left on counter tops after cooking. Always have emergency numbers including poison control on hand and familiarize yourself with first aid for choking and spice-related irritations.

---

🐞 Astonishingly, over a quarter of imported spices, like chili powder and turmeric, used in American kitchens contain dangerous lead levels. **Studies show that just a few bites can raise preschool children's blood lead by 25–30%, driving some toddlers above the 10 µg/dL danger level.** In one North Carolina study, nearly 29% of spices found in homes of lead-poisoned kids were contaminated. It's a hidden hazard in everyday cooking. *-National Library of Medicine*

---

<u>Kitchen</u>
Infant/Non-mobile: (Birth - 6 months)
→ **Infant crawl/roll: (5 months - 1 year)**
Toddler/Pre-school: (1 year - 4 years)
School-age: (5 years - 6+ years)

# SIPPY CUP SAFETY

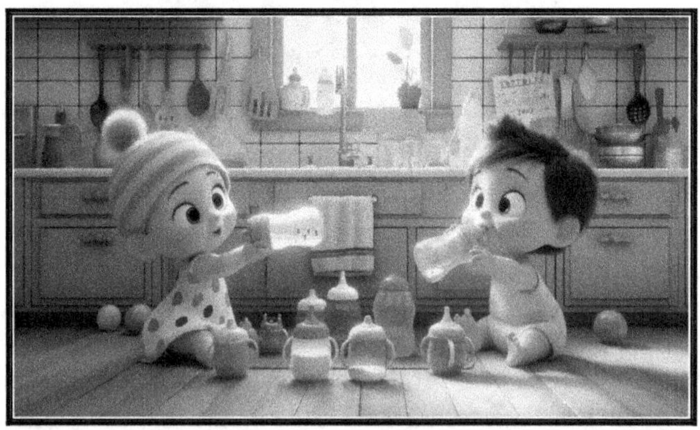

**Choose sippy cups made from safe materials like BPA-free plastic, stainless steel, or silicone, avoiding harmful chemicals. Opt for simple designs with no small detachable parts posing choking hazards.** Cups with one-piece spouts or valves are safer. Ensure lids fit tightly and securely, preventing spills and making it harder for children to open. Choose cups that are easy for children to handle with handles or grip-friendly designs and easy to disassemble and clean thoroughly.

Regularly inspect for wear and tear, replacing cups with cracks, broken parts, or damage.

**Fill only with age-appropriate drinks, avoiding sugary drinks, carbonated beverages, or hot liquids.** Always supervise children using sippy cups, especially younger ones. As children grow, transition them to open cups when appropriate to develop proper drinking skills.

<u>**Kitchen**</u>
Infant/Non-mobile: (Birth - 6 months)
→ **Infant crawl/roll: (5 months - 1 year)**
→ **Toddler/Pre-school: (1 year - 4 years)**
School-age: (5 years - 6+ years)

# Doggy Door Concerns

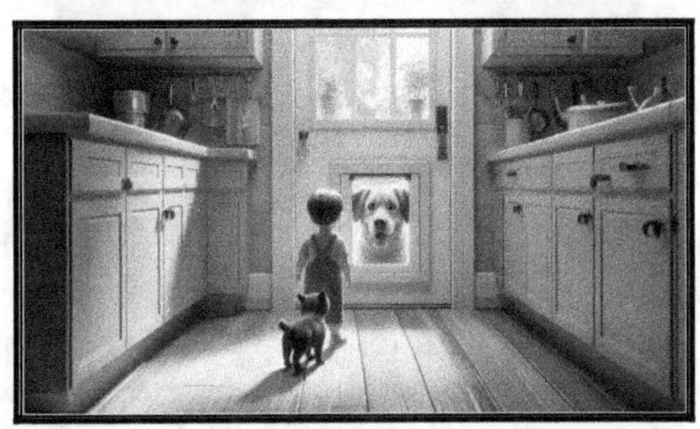

**Install a lockable pet door with a manual lock or electronic door operating with a sensor on your pet's collar, unlocking only when detecting your pet.** Ensure the opening is just large enough for your dog but too small for your child to crawl through. For larger dogs, install the door at a higher position accessible to your pet but out of reach for your child. **Use a solid cover with child-resistant locking mechanism over the doggy door when not in use. Install a child safety gate at the kitchen entrance restricting access, with some gates including smaller pet doors at the bottom.** Add audible alarms that sound when the door is used or motion-activated sensors near the door. **Explain to children that the doggy door is only for pets and not safe for them to use.** Keep a close eye on children near the kitchen or doggy door area. Consider a one-way pet door allowing your dog inside but requiring manual assistance to go outside. Regularly inspect the door ensuring locks and mechanisms function properly. If feasible, relocate the door to a less accessible area or use a door fitting into a sliding door or window out of children's reach. **Ensure the outdoor area is safe for your pet and not accessible to your child.**

# Kitty Litter Safety

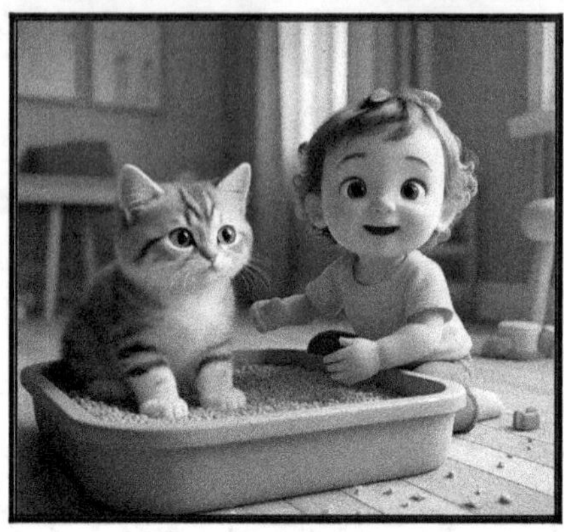

**Chose clumping or non-clumping litter safe for both cats and children, avoiding litter with added chemicals or fragrances.** Select a well-ventilated, low-traffic location for the litter box that's easily accessible for cats yet out of children's reach. Use covered or hooded litter boxes to prevent children from accessing litter, ensuring the cover is easy for cats to use. Instruct children on proper hand hygiene after handling cats or being near the litter box. Always supervise interactions between children and the litter box area, discouraging playing with or touching litter. Consider childproof enclosures or gates around the litter box area. Choose litter that minimizes tracking and use litter mats around the box. Maintain a consistent cleaning schedule to minimize odors and prevent bacteria spread.

**Consider natural or biodegradable litters made from corn, wheat, or pine as safer alternatives.** Store extra bags in secure, out-of-reach locations. Teach children to properly dispose of litter waste by sealing in bags and placing in outdoor trash. Monitor for allergies or sensitivities related to cat litter.

# SMOKE DETECTORS

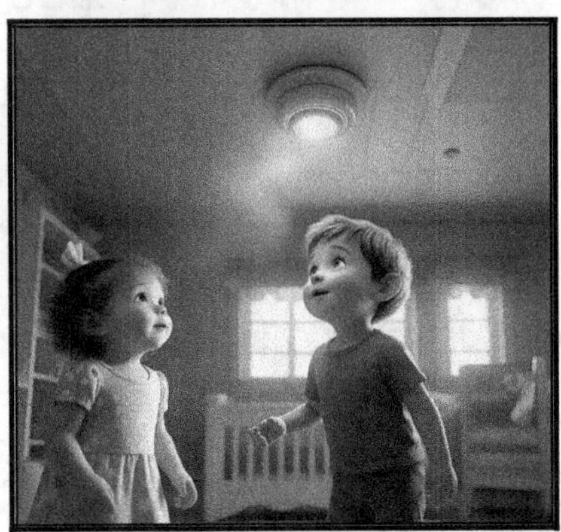

**Over 700 children are treated annually for fire-related injuries including burns and smoke inhalation.** Install smoke detectors on every level of your home including the basement. Place detectors in hallways outside bedrooms and inside rooms where people sleep. Keep detectors at least 10 feet from cooking appliances. Test batteries monthly using the test button. Replace batteries twice a year, such as when adjusting clocks for daylight saving time. Replace batteries immediately when hearing a chirping sound indicating low battery. Use a vacuum cleaner to remove dust from detectors' exteriors every six months. Wired detectors have signal lights flashing periodically indicating operation and often have battery backups needing checking and replacing. Special detectors with strobe lights and bed shakers are available for the hearing impaired. Smart detectors can send alerts to your phone indicating which room has danger. Consider interconnected systems so when one goes off, they all do. Check expiration dates and replace units past their useful life, generally 10 years.

---

# Carbon Monoxide (CO): The Silent Danger

**Approximately 400 cases of carbon monoxide poisoning in children occur annually in the U.S., often due to faulty heating systems or improper generator use.**

Install carbon monoxide detectors near sleeping areas and in communal spaces like living rooms and kitchens. Test detectors monthly and replace batteries at least twice a year or immediately if a low-battery warning sounds. Ensure all fuel-burning appliances are adequately ventilated with vents and flues free from blockages. Never use outdoor appliances like grills or generators inside the home. An orange flame indicates inefficient burning and possible CO production, requiring immediate appliance shutdown and technician consultation. A blue flame typically signifies efficient combustion but regular maintenance remains essential. Schedule annual inspections with certified technicians. Regularly inspect flues and chimneys for obstructions like plants, nests, or debris. Never leave hot grills unattended and install latches, locks, anchors, protective bumpers, and place grills away from combustible materials. Install ventilation systems tailored to specific appliances and regularly clean vents. Regularly inspect electrical cords and plugs for wear and ensure gas appliances have proper ventilation. For landlords, provide functional detectors, conduct regular inspections, ensure appliances meet safety standards, address maintenance concerns promptly, and provide clear usage instructions with emergency contact information. Ensure proper roof ventilation in attics and never leave cars running in garages. Install CO detectors with low-level indicators in garages.

---

<u>**Kitchen**</u>
→ **Infant/Non-mobile: (Birth - 6 months)**
→ **Infant crawl/roll: (5 months - 1 year)**
→ **Toddler/Pre-school: (1 year - 4 years)**
→ **School-age: (5 years - 6+ years)**

# First Aid Kits Should Include...

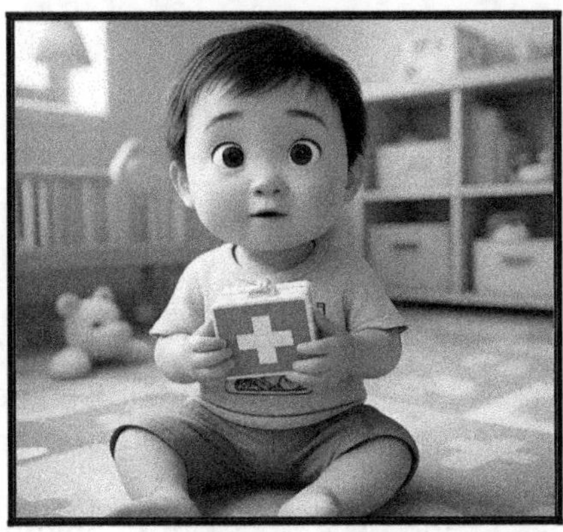

Include adhesive bandages in different sizes, sterile gauze pads and adhesive tape, antiseptic wipes or solution, tweezers, scissors, instant cold packs, elastic bandages, cotton balls and swabs, a thermometer, non-latex disposable gloves, CPR face shield or barrier device, pain relievers and antihistamines, oral re-hydration solution or electrolyte packets, a first aid manual or instruction booklet, and emergency contact information including phone numbers for your family doctor, pediatrician, and local emergency services. Check your kit regularly, replacing expired or used items, and tailor contents to your family's specific needs and activities.

---

<u>**Kitchen**</u>
Infant/Non-mobile: (Birth - 6 months)
→ **Infant crawl/roll: (5 months - 1 year)**
→ **Toddler/Pre-school: (1 year - 4 years)**
→ **School-age: (5 years - 6+ years)**

# Medicine Safety

**Store medicines in childproof containers out of children's reach and supervise intake of multivitamins or gummy supplements to prevent them from mistaking them for candies.** Always adhere to dosing instructions and avoid referring to medicine as candy. In case of suspected overdose, seek immediate medical help. Never give honey to infants under one year as it can lead to infant botulism due to underdeveloped digestive systems. Symptoms like weakness and difficulty swallowing require immediate medical attention. Maintain separate storage for medications and honey to avoid confusion. Consult healthcare providers before introducing new medications or supplements. Dispose of expired or unused medications responsibly.

---

<u>**Kitchen**</u>
Infant/Non-mobile: (Birth - 6 months)
→ **Infant crawl/roll: (5 months - 1 year)**
→ **Toddler/Pre-school: (1 year - 4 years)**
→ **School-age: (5 years - 6+ years)**

# MEALTIME SAFETY

**Nearly 7,500 toddlers ages 0-3 are rushed to ERs annually after choking on foods like hot dogs, grapes, or hard candy.** About 20 kids daily. Tragically, food choking causes over 60 deaths annually in children under six, with up to 90% of meat and candy-related choking injuries and nearly all fatalities happening at the dinner table. Always place hot dishes and beverages out of children's reach and avoid handling them while holding a child. Never pass hot items over children's heads. Avoid sporks as they can shatter, posing choking risks. Choose unbreakable plates like paper or plastic over ceramic. Cut high-risk foods like grapes, hot dogs, nuts, and popcorn into safe, non-round pieces, never serving them to children under four. Ensure children remain seated while eating and discourage walking or playing with food in mouths. Assess the size and age-appropriateness of small toys or trinkets before allowing children to play with them. Nothing replaces attentive supervision during mealtimes, even if an older sibling is assisting.

---

🦉 Every year in the U.S., nearly 7,500 toddlers (ages 0–3) are rushed to emergency rooms after choking on foods like hot dogs, grapes, or hard candy. About 20 kids every day. Tragically, food choking also causes **over 60 deaths** annually in children under six. Experts say up to **90%** of meat- and candy-related choking injuries. Nearly all fatalities happen at the dinner table. *(National Library of Medicine)*

---

# Baby Bottle Tooth Decay

**Baby Bottle Tooth Decay can lead to cavities and dental problems in baby teeth, causing pain and affecting oral health and development.** Avoid letting babies fall asleep with bottles in their mouths as prolonged exposure to sugary liquids during sleep is particularly damaging. If babies need bottles to soothe them to sleep, fill with water rather than sugary drinks. Introduce fruit juice in moderation, preferably during mealtime, avoiding bottles or sippy cups for extended periods.

**Gently wipe gums with a clean, damp cloth after feeding before teeth erupt. Once teeth appear, use a soft, age-appropriate toothbrush.** Schedule baby's first dental visit around their first birthday or within six months after their first tooth appears. Limit sugary snacks and drinks between meals, opting for healthier options. Show good oral hygiene habits by brushing and flossing regularly as children imitate parents.

**Discuss with pediatricians or dentists whether fluoride supplements or fluoride toothpaste are recommended based on age and water supply fluoride content.** Avoid sharing utensils or cleaning pacifiers with your mouth as this transfers harmful bacteria.

---



# A Deep Dive into Charcoal vs. Ipecac for Poisoning

Activated charcoal's porous structure absorbs toxins, preventing them from entering the bloodstream. It's particularly effective for medications, heavy metals, and certain plant toxins. Administer orally or through nasogastric tube as soon as possible after ingestion, ideally within an hour. Ipecac syrup was once common for poisoning, inducing vomiting to expel ingested substances. However, it has drawbacks including aspiration risk where stomach contents are inhaled into lungs potentially causing pneumonia, limited effectiveness for certain poisons, difficulty inducing vomiting in some individuals, and dehydration from repeated vomiting. Modern poison treatment includes supportive care addressing symptoms, antitoxins for specific poisonings, and dialysis in severe cases. The best action for poisoning emergencies is calling 911 or local poison control for specific advice based on poison type and symptoms. Do not attempt home treatment without medical advice.

---

**Kitchen**
Infant/Non-mobile: (Birth - 6 months)
Infant crawl/roll: (5 months - 1 year)
→ **Toddler/Pre-school: (1 year - 4 years)**
→ **School-age: (5 years - 6+ years)**

# Matches/Lighters

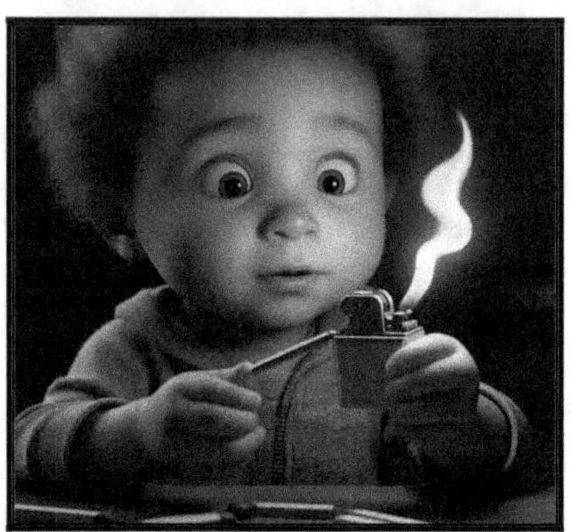

**Store matches in secure, locked locations out of children's reach and sight, using high cabinets or locked drawers.** Opt for safety matches that can only be struck on specific surfaces. If using large matchboxes with built-in strikers, keep out of reach or remove strikers and store separately. Place warning labels on or near storage areas.

**Educate children about fire dangers, explaining matches are not toys and only for adults.** Always supervise children when matches are used and never leave them unattended. Keep lighters out of reach and use child-resistant lighters with safety mechanisms. Set a good example by demonstrating responsible fire safety practices. Emphasize never playing with fire or lighting matches without adult supervision. Create a fire escape plan and practice it regularly. Ensure matches and lighters are safely stored during parties.

---

<u>Kitchen</u>
→ Infant/Non-mobile: (Birth - 6 months)
→ Infant crawl/roll: (5 months - 1 year)
→ Toddler/Pre-school: (1 year - 4 years)
→ School-age: (5 years - 6+ years)

# Fire Extinguishers

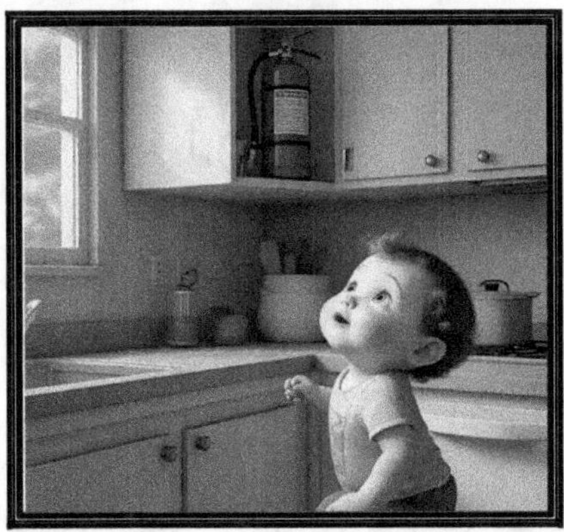

**Perform monthly inspections checking if extinguishers are easily accessible, fully charged, with correct pressure.** Examine nozzles for obstructions and verify pin and tamper seals are intact. Look for wear like dents, leaks, rust, or chemical deposits. Keep extinguishers clean and free from corrosive chemicals, oils, or debris. Fire extinguishers require hydrostatic testing after certain years to check for weaknesses or flaws.
**Consult owner's manuals, labels, or manufacturer guidelines for testing schedules.** Consider fire safety training to learn proper operation. Teach all family members how to use extinguishers and practice fire safety drills regularly. Baking soda can tackle grease fires on stoves by pouring directly over flames to smother them. Fire blankets can slow or put out small kitchen fires but aren't suitable for large or intense fires.

---

<u>Kitchen</u>
→ Infant/Non-mobile: (Birth - 6 months)
→ Infant crawl/roll: (5 months - 1 year)
→ Toddler/Pre-school: (1 year - 4 years)
→ School-age: (5 years - 6+ years)

# Emergency phone Numbers

**Save these numbers in cell and home phones:** Emergency services (911 in the U.S.) for life-threatening situations, pediatrician or primary care doctor, Poison Control Center, trusted family members or neighbors for emergencies, school or childcare facility, home address (especially if young children don't know it yet), nearest hospital, non-emergency police line, and trusted babysitters or caregivers. Ensure children know how to call for help in emergencies and understand the importance of these numbers.

---

<u>**Kitchen**</u>
Infant/Non-mobile: (Birth - 6 months)
→ **Infant crawl/roll: (5 months - 1 year)**
→ **Toddler/Pre-school: (1 year - 4 years)**
→ **School-age: (5 years - 6+ years)**

# PLASTIC BAGS

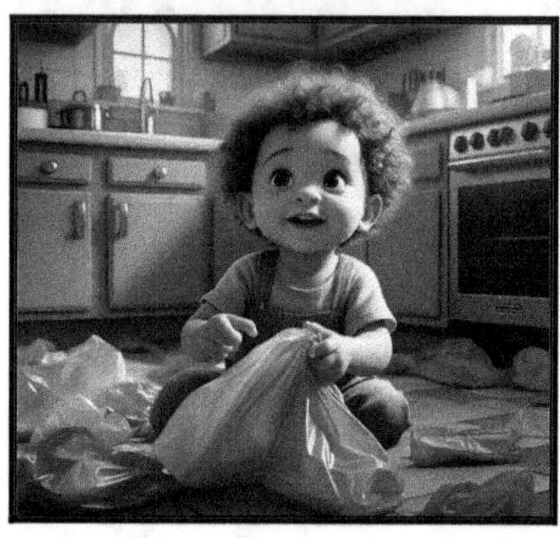

**Unintentional suffocation causes 1,200 child deaths annually, frequently from unsafe sleep environments or household items.** Store plastic bags in secure places out of young children's reach. Avoid leaving them on counter tops, tables, or floors. Promptly dispose in designated recycling bins or trash cans with secure lids after use. Never use plastic bags as mattress covers or bedding protectors as they're not breathable and can create suffocation risks. **Teach children about plastic bag dangers and the importance of not playing with or putting them over heads or faces.** Use reusable bags made from cloth or eco-friendly materials. Childproof storage areas containing plastic bags with safety latches or locks. Always supervise young children during playtime. Be cautious with dry-cleaning bags, immediately disposing of them safely or keeping out of reach.

---

<u>**Kitchen**</u>
→ **Infant/Non-mobile: (Birth - 6 months)**
→ **Infant crawl/roll: (5 months - 1 year)**
→ **Toddler/Pre-school: (1 year - 4 years)**
→ **School-age: (5 years - 6+ years)**

# Green Cleaning Benefits

**Indoor air can be two to five times more contaminated than outdoor air largely due to chemical-laden cleaning products.**

Childhood asthma prevalence has increased significantly in the past two decades, with some cleaning products acting as triggers. The average home contains approximately 25 gallons of hazardous chemicals, with significant portions in cleaning products.

**About 70% of all poisonings occur in the home, with children at higher risk.** Choose non-toxic, eco-friendly cleaning brands with simple, natural ingredients like vinegar and baking soda. Make DIY cleaning solutions using vinegar, baking soda, lemon, and essential oils. Ensure proper ventilation by opening windows and doors when using cleaning products. Store all cleaning supplies in locked cabinets or high shelves out of children's reach. Install childproof locks on cabinet doors. Never transfer cleaning supplies into containers resembling food or drink containers. Choose products in child-resistant packaging. Consider child-safe, eco-friendly products free from harsh chemicals. Never leave cleaning supplies unattended and keep children away while cleaning. Dispose of empty containers properly, rinsing before recycling. Educate older siblings about keeping supplies away from younger siblings.

---

<u>**Kitchen**</u>
Infant/Non-mobile: (Birth - 6 months)
Infant crawl/roll: (5 months - 1 year)
→ **Toddler/Pre-school: (1 year - 4 years)**
→ **School-age: (5 years - 6+ years)**

# The Dangers of Switching Containers and Labels

**More than 4,500 poisoning incidents annually** involve dangerous household chemicals mistakenly stored in unmarked or food/beverage containers, resulting in almost 9,400 ER visits and nearly 1,900 hospitalizations. In one example, 94 children were exposed in four months to brightly colored cleaners in juice-like bottles. Original containers provide essential information including usage instructions, ingredients, and warnings. Switching containers loses this vital information. Children are naturally curious and might be attracted to familiar-looking containers. **Transferring medications to unmarked or**

**incorrectly labeled containers can lead to overdoses or adverse reactions.** Storing cleaning agents in food or drink containers is especially misleading. Many medications and toxic products come in child-resistant packaging. Transferring bypasses these safety features. Even emptied containers might have residues, and mixing substances can lead to dangerous chemical reactions or increased toxicity. In emergencies, having original containers provides crucial information to poison control or medical professionals. **Misidentification can delay treatment.** Always store cleaning supplies, medications, and harmful substances in locked cabinets or out of reach. Teach children about dangers of consuming unknown substances. Periodically review and declutter storage areas ensuring all items are in original containers. When disposing of empty containers, rinse and render them unusable.

---

*🍎 Each year in the U.S., more than **4,500 poisoning incidents involve dangerous household chemicals mistakenly stored in unmarked or food/beverage containers.** These errors result in almost **9,400 ER visits** and nearly **1,900 hospitalizations** annually. In one notable example, 94 children were exposed in just four months to brightly colored cleaners decanted into juice-like bottles. (The American Association of Poison Control Centers (AAPCC))*

---

<u>Kitchen</u>
Infant/Non-mobile: (Birth - 6 months)
Infant crawl/roll: (5 months - 1 year)
→**Toddler/Pre-school: (1 year - 4 years)**
→**School-age: (5 years - 6+ years)**

# Duct Tape

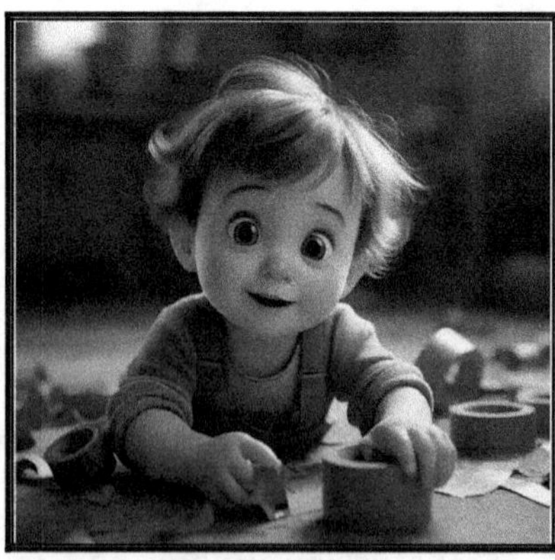

Use duct tape to keep cords and cables neatly fastened and out of reach, preventing tripping hazards and keeping hands away from electrical items. Apply layers to temporarily soften sharp edges, though it's a quick fix, not permanent. Use it to temporarily secure cabinets or drawers in a pinch, but invest in proper childproof locks for long-term safety. Attach it to create makeshift barriers temporarily blocking off areas. Sometimes it can fix broken toys or baby-proofing equipment. However, duct tape should never be used as a permanent childproofing solution. For comprehensive childproofing, rely on purpose-built safety products adhering to safety standards like baby gates, outlet covers, cabinet locks, and corner protectors.

---

<u>**Kitchen**</u>
Infant/Non-mobile: (Birth - 6 months)
→ **Infant crawl/roll: (5 months - 1 year)**
→ **Toddler/Pre-school: (1 year - 4 years)**
→ **School-age: (5 years - 6+ years)**

# MAGNET CONCERNS

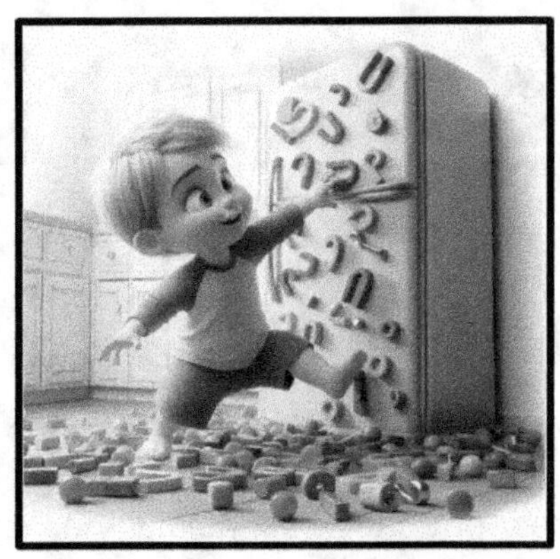

**Always supervise children playing with toys containing magnets.** Ensure toys are age-appropriate following packaging recommendations. Frequently inspect toys for wear and tear, repairing or discarding broken toys. Place refrigerator magnets high where young children can't reach them. Opt for larger, child-friendly magnets that can't be easily swallowed. Store magnetic jewelry in locked jewelry boxes or out of reach. Educate older children about swallowing dangers. **If using magnetic locks for cabinets, place them high up and periodically check mechanisms work correctly.** Store magnetic desk toys in locked drawers or high shelves when not in use. Ensure devices like speakers are securely placed on shelves or stands. Use cord organizers for charging cables with magnetic connectors. Store craft supplies including magnets in dedicated containers with secure lids. Clean workspaces immediately after projects. Store magnetic tools in locked toolboxes and ensure workspaces are off-limits to children or closely supervised. Be aware of magnet ingestion symptoms like abdominal pain, nausea, or vomiting, seeking medical attention immediately if suspected. Regularly remind children of dangers and periodically inspect homes for loose or stray magnets.

---

<u>**Kitchen**</u>
Infant/Non-mobile: (Birth - 6 months)
Infant crawl/roll: (5 months - 1 year)
→ **Toddler/Pre-school: (1 year - 4 years)**
→ **School-age: (5 years - 6+ years)**

# Purse/Handbags

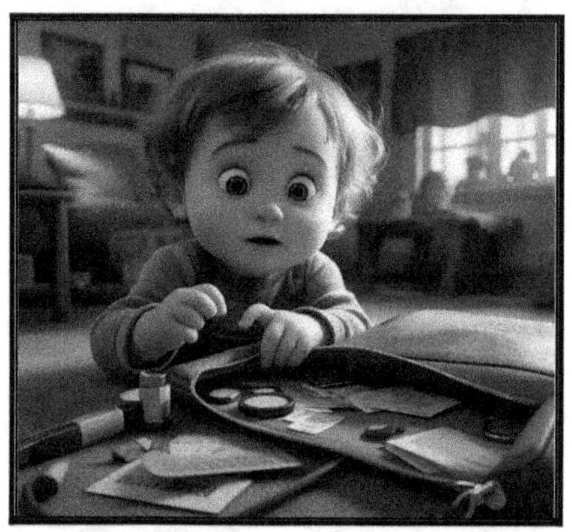

**Use child-resistant pill cases for medications or supplements, remembering child-resistant doesn't mean childproof.** Store cosmetics in zippered pouches, especially nail polish, perfume, or makeup removers. Some lipsticks contain elements that shouldn't be ingested in large amounts. Store sharp items like scissors, nail files, or tweezers in protective sheaths or cases in separate zippered pouches. Use secure coin purses for loose change as coins are choking hazards. Store small jewelry in jewelry pouches or zippered compartments. Ensure all buttons or decorative elements are secure. Hand sanitizers contain high alcohol levels, so use childproof bottles or keep in zipped compartments. **Store electronics in zipped compartments and ensure battery compartments are securely closed.** Wrap cords securely in pouches. If carrying snacks, ensure they're age-appropriate and not choking hazards. Ensure beverages have secure caps. Use key holders or pouches to prevent sharp edges from being accessible. Avoid too many small or detachable key chains. If carrying mini first aid kits, ensure antiseptics are sealed and out of reach. Keep emergency contact lists in purses. When at home, store purses in consistent, out-of-reach locations. Periodically empty and clean out purses removing expired items, hazards, or unnecessary objects. As children grow, educate them about dangers and teach them not to go through bags without permission.

---

<u>**Kitchen**</u>
Infant/Non-mobile: (Birth - 6 months)
Infant crawl/roll: (5 months - 1 year)
→ **Toddler/Pre-school: (1 year - 4 years)**
→ **School-age: (5 years - 6+ years)**

# ALUMINUM FOIL, PLASTIC WRAP, WAX PAPER, AND PARCHMENT PAPER

**Keep these materials out of children's reach in locked or high cabinets.** Avoid storing in low drawers or on accessible counter tops. Be cautious while cutting or tearing, keeping sharp edges and blades out of reach. Promptly dispose of used materials in secure trash bins. Don't leave them lying around. Always supervise children when using these materials in food preparation. Avoid letting children play with them as they pose choking hazards. Don't wrap small objects or toys in these materials as children might mistake them for edible items. Educate older children about potential hazards and the importance of keeping them away from younger siblings. If stored in cabinets within children's reach, use childproof locks.

---

<u>**Kitchen**</u>
→ **Infant/Non-mobile: (Birth - 6 months)**
→ **Infant crawl/roll: (5 months - 1 year)**
→ **Toddler/Pre-school: (1 year - 4 years)**
→ **School-age: (5 years - 6+ years)**

# FUSE BOX CONCERNS

**Invest in lockable fuse box covers or panels with locks and keys ensuring only adults can access fuses and electrical components.** If possible, relocate fuse boxes to out-of-reach areas like locked utility rooms or basements. Place warning labels on or near fuse boxes reminding adults of their importance. Teach children about dangers of playing with electrical components and the importance of leaving fuse boxes alone. Ensure any cords or wires around fuse boxes are securely fastened and out of reach. Periodically check for loose or damaged components, promptly addressing issues. If adults need to access, ensure children are supervised and kept away. Consider having professional electricians inspect if unsure about safety.

---

❦ Fuses are very safe only if used correctly. Because they are mechanical, people often make dangerous mistakes:

**Never "Penny" a Fuse:** There is an old, dangerous myth about putting a copper penny behind a blown fuse to get the power back on. This is a death trap. It bypasses the safety mechanism, allowing the wires to melt and start a fire.

**Match the Amps:** If a 15-amp fuse blows, do not replace it with a 20-amp or 30-amp fuse. This is called "over-fusing." The wires in the wall are only rated for 15 amps; if you put in a 20-amp fuse, the wires will melt before the fuse does.

**Check for "Scorching":** If the glass on a fuse is dark or cloudy, it blew from a short circuit (sudden surge). If the metal strip is just broken, it likely blew from an overload (too many gadgets).

---

**Kitchen**
Infant/Non-mobile: (Birth - 6 months)
Infant crawl/roll: (5 months - 1 year)
→ **Toddler/Pre-school: (1 year - 4 years)**
→ **School-age: (5 years - 6+ years)**

# Pantry Concerns

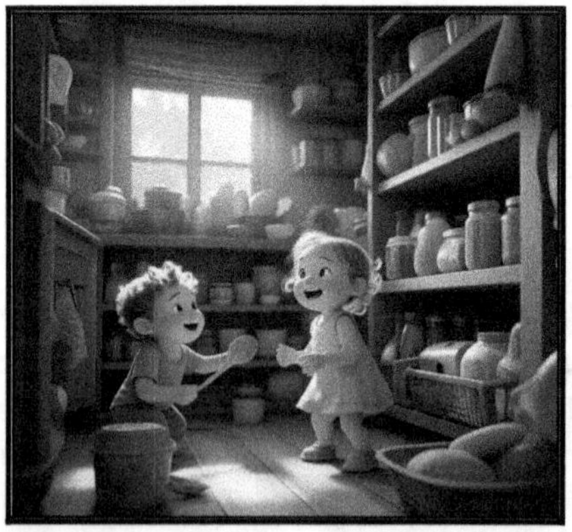

**Install childproof cabinet locks on pantry doors preventing easy access.** Store potentially dangerous items like cleaning products, chemicals, sharp utensils, and breakable items on higher shelves out of reach. Place heavy items like large kitchen appliances or bulk containers where they're stable and can't be pulled down. Use childproof storage bins or containers for small items like snacks, grains, and baking ingredients, ensuring they're tightly closed and placed on higher shelves.

**Keep toxic or harmful substances like medicine or alcohol in locked storage separate from the pantry.** Check for small items posing choking hazards like small candies or nuts, storing them in childproof containers or avoiding keeping them in the pantry. Teach children about pantry safety, explaining why certain items are off-limits. If storing cleaning supplies in the pantry, ensure they're in child-resistant containers on higher shelves. Regularly inspect for potential hazards, damaged containers, or expired products, disposing of expired items promptly.

---

<u>**Kitchen**</u>
Infant/Non-mobile: (Birth - 6 months)
Infant crawl/roll: (5 months - 1 year)
→ **Toddler/Pre-school: (1 year - 4 years)**
→ **School-age: (5 years - 6+ years)**

# GROCERY BAGS

Store bags in high, locked cupboards or pantry organizers mounted on door insides. Use wall-mounted bag holders keeping them organized and hard to pull out. Consider switching to reusable cloth bags that are less likely to cause harm and don't pose suffocation risks. Explain that grocery bags are not toys and should be left alone.

---

❦ To prevent both suffocation and accidental ingestion of microplastics, treat plastic grocery bags as high-level bio hazards by storing them in a wall-mounted, locking steel dispenser located entirely outside the kitchen environment, such as a high shelf in a locked garage. For an even more extreme approach, *the American Academy of Pediatrics (AAP)* recommends a total transition to short-handled, heavy-duty canvas totes to eliminate the strangulation risk posed by the thin, stretchy handles of standard plastic bags.

---

# |Ch. 4| Dining Room

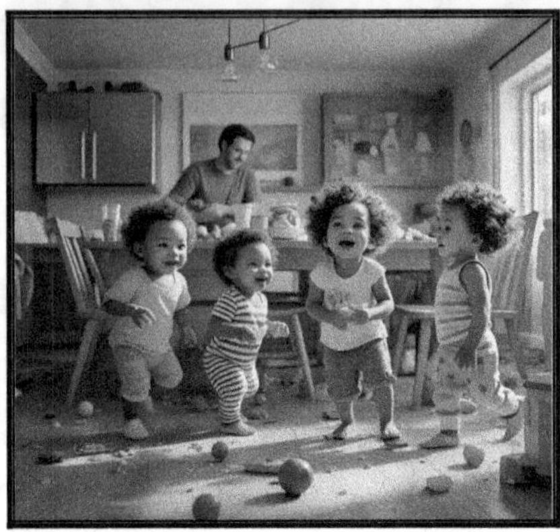

**Introduction:** Childproofing a dining room is crucial to ensuring a safe environment for young children. Often bustling with activity, this space contains several elements that might pose risks to curious little ones. To initiate childproofing, it is essential to identify and mitigate potential hazards, which could include securing unstable objects and restricting access to certain areas. Employing safety measures such as using child-friendly furniture and installing protective barriers can be beneficial. It is important to approach childproofing as an ongoing task, adapting strategies as children grow and their abilities evolve. This proactive approach helps in fostering a safe and enjoyable dining space for the entire family.

---

**<u>Dining room</u>**

Infant/Non-mobile: (Birth - 6 months)

→ **Infant crawl/roll: (5 months - 1 year)**

→ **Toddler/Pre-school: (1 year - 4 years)**

→ **School-age: (5 years - 6+ years)**

## PLACEMATS VS TABLECLOTHS

Place mats and tablecloths both have their pros and cons. Place mats offer stability, easy cleaning, and less risk of pulling, while tablecloths provide comprehensive coverage, soften impacts, and enhance the aesthetic appeal of your dining area. However, tablecloths are more prone to stains and require more maintenance. The best choice between the two depends on your family's specific needs, including the age of your children, the layout of your dining area, and your personal preferences.

<u>**Dining room**</u>
Infant/Non-mobile: (Birth - 6 months)
→ **Infant crawl/roll: (5 months - 1 year)**
→ **Toddler/Pre-school: (1 year - 4 years)**
→ **School-age: (5 years - 6+ years)**

# Unfinished Furniture

The rough and uneven surfaces typical of unfinished furniture can be a source of splinters, potentially causing painful wounds and infections in tender young skin. Moreover, these pieces of furniture may lack the stability and robustness found in finished products, increasing the risk of tipping or collapsing under the weight of a climbing child, leading to serious injuries. Additionally, unfinished furniture can be more susceptible to harboring bacteria and mold, as the lack of a protective sealant allows for the easier penetration of moisture and germs, creating an unhealthy environment for little ones who are prone to putting their mouths on surfaces. Furthermore, the materials used in the construction of such furniture might contain harmful chemicals or toxins that can be easily ingested or inhaled by children, posing a risk to their developing systems. Therefore, when considering the safety of a child-friendly home, it's prudent to meticulously evaluate the potential hazards associated with unfinished furniture.

---

<u>**Dining room**</u>
Infant/Non-mobile: (Birth - 6 months)
Infant crawl/roll: (5 months - 1 year)
→ **Toddler/Pre-school: (1 year - 4 years)**
→ **School-age: (5 years - 6+ years)**

# Secure Pictures to the Wall

**Securing pictures and other wall hangings is a critical aspect of childproofing.** Brimming with curiosity and energy, little ones may be tempted to tug at or climb on protruding frames, risking damage to the artwork and potentially serious injuries from falls or broken glass. Moreover, the heavy weight of some frames can cause substantial harm if they were to fall on a child. To mitigate these risks, it's advisable to use sturdy wall anchors and hooks that can bear significant weight, ensuring a firm hold. Additionally, placing pictures out of the reach of children and opting for shatterproof acrylic glass instead of traditional glass can further enhance safety. Regular checks to ensure the stability of these hangings can prevent accidents, maintaining a safe and harmonious home environment.

---

# Secure China and Utensils

When it comes to protecting your fine china, the key is elevation and security. **Store your china on high shelves or cabinets** that are completely out of reach of young children, making sure these storage areas are sturdy enough to bear the weight without any risk of collapse. **Invest in high-quality childproof cabinet locks** that can withstand determined tugging and pulling, and make it a habit to regularly inspect these locks to ensure they haven't loosened over time. Line your shelves with thick non-slip mats that provide cushioning and prevent china from shifting if the cabinet gets bumped. If you have glass-fronted cabinets, ensure the glass is tempered to prevent shattering, and consider adding safety film that holds the glass together if it breaks. For freestanding cabinets, use furniture straps or brackets to anchor them securely to the wall, preventing any tipping hazards.

**For utensils, especially sharp ones, drawer locks are your first line of defense.** Equip all drawers containing utensils with childproof locks that are durable and regularly inspected for wear and tear. For drawers with particularly sharp utensils like knives, consider double-locking systems for extra security. Use utensil organizers with tight compartments to segregate items, making it harder for small hands to grasp dangerous objects while keeping sharp edges contained. Consider using magnetic strips mounted high on walls for knives and sharp utensils, ensuring the magnetic strength is adequate to hold the weight securely. Dedicate specific drawers or compartments solely for sharp utensils so children can't accidentally access them when reaching for other items. When storing utensils in organizers or holders, always ensure that sharp or pointed ends face downward so that if a child does manage to reach, they touch the blunt end first.

---

**Dining Room**
Infant/Non-mobile: (Birth - 6 months)
Infant crawl/roll: (5 months - 1 year)
→ **Toddler/Pre-school: (1 year - 4 years)**
→ **School-age: (5 years - 6+ years)**

# Ensuring Mealtime Safety for Children

**Mealtime safety involves a comprehensive series of precautionary measures combined with vigilant supervision.** Keeping hot dishes and beverages well away from children is absolutely essential to prevent burns and spills that can cause serious injuries. Choose safe utensils and unbreakable plates to minimize the risk of injuries from broken dishes, which can create sharp edges that are particularly dangerous for little hands. Be cautious about your food choices for children, avoiding high-risk foods that pose choking hazards or carefully cutting them into safe, non-round pieces that are easier to swallow. It's also important to scrutinize the small toys or trinkets that often come with children's meals or purchases, ensuring they are age-appropriate to prevent choking hazards. Despite taking all these precautions, constant supervision during mealtimes remains irreplaceable, guaranteeing the safety of young children while fostering healthy eating habits and providing peace of mind for caregivers.

---

**Dining room**
Infant/Non-mobile: (Birth - 6 months)
→ **Infant crawl/roll: (5 months - 1 year)**
→ **Toddler/Pre-school: (1 year - 4 years)**
→ **School-age: (5 years - 6+ years)**

# Plant Safety

Having plants in your home adds beauty but also poses some risks that require careful childproofing attention. Many common houseplants like philodendrons, pothos, and dieffenbachia contain harmful toxins that can cause nausea, mouth irritation, and other uncomfortable symptoms if ingested, which is especially concerning for curious kids and pets who explore with their mouths. Cacti and succulents present their own dangers with painful thorns that can injure small hands, while heavy pots can tip over and crush little fingers during exploration. The safest approach is to keep all plants entirely out of reach of children by placing them on high shelves or in locked planters where curious hands can't access them. Make sure hanging plants are securely mounted and cannot be pulled down, and isolate plants with thorns in areas where children don't play.

<u>**Dining room**</u>
Infant/Non-mobile: (Birth - 6 months)
Infant crawl/roll: (5 months - 1 year)
**Toddler/Pre-school: (1 year - 4 years)**
**School-age: (5 years - 6+ years)**

# Secure Throw Rugs

**Throw rugs pose significant safety risks for young children and require careful attention when childproofing your home.** Loose rugs are major tripping hazards that can cause falls and injuries, particularly when children are running or playing enthusiastically. The best approach is actually to remove small throw rugs altogether during the years when children are most active and unsteady on their feet. If you do use rugs, choose those with non-slip backing or use rug pads and double-sided tape to firmly secure rugs against slipping. Never place rugs on top of each other, as this creates an even greater tripping hazard. Inspect the edges regularly to ensure they remain flat and haven't started to curl up, which commonly happens with wear. **For high-traffic areas where rugs are necessary, tightly woven low-pile rugs are best because they lay flatter and are less likely to catch little feet.** Taking these precautions with throw rugs by anchoring them firmly or removing them creates a safer play environment for kids, with the ultimate goal being to minimize hazards throughout your home.

---

<u>**Dining room**</u>
Infant/Non-mobile: (Birth - 6 months)
→ **Infant crawl/roll: (5 months - 1 year)**
→ **Toddler/Pre-school: (1 year - 4 years)**
→ **School-age: (5 years - 6+ years)**

# Floor Lamps

**To properly childproof a floor lamp, start by making sure it has a heavy, stable base that won't easily tip over, and place it strategically in a corner or against a wall rather than in open spaces where children play.** You can also secure the lamp to the wall using a lamp anchor or cable tie for extra stability, preventing it from being pulled over during active play. Use a childproof lamp cord cover to prevent children from chewing on the cord, which presents both electrical and choking hazards. If you have a cordless floor lamp, keep it out of reach of children or place it in a playpen or gated area where little hands can't access it during unsupervised moments.

# OUTLET COVERS

**You have several effective options for childproofing electric outlets to keep curious fingers safe.** Outlet plugs are simple devices that insert directly into the outlet and block access to the prongs, making them a quick first line of defense. Outlet covers fit over the entire outlet and are more difficult for children to remove than simple plugs, providing better protection for determined explorers. The most secure option is tamper-resistant outlets, which have built-in shutters that automatically prevent children from inserting objects into the outlet, providing protection even when the outlet is in use. According to the Electrical Safety Foundation International, approximately 2,400 children in the United States are treated for electrical outlet-related injuries each year, making this an essential safety measure that shouldn't be overlooked.

**Notes:**

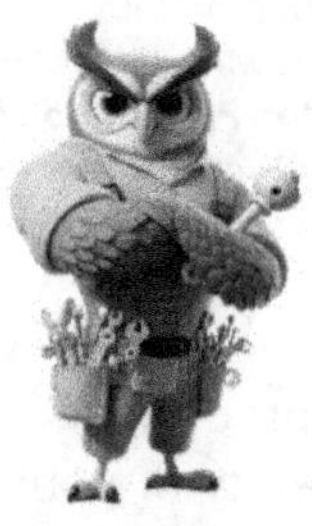

 # Hallways/Stairways

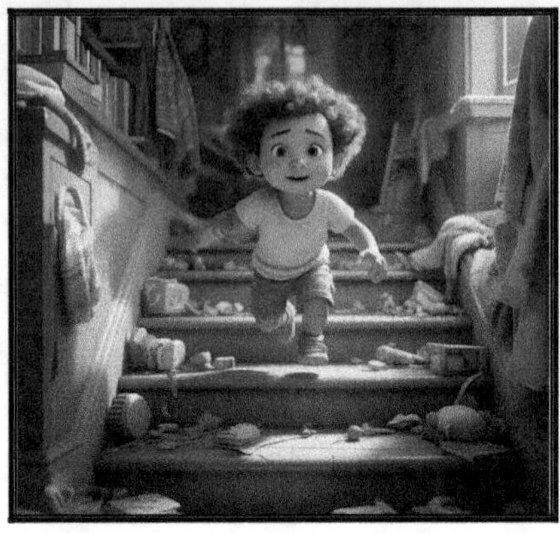

**Introduction**: These transitional areas of your home can often be overlooked during childproofing efforts, yet they harbor numerous potential hazards that can lead to slips, trips, and falls, especially for children between the ages of zero and six who are just learning to navigate their surroundings confidently. From securing loose rugs to installing safety gates at both the top and bottom of staircases, taking precautionary measures in these spaces is absolutely vital for preventing serious injuries. Additionally, ensuring that hallways are well-lit and free from clutter, combined with installing sturdy handrails that children can reach, can further safeguard your little explorers from potential accidents. The statistics are sobering: staircase-related injuries account for over 300,000 emergency room visits annually for children in the United States, often due to falls or entrapment, with approximately 1,076,558 people total suffering from staircase-related injuries each year. Young children and elderly people are the most vulnerable, with a child under five years old being treated for a stair-related injury approximately every six minutes.

---

**Hallways/Stairways**
Infant/Non-mobile: (Birth - 6 months)
Infant crawl/roll: (5 months - 1 year)
→ **Toddler/Pre-school: (1 year - 4 years)**
→ **School-age: (5 years - 6+ years)**

# DOORKNOB CONCERNS

Childproofing all possible doors in your house is a critical step in ensuring the safety of young children, as each type of door presents unique risks that require proactive solutions. A secure home begins with thoughtful planning and the right safety tools to prevent accidents and give caregivers genuine peace of mind.

**Front and back doors, being the primary entry and exit points**, require especially stringent safety measures to prevent wandering. Installing high-placed deadbolts that are well out of a child's reach is one of the most effective ways to prevent them from unlocking doors and wandering outside unsupervised. Door alarms are also essential because they alert you immediately if a door is opened, giving you precious time to respond before a child exits unnoticed into potentially dangerous situations. If your doors have glass panels, make sure they are made of safety glass, which is specifically designed to resist shattering and minimize injury in case of breakage.

**Interior doors, such as those leading to bedrooms, bathrooms, and laundry rooms, also need careful attention because children can access hazardous items,** fall into water, or accidentally lock themselves in. To mitigate these risks, use doorknob covers that are difficult for small hands to twist and open effectively. Finger pinch guards are a must-have to protect tiny fingers from getting caught in the door hinge, which can cause extremely painful injuries. Door stoppers can also help by preventing doors from slamming shut suddenly, which could cause injury to children who are nearby.

**Sliding doors, often found leading to patios or balconies, require different childproofing strategies than standard doors.** Install sliding door locks at the top of the frame to prevent young children from opening them and accessing outdoor areas unsupervised. To improve safety further, apply shatter-resistant window film to the glass, which minimizes injury if the door is accidentally broken. Additionally, installing safety bars ensures the door cannot be forced open easily, adding an extra layer of security against unauthorized access.

**Garage doors pose another serious hazard because garages often contain tools, chemicals, and vehicles that are extremely dangerous for children.** Store remote controls for garage doors out of reach to avoid unintentional operation that could trap or injure a child. It's vital to install safety sensors that detect obstructions and automatically reverse the door's motion to prevent injury. For extra protection, use childproofing straps on emergency release levers so that children can't operate them manually and accidentally open the door.

**Closet doors, though seemingly harmless, can pose hidden risks that many parents overlook.** Children may attempt to climb or play inside closets, leading to potential injury or entrapment among stored items. For bi-fold closet doors, install bi-fold door locks to prevent pinching or unintended access to potentially dangerous contents. Magnetic locks are another excellent option because they can only be opened with a magnetic key, effectively keeping dangerous contents completely out of reach.

**In addition to these physical measures, don't overlook general safety practices that reinforce physical childproofing.** Teach children early about the dangers of unsupervised access to certain areas, as awareness is a powerful tool in preventing accidents. Most importantly, supervise young children closely, especially around doors that could lead to hazards, combining education with vigilant oversight for maximum safety.

---

**Hallways/Stairways**
Infant/Non-mobile: (Birth - 6 months)
Infant crawl/roll: (5 months - 1 year)
→ **Toddler/Pre-school: (1 year - 4 years)**
→ **School-age: (5 years - 6+ years)**

# Night Lights

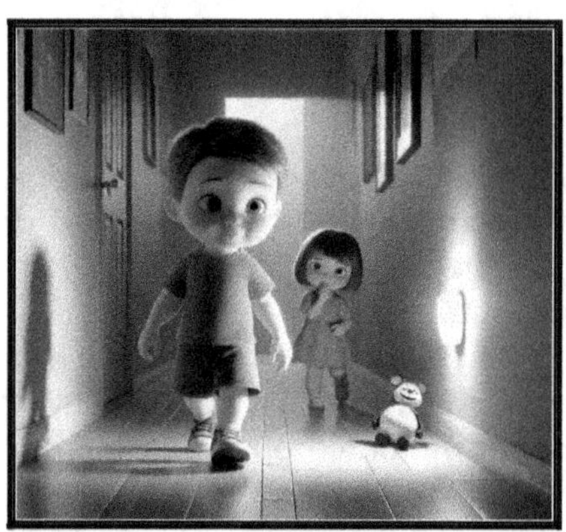

There are various hallway nightlight options available to suit different preferences and needs throughout your home. Plug-in nightlights are simple and easy to use, plugging directly into a wall outlet to provide gentle illumination, with many featuring sensors that automatically turn the light on when it gets dark and off when it's bright. LED nightlights are energy-efficient and long-lasting, coming in various shapes and designs, including ones that resemble stars, animals, or decorative elements, adding a touch of fun and aesthetics to the hallway. Motion-activated nightlights turn on when they detect movement, making them ideal for hallways used primarily at night while conserving energy by only activating when needed. Battery-operated nightlights offer flexibility in placement since they don't require an electrical outlet, making them convenient for areas without easy access to outlets.

**Wall-mounted nightlights** can be permanently fixed to the wall, providing a stable and constant source of light in the hallway. Rechargeable nightlights are eco-friendly and cost-effective, able to be charged using a USB cable or a docking station and providing illumination without the need for disposable batteries.

**Projector nightlights** create a soothing ambiance by projecting patterns or images on the walls or ceiling, with some including lullabies or nature sounds to help children sleep peacefully. Smart nightlights can be controlled through smartphone apps or voice commands, allowing you to adjust brightness, color, and scheduling according to your preferences.

**Glow-in-the-dark nightlights** absorb light during the day and emit a soft glow at night, beneficial during power outages or for a subtle glow without using electricity. Portable nightlights are small and lightweight, making them easy to carry around the house and handy for children who might need extra light in the hallway or their bedroom. When choosing a hallway nightlight, consider factors such as brightness levels, energy efficiency, ease of use, and safety features, selecting a nightlight that complements your hallway decor and meets your family's specific needs.

---

🌱 **Nightlights are among the top three "portable lighting" products involved in home fire incidents, but unlike floor lamps, nearly 100% of nightlight hazards are attributed to total fixture failure (internal short-circuiting) rather than user error** (like using the wrong bulb). The Shock Factor: Most parents assume a fire starts because a child "messed" with the light. In reality, nightlights are frequently left on for 10–12 hours straight in poorly ventilated corners behind curtains or furniture, causing them to smolder, melt, or ignite without any external interference. *U.S. Consumer Product Safety Commission (CPS), "Hazards Related to Electric Lighting Products."*

---

# The Gate Keeper (Gate Safety)

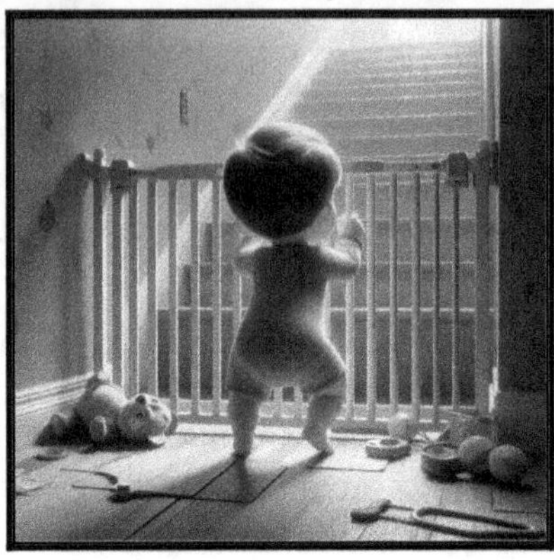

**Childproofing with a gate for the stairs is absolutely crucial in creating a safe environment for young children and pets, as stair gates act as protective barriers to prevent access to staircases.** Choose the right gate by selecting a stair gate that fits the width of your staircase and is appropriate for your specific needs, understanding that there are two main types: pressure-mounted gates that are convenient for easy installation, and hardware-mounted gates that offer a more secure and permanent solution.

**Measure the staircase opening carefully where you plan to install the gate,** ensuring that the gate you choose is adjustable to fit the width of your stairs precisely. It's essential to install gates at both the top and bottom of the staircase to completely childproof the area and prevent access from either direction. Follow the manufacturer's installation instructions carefully, as improper installation can seriously compromise the gate's effectiveness and safety.

**Position the gate correctly at the top or bottom of the stairs,** depending on where you want to restrict access, ensuring the gate is securely attached and leveled to function properly. Use hardware-mounted gates specifically for the top of stairs, as this is critically important for added safety since pressure-mounted gates may not be suitable for this area because they could potentially dislodge under pressure.

**Check that the gate's latching mechanism works correctly** and is child resistant, designed to be easy for adults to open and close but challenging for young children to figure out. Regularly inspect the gate periodically for signs of wear, damage, or loose components, addressing any issues immediately to maintain the gate's effectiveness.

Even with stair gates in place, always supervise children and pets when they are near the stairs, and educate family members and caregivers about the importance of always using the gate and keeping it closed. Remove clutter from the stairway area, including toys and objects that could pose a tripping hazard. If your staircases are wider than standard, consider using extra-wide gates that can extend to cover larger openings effectively.

---

**Hallways/Stairways**
Infant/Non-mobile: (Birth - 6 months)
Infant crawl/roll: (5 months - 1 year)
→ **Toddler/Pre-school: (1 year - 4 years)**
→ **School-age: (5 years - 6+ years)**

# Stairway Traction

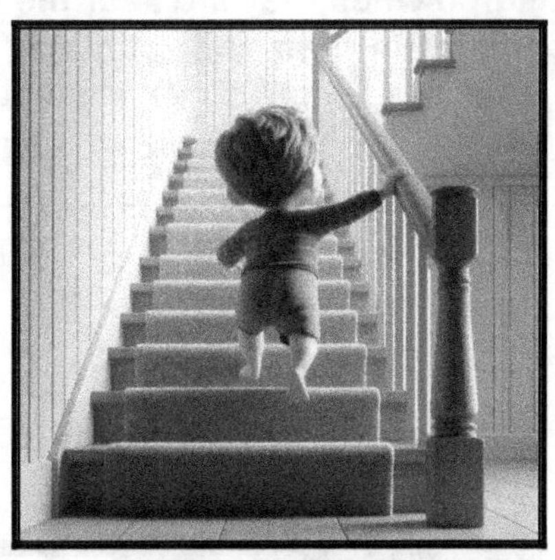

**Childproofing stairs includes ensuring they are safe and secure to prevent slips and falls, especially for young children who are still developing coordination**. Making stairs anti-slip is an essential step in enhancing stair safety throughout your home. Install non-slip treads or stair mats on each step, as these adhesive mats provide a textured surface that improves traction and significantly reduces the risk of slipping. Covering the stairs with carpeting or runners can add an extra layer of slip resistance, but for optimal safety, choose a carpet with a low pile and a non-slip backing that won't bunch up or create additional hazards. Ensure that handrails are securely attached on both sides of the staircase, as handrails provide essential support and stability while climbing the stairs, reducing the risk of accidents considerably.

Proper lighting in the stairway is essential for visibility, so install bright and energy-efficient lighting to ensure that each step is well-illuminated, even at night when visibility is naturally reduced.** Keep the stairway area free from clutter, toys, and other items that could become tripping hazards during daily use. You can also apply slip-resistant paint or coatings to wooden or concrete stairs to improve traction beyond what natural materials provide.

**Keep stair edges clearly marked with contrasting colors or reflective strips to make them more visible, which is especially helpful for young children who are still learning depth perception.** Teach children safe stair habits, such as always using the handrail, walking instead of running, and paying attention while climbing or descending. Regularly inspect the stairs for any loose or damaged treads, handrails, or carpeting, and repair or replace any worn-out or damaged parts promptly to maintain safety. Install stair gates at the top and bottom of the stairs to prevent young children from accessing the staircase unsupervised, combining multiple safety measures for maximum protection.

**Always supervise children when they are near the stairs, especially if they are not yet confident in their stair-climbing abilities.** Consider installing stair nosing, which is a protruding edge that provides additional grip, on the front of each stair to enhance slip resistance further.

---

**Hallways/Stairways**
Infant/Non-mobile: (Birth - 6 months)
Infant crawl/roll: (5 months - 1 year)
→ **Toddler/Pre-school: (1 year - 4 years)**
→ **School-age: (5 years - 6+ years)**

# BANISTERS

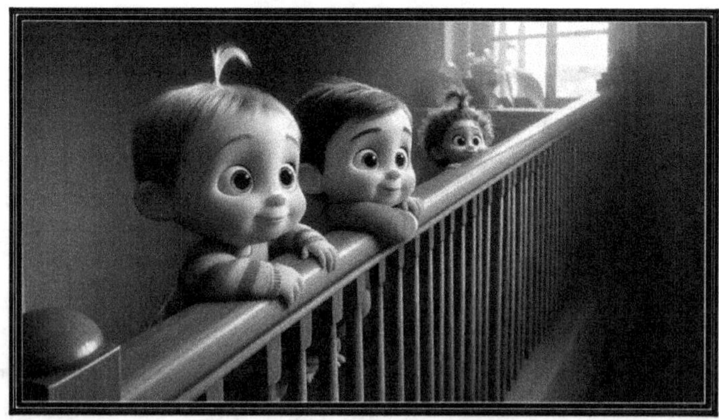

**Childproofing the banister is essential to create a safe environment**

for children, especially toddlers and young explorers who are naturally curious about climbing. Install a safety gate at the top and bottom of the stairs to prevent children from accessing the banister and staircase when unsupervised, choosing a gate that is specifically designed for use with banisters. Add baluster guards or netting that can be attached to the banister to create a barrier that prevents children from sticking their arms or legs between the balusters, helping to prevent entrapment or climbing attempts. Regularly inspect the banister for any loose or wobbly balusters and secure them firmly to prevent accidents.

Use cushioned padding on the banister to soften any potential impact if a child accidentally bumps into it during play or while learning to navigate stairs. Consider using childproofing covers or guards designed specifically for banisters, as these covers are typically made of durable materials and prevent children from easily dislodging or tampering with the banister.

Remove furniture or other items away from the banister that could act as a climbing aid for children to access higher areas. Regularly check the banister for any splinters or rough edges and sand down any rough areas to prevent injuries to tender skin.

Educate children about the banister's purpose as a safety feature and instruct them not to play or climb on it, reinforcing these lessons regularly. Ensure that handrails are securely attached on both sides of the staircase to provide stability and support while climbing or descending. Always supervise children when they are near the banister and stairs, especially if they are not yet confident in using the stairs independently. If you have carpeting or rugs on the stairs, make sure they are securely fastened to the steps to prevent tripping hazards. Periodically inspect the banister for any signs of wear or damage and address any issues promptly to maintain safety.

---

**Hallways/Stairways**
Infant/Non-mobile: (Birth - 6 months)
Infant crawl/roll: (5 months - 1 year)
→ **Toddler/Pre-school: (1 year - 4 years)**
→ **School-age: (5 years - 6+ years)**

# RAILS ON BOTH SIDES OF STAIRS

**Having handrails on both sides of stairs is not only a safety measure for general use but also an important aspect of childproofing your home effectively.** Children, especially toddlers and young kids, are still developing their balance and coordination, so having handrails on both sides of the stairs provides them with enhanced stability and support, significantly reducing the risk of slips and falls. Handrails help guide children along the staircase, preventing them from veering off the steps or losing their footing during navigation. With handrails on both sides, children can use both hands to hold onto the rails while climbing up or down the stairs, enabling them to move more comfortably and confidently. As children become more confident in using the stairs independently, the presence of handrails on both sides gives them the freedom to navigate the staircase with minimal assistance while still maintaining safety.

While stair gates are essential to block access to stairs when not supervised, having handrails on both sides provides an added layer of protection when children are using the stairs under adult supervision. In emergencies, children can rely on the handrails to help them safely evacuate the building, providing additional support and guidance during stressful situations. With handrails on both sides, children are less likely to place toys or other objects on the stairs because their hands are occupied, reducing the risk of tripping hazards.

**Handrails on both sides benefit not only children but also adults and elderly individuals, making the staircase safer for everyone in the household.** When childproofing stairs, ensure that the handrails are securely attached to the wall or balustrade and regularly inspect them for any signs of wear or damage, promptly addressing any issues to maintain their effectiveness in providing a safe and child-friendly staircase.

---

**Hallways/Stairways**
Infant/Non-mobile: (Birth - 6 months)
Infant crawl/roll: (5 months - 1 year)
→ **Toddler/Pre-school: (1 year - 4 years)**
→ **School-age: (5 years - 6+ years)**

# INSTALL A "JR. HANDRAIL"

**Adding a lower stair handrail specifically designed for children is a great way to further enhance safety on the staircase and encourage their independence as they grow.** A lower handrail allows children to have a secure grip and support while climbing or descending the stairs, making the stairway more accessible and less intimidating for them. Measure and mark the height at which you want to install the lower handrail, with the ideal height being around 24 to 28 inches from the ground, which is suitable for children's reach.

**Select a child-friendly handrail that is sturdy, smooth, and appropriately sized for small hands, with options available in wood, metal, or plastic depending on your preference and decor.** Prepare the handrail by cutting it to the desired length using a saw, making sure it fits the width of the staircase precisely. Attach mounting brackets to the wall at the marked height, using screws and anchors suitable for your wall type to secure the brackets firmly. Install the handrail by sliding it into the mounted brackets and ensuring it is level, using a level tool to double-check its horizontal alignment. Secure the handrail using screws to attach it firmly to the brackets, ensuring it can support a child's weight. Smooth any rough edges or corners of the handrail if necessary by sanding them down to ensure it is safe for children to hold. You can optionally paint or finish the handrail if you want to add a decorative touch or match it with your decor. **Educate children on how to use the lower handrail safely and encourage them to hold onto it while going up and down the stairs.** Always supervise children when they are using the stairs, especially when they are still learning to climb independently.

---

**Hallways/Stairways**
Infant/Non-mobile: (Birth - 6 months)
Infant crawl/roll: (5 months - 1 year)
→ **Toddler/Pre-school: (1 year - 4 years)**
→ **School-age: (5 years - 6+ years)**

# Banister Guard on the Outside of Stairs to Prevent Climbing

Adding a banister guard to the portion of the staircase ending in a newel post is an important safety precaution, especially if young children can use the newel post as a foothold to climb over the banister. A banister guard serves as an additional barrier that prevents children from accessing the space between the newel post and the banister, reducing the risk of climbing and potential falls. Measure the length and height of the space between the newel post and the banister where you plan to install the guard carefully. Choose a banister guard that is designed to fit the measurements of the area and is made of sturdy, child-safe materials that can withstand pulling and tugging. Install the banister guard by attaching it to the banister and newel post securely using screws or other provided fasteners, making sure the guard is firmly in place and cannot be easily dislodged. Check carefully that there are no gaps or openings between the banister guard and the newel post or banister where a child's foot or hand could get caught. If the banister guard has any sharp edges or rough surfaces, consider sanding them down to ensure it is safe for children. **Periodically inspect the banister guard** to ensure it remains securely attached and free from any damage or wear. Teach children about the purpose of the banister guard and instruct them not to climb on or over the banister, reinforcing this message regularly. Always supervise children when they are near the stairs, even with the banister guard in place.

---



# BEADED CURTAINS

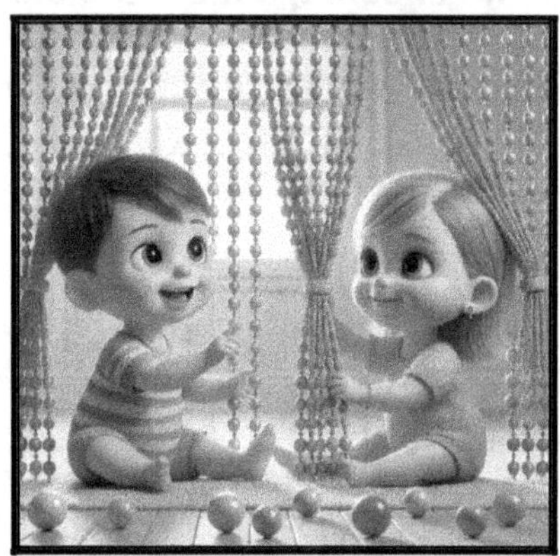

**Beaded curtains can pose a significant safety hazard to young children despite their decorative appeal.** Their small size and colorful appearance make them highly attractive to curious toddlers and infants who are drawn to bright, interesting objects. However, the beads can be easily pulled and ingested, leading to choking or other serious injuries.

**Choose shorter curtains that hang well out of reach of young children, which prevents them from accessing the beads and reduces the risk of accidents.** Consider replacing the beads with soft, fabric strands, which are less enticing to pull and less dangerous if a child becomes tangled. Install a latch or hook to tie the curtain out of the way when not in use, preventing children from accidentally pulling on the curtain and becoming entangled.

---

# |Ch. 6| Children's Bedroom

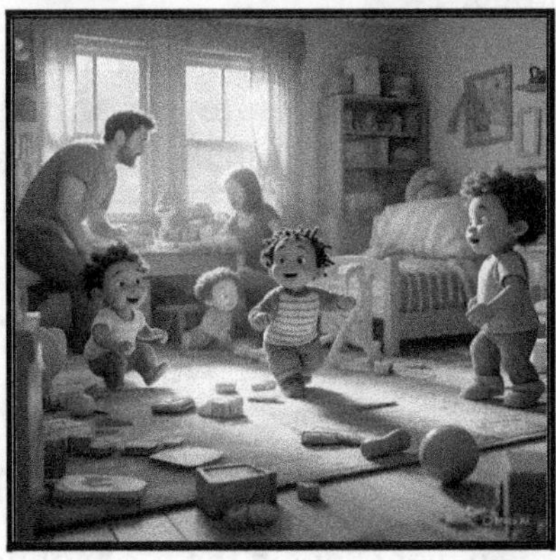

**Introduction**: A man's house is his castle; that makes the child's room the tower. Or the Great Hall. Or the dungeon. It depends on the child. Anyway, young toddlers have little say in their environment, but as they grow, their wants and needs are going to change. We're going to address the beginning phases and let you guys take it from there.

---

**Children's Bedroom**
Infant/Non-mobile: (Birth - 6 months)
Infant crawl/roll: (5 months - 1 year)
→ **Toddler/Pre-school: (1 year - 4 years)**
School-age: (5 years - 6+ years)

# KIDDO'S FIRST BED

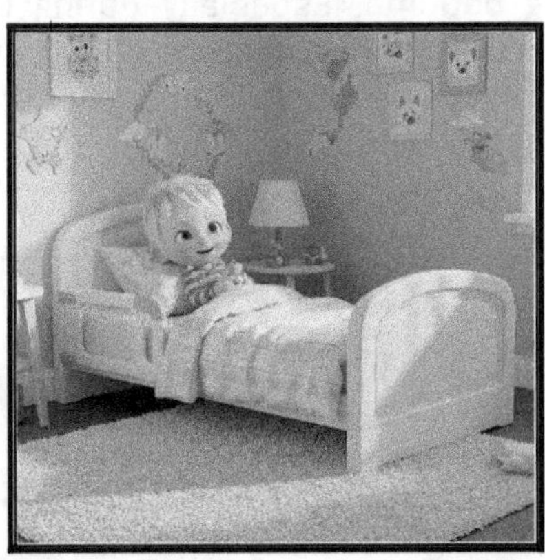

Transitioning a child from a crib to their first real bed is an exciting milestone that marks growing independence, but it's essential to childproof the new bed to ensure their safety during this transition. Install sturdy guardrails on both sides of the bed to prevent the child from accidentally rolling off during sleep, which is common as children adjust to more sleeping space.

**Choose a low-profile bed frame to reduce the risk of injury in case of accidental falls, as being closer to the ground minimizes impact.** Ensure the mattress fits snugly within the bed frame, leaving no gaps that could pose an entrapment hazard where limbs could get stuck.

**Use appropriately sized and firm bedding to reduce the risk of suffocation, and avoid pillows and heavy blankets for children under the age of one.** Opt for child-friendly and age-appropriate bedding designs without small parts that could detach and become a choking hazard. Keep the area around the bed clear of toys, cords, and other potential tripping hazards that could cause falls during nighttime bathroom trips. Place a night light in the room or hallway to provide a dim glow and reduce the risk of trips and falls during nighttime visits to the bathroom.

**Make sure any nearby furniture, such as dressers or shelves, is securely anchored to the wall to prevent tipping hazards if climbed on.** Cover electrical outlets near the bed with childproof outlet covers to prevent the child from inserting objects into them. If the bed is near a window, install window guards or use window stops to prevent the child from falling out or accessing cords or blinds.

**Secure cords from window blinds or curtains out of the child's reach to prevent strangulation hazards.** Teach your child about safe behavior in their new bed, such as not jumping on it, not using it as a play area, and staying in bed during bedtime. Especially during the initial transition period, supervise your child during naptime and bedtime to ensure they are adjusting well to the new bed. Childproof the entire bedroom by using outlet covers, securing furniture, and removing or securing any potential hazards throughout the space.

---

**Notes:**

# BUNK BED CONCERNS

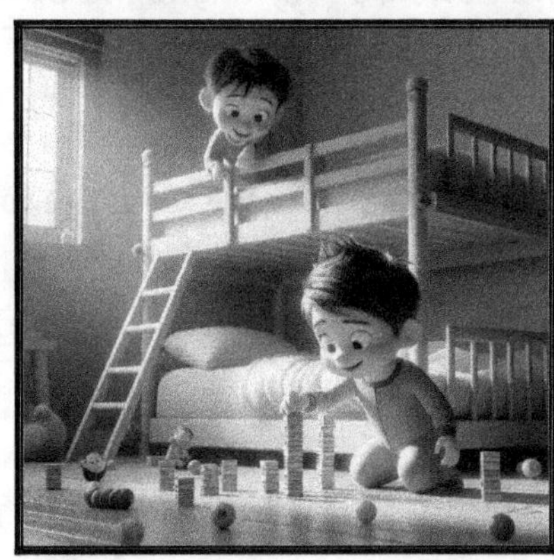

Using a bunk bed comes with certain safety considerations, and **it's generally recommended that children be at least six years old before using one due to developmental factors.** Children under six years old may not have the physical coordination and cognitive skills needed to safely navigate a bunk bed, especially the top bunk which requires climbing and balance. The top bunk is specifically not recommended for children under six due to the significant risk of falls and injuries from the height.

**Older children using the top bunk should be mature enough to understand safety rules and follow them consistently.** Both the top and bottom bunks should have sturdy guardrails on all sides to prevent accidental falls during sleep when children move around unconsciously. Ensure that the mattress fits snugly within the bed frame, with no gaps between the mattress and the guardrails where a child could become trapped.

**Choose a bunk bed with sturdy and durable construction to prevent the risk of collapse or other structural failures that could cause serious injury.** If the bunk bed has a ladder or stairs for access to the top bunk, make sure it is secure, slip-resistant, and properly attached to the bed frame. Place the bunk bed away from ceiling fans, light fixtures, or any other potential hazards that could be struck during play.

**Teach children that bunk beds are not for jumping or playing on, as rough play can lead to serious injuries from falls.** Follow the manufacturer's instructions carefully when assembling the bunk bed to ensure it is stable and safe for use.

**Use high-quality, appropriately sized mattresses with good support for growing bodies.** Avoid hanging items such as ropes, belts, or cords from the bunk bed, as they can pose strangulation hazards.

**Regularly inspect the bunk bed for any signs of wear, loose parts, or damage, and make necessary repairs promptly.** Encourage children to sleep alone on the top bunk and avoid allowing multiple children to sleep on the same level.

**Teach children how to safely evacuate from the top bunk** in case of an emergency like a fire. Always supervise children around bunk beds, especially during playtime, to ensure their safety.

---

**Children's Bedroom**
Infant/Non-mobile: (Birth - 6 months)
Infant crawl/roll: (5 months - 1 year)
→ **Toddler/Pre-school: (1 year - 4 years)**
→ **School-age: (5 years - 6+ years)**

# Clutter Concerns

**Removing clutter from bedroom floors regularly is essential to keep your child safe and maintain a healthy environment.** Clutter on the bedroom floor creates tripping hazards that can lead to falls and injuries, particularly when children are moving around in dim light or rushing to play. Regularly cleaning and organizing the floor space minimizes the risk of accidents significantly. Keeping the bedroom floor clean helps maintain a hygienic living environment, as clutter can collect dust, dirt, and allergens that can trigger allergies or respiratory issues in sensitive children. A clean and organized bedroom fosters better focus and productivity for children, allowing them to find their belongings easily and reducing distractions during homework or quiet time. Encouraging children to clean their bedroom floors helps instill a sense of responsibility for their personal space and belongings, teaching valuable life skills.

**A clean and tidy bedroom can boost a child's self-esteem and create a sense of pride in taking care of their space.** Teaching children to keep their bedroom floors clean instills good habits that they can carry into adulthood, leading to a more organized and clutter-free life overall. Clearing clutter from the floor creates more play space, allowing children to engage in activities without obstacles or safety concerns. A clutter-free bedroom promotes a relaxing and peaceful sleep environment, which is crucial for a child's physical and emotional well-being. Removing clutter and regularly cleaning the floor reduces dust accumulation, leading to better indoor air quality and fewer allergens. Cleaning their bedroom floor requires children to decide what items are essential and what can be put away or donated, teaching them valuable prioritization skills.

Set a regular cleaning schedule to make it a routine part of their daily or weekly chores, making cleaning fun by turning it into a game or playing music while they tidy up, offering praise and positive reinforcement when they complete the task, and providing storage solutions such as shelves, bins, and drawers to help keep belongings organized. Lead by example and maintain a clean and clutter-free environment in shared living spaces.

---

**Children's Bedroom**
Infant/Non-mobile: (Birth - 6 months)
Infant crawl/roll: (5 months - 1 year)
→ **Toddler/Pre-school: (1 year - 4 years)**
→ **School-age: (5 years - 6+ years)**

# FLASHLIGHT IMPORTANCE

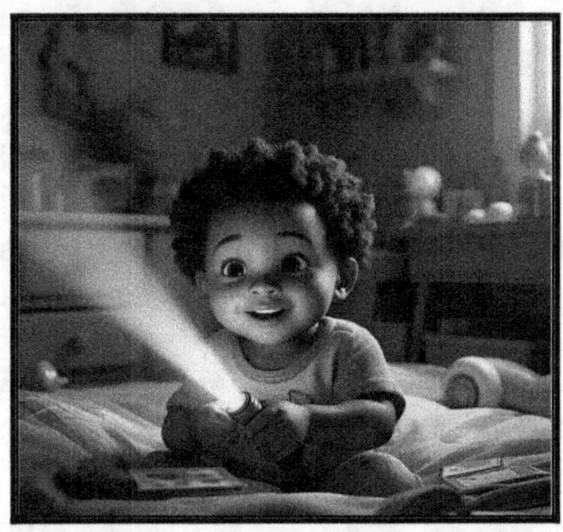

**Having a flashlight in the bedroom can be beneficial for children for various important reasons.** In the event of a power outage, a flashlight can provide a reliable source of light, ensuring that the child feels safe and secure during a potentially scary situation. Some children may feel uneasy or afraid of the dark, and having a flashlight nearby can offer a sense of comfort and control, allowing them to turn on the light whenever they feel anxious. A flashlight allows the child to move around the bedroom or go to the bathroom without turning on the main room light, which could disrupt their sleep or wake up other family members unnecessarily. A flashlight can add an element of fun during playtime or imaginative play in the bedroom, allowing the child to create shadow puppets or explore different lighting effects. Teaching children about the purpose and proper use of a flashlight can be part of emergency preparedness education, as they can learn how to use it during power outages or other emergencies. Having a flashlight encourages problem-solving skills as children learn to handle and use the device responsibly. A flashlight can be used as an educational tool to teach children about light, shadows, and how light travels through space. When introducing a flashlight to a child's bedroom, choose a child-friendly, durable, and easy-to-use flashlight suitable for their age and ensure the flashlight is always in working order by regularly checking and changing the batteries. Discuss the proper use of the flashlight and when it's appropriate to use it, such as during power outages or when moving around the room at night, and establish clear rules, such as not shining the light directly into someone's eyes or using it as a toy.

---

**Children's Bedroom**
Infant/Non-mobile: (Birth - 6 months)
Infant crawl/roll: (5 months - 1 year)
→ **Toddler/Pre-school: (1 year - 4 years)**
→ **School-age: (5 years - 6+ years)**

# Emergency Escape Plan

**Having an emergency plan is of utmost importance for the safety and well-being of individuals and families in case of crisis.** An emergency plan ensures that everyone in the household knows what to do in case of a crisis, reducing panic and confusion during high-stress situations when clear thinking is most needed. With a well-thought-out plan, individuals can respond promptly and take appropriate actions, potentially preventing injuries or further damage. An emergency plan includes an evacuation strategy, indicating safe routes and assembly points in case the family needs to leave the home quickly.

The plan outlines how family members will communicate with each other during an emergency, ensuring everyone is accounted for and safe. The plan includes important contact information for emergency services, neighbors, relatives, and other relevant individuals who can assist.

**For families with specific medical needs**, an emergency plan can include information about necessary medications, medical equipment, and contact details for healthcare providers. The plan identifies the location of safety equipment such as fire extinguishers, first aid kits, and flashlights, enabling swift access when needed.

**Regularly reviewing and practicing the emergency plan with all family members ensures everyone is familiar with the procedures and can**

**act confidently during an actual emergency.** An emergency plan can be adapted to address different types of emergencies with unique challenges and response measures based on the type of emergency, whether fire, natural disaster, or other crisis. Having an emergency plan in place provides peace of mind, knowing that everyone in the family is prepared for unforeseen circumstances.

**To create an effective emergency plan, involve all family members** in the planning process and make sure they understand their roles and responsibilities, establish meeting points and communication methods in case family members are separated during an emergency, review and update the plan regularly especially as family dynamics change or new risks emerge, practice evacuation drills and other emergency procedures to reinforce preparedness, and keep important documents such as identification, insurance policies, and medical records in a safe and easily accessible place.

---

**Children's Bedroom**
Infant/Non-mobile: (Birth - 6 months)
Infant crawl/roll: (5 months - 1 year)
→ **Toddler/Pre-school: (1 year - 4 years)**
→ **School-age: (5 years - 6+ years)**

# Nightlights

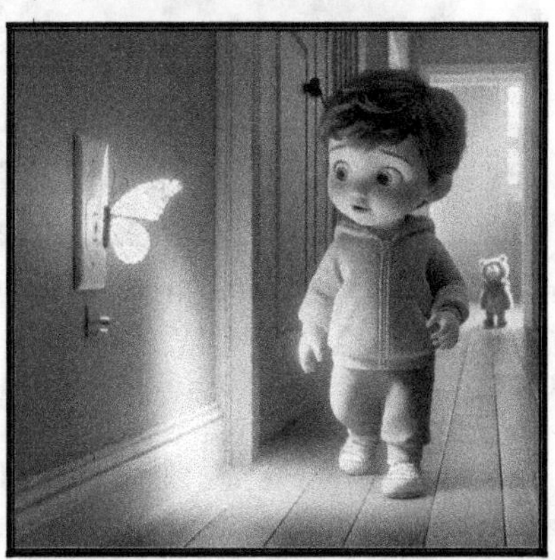

Nightlights come in various types to cater to different needs and preferences throughout your child's bedroom. **Plug-in nightlights** are straightforward to use and often feature sensors for automatic operation. **LED nightlights** are known for their energy efficiency and decorative designs. Motion-activated nightlights are energy-saving as they light up only upon detecting movement. **Battery-operated** ones offer placement flexibility without requiring electrical outlets. Wall-mounted nightlights provide constant illumination. **Rechargeable** ones are an eco-friendly option that can be charged via USB. Projector nightlights create a calming atmosphere with visual projections and sometimes include soothing sounds. Smart nightlights allow customization through apps or voice commands. **Glow-in-the-dark** variants offer a gentle, electricity-free glow that's useful during power outages. Portable nightlights are convenient for children who need a movable light source. When selecting a nightlight, consider its brightness, energy efficiency, user-friendliness, safety features, and how well it matches your bedroom decor and meets your family's needs.

---

**<u>Children's Bedroom</u>**
Infant/Non-mobile: (Birth - 6 months)
Infant crawl/roll: (5 months - 1 year)
→ **Toddler/Pre-school: (1 year - 4 years)**
→ **School-age: (5 years - 6+ years)**

# ELECTRIC BLANKETS

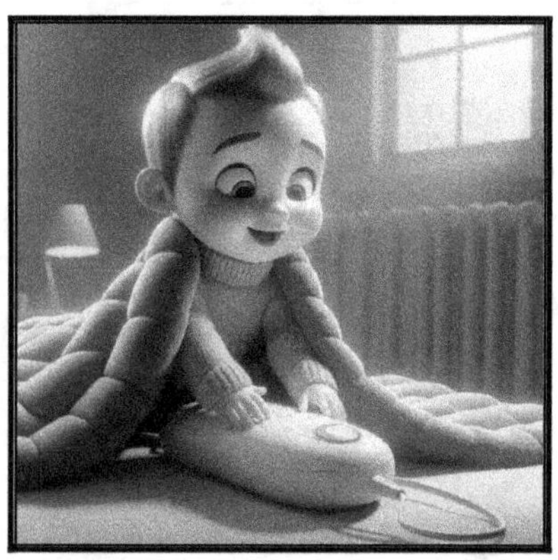

**Each year, over 1,500 children suffer burns or electrical injuries from electric blankets, making proper safety precautions essential.** Avoid using electric blankets for infants and very young children entirely, and if used for older children, make sure they are old enough to understand and follow safety guidelines. Regularly inspect the electric blanket for signs of wear, damage, or frayed cords, and follow the manufacturer's guidelines for maintenance and care.

**Purchase electric blankets only from reputable manufacturers and look for safety certifications or approval from recognized organizations.** Follow the manufacturer's instructions regarding safe usage and temperature settings carefully, and never turn an electric blanket on when not in use or while sleeping. Keep the electric blanket away from water or liquids, and never use the blanket if it is wet.
**Ensure that cords and controllers are securely attached to the**

**blanket and out of reach of young children.** Some electric blankets have safety features like automatic shut-off timers, which can provide added protection against overheating. If using an electric blanket for an older child, supervise them during its use, especially if they are using it for the first time. Remove the electric blanket from the bed before bedtime or naps to avoid accidental overheating or entanglement during sleep.

**Teach older children about the safe and responsible use of electric blankets, emphasizing the importance of turning them off when not needed.** Remember that electric blankets are not recommended for cribs or toddler beds due to the risk of suffocation, overheating, and entanglement, so always prioritize safety when using electric blankets and consider alternative heating methods for young children or infants.

---

<u>**Children's Bedroom**</u>
Infant/Non-mobile: (Birth - 6 months)
Infant crawl/roll: (5 months - 1 year)
→ **Toddler/Pre-school: (1 year - 4 years)**
→ **School-age: (5 years - 6+ years)**

# Toy Chest Safety

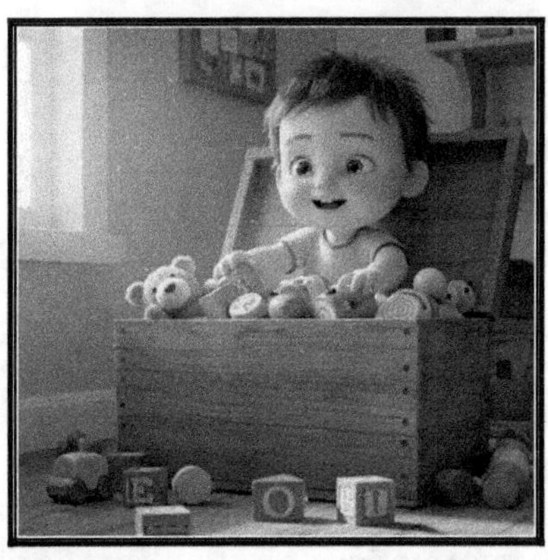

Childproofing a toy chest is essential to ensure the safety of children who interact with it regularly. **Over 50,000 children suffer minor to severe injuries each year from overheating toys and electronic devices, while according to the CPS**, in 2022 there were 11 toy-related fatalities among children aged one to 14 years old, and **approximately 209,500 toy-related injuries were treated in US hospital emergency departments, with 38% of the injuries involving children aged four or younger**. Choose a toy chest made of sturdy, non-toxic materials with smooth edges and no sharp corners, ensuring there are no small parts or choking hazards on the chest's exterior. Opt for a toy chest with safety hinges that prevent the lid from slamming shut, as these hinges should hold the lid in an open position, allowing for safe access to toys. If possible, choose a toy chest with a slow-close lid feature that gently closes the lid without sudden movements, reducing the risk of accidental finger pinching. Avoid toy chests with locks that can accidentally trap a child inside, as the chest should be easy for a child to open from the inside. Ensure the toy chest has holes or gaps to allow for airflow and prevent suffocation if a child climbs inside. If the toy chest is tall or top-heavy, anchor it securely to the wall to prevent tipping over if a child tries to climb on it. If the toy chest has a latch or lock, install a childproof latch that prevents young children from opening it without adult assistance. Be mindful of the toy chest's weight limit and don't overload it with too many heavy items, as this could cause instability.

**Place the toy chest in a safe location away from heavy furniture or areas where children run and play to avoid accidental collisions.** Regularly clean and organize the toy chest, removing broken or unsafe toys and ensuring that all toys are age-appropriate and free of hazards. Teach children about the proper use of the toy chest, such as avoiding climbing inside and closing the lid gently. If you have concerns about lid safety, consider removing the lid altogether and using the toy chest as an open storage container.

---

<u>Children's Bedroom</u>
→ **Infant/Non-mobile: (Birth - 6 months)**
→ **Infant crawl/roll: (5 months - 1 year)**
→ **Toddler/Pre-school: (1 year - 4 years)**
→ **School-age: (5 years - 6+ years)**

# Recalled Toys

The Consumer Product Safety Commission website at cpsc.gov is the primary authority responsible for monitoring and issuing recalls for unsafe products, including toys, and visiting their official website provides up-to-date information on toy recalls. Sign up for email subscriptions from the CPS or other reputable consumer safety organizations, as they often send out alerts and notifications about product recalls, including toys. Check the websites of toy manufacturers regularly for announcements and recall information, as reputable manufacturers will often publish recall notices on their websites to inform consumers. Some retailers may notify customers if they have purchased a recalled product, so ensure the retailer has your contact information when making purchases. Stay connected with nonprofit organizations focusing on child safety and consumer product recalls, as they may share recall information through their websites, newsletters, or social media channels. Local government agencies and health departments may share information about product recalls, including toys, through their official websites or social media accounts. **Follow reputable safety organizations, consumer protection agencies, and the CPS on social media platforms, as they often share recall information and safety tips with their followers.** Watch news outlets for reports about toy recalls, as major news networks often cover significant product recalls to alert the public. Join online forums and parenting groups where parents discuss child safety topics, as members may share recall information and safety tips with the community. Some mobile apps and services offer alerts and notifications for product recalls, so check if there are any apps specifically dedicated to child safety and product recalls. Remember that prompt action is crucial if you learn about a toy recall, so follow the instructions provided by the CPS or the manufacturer on safely returning or disposing of the recalled toy.

---

**Child's Bedroom**
Infant/Non-mobile: (Birth - 6 months)
Infant crawl/roll: (5 months - 1 year)
→ **Toddler/Pre-school: (1 year - 4 years)**
→ **School-age: (5 years - 6+ years)**

# HEADPHONE SAFETY

Headphone use among children can raise several concerns related to their safety, hearing health, and overall well-being. Children's ears are more sensitive and prone to damage from loud sounds, as prolonged exposure to high-volume levels through headphones can lead to hearing loss and other auditory issues.

**Children may not be aware of the appropriate volume levels when using headphones and may inadvertently expose themselves to dangerously loud sound levels without proper supervision or volume-limiting features.** Wearing headphones can make children less aware of their surroundings, leading to safety risks, especially when crossing streets, playing near traffic, or participating in outdoor activities. Overusing headphones can lead to social isolation, as children may become less engaged with their immediate environment and interactions with others. Children may access inappropriate or harmful content through headphones, especially if not properly monitored by parents or caregivers. Ill-fitting or poorly designed headphones can cause discomfort or pressure on a child's ears, leading to pain or irritation.

**Headphone cords can pose a strangulation risk**, especially for younger children or those who are not aware of the potential hazard. Listening to music or other audio content through headphones before bedtime can disrupt sleep patterns and impact the quality of rest.

**To promote safe headphone use, encourage responsible headphone use and set clear guidelines regarding volume levels and content access, consider using headphones with built-in volume-limiting features** to protect children's hearing, choose well-fitting, comfortable headphones designed specifically for children to minimize physical discomfort, supervise younger children when using headphones and limit their usage time, educate children about the importance of taking breaks from headphone use to rest their ears, opt for wireless or cordless headphones to reduce the risk of entanglement and strangulation, encourage children to be aware of their surroundings especially when wearing headphones in public places, and use parental controls and content filters on devices to restrict access to age-appropriate content.

---

**Children's Bedroom**
Infant/Non-mobile: (Birth - 6 months)
Infant crawl/roll: (5 months - 1 year)
→ **Toddler/Pre-school: (1 year - 4 years)**
→ **School-age: (5 years - 6+ years)**

# Hang Things Up on the Wall Properly

**When hanging things in a kids' bedroom, using tacks and nails should be done with caution and consideration for safety.** Small tacks or nails can be a choking hazard for young children, so avoid using small tacks or nails that can be easily removed and swallowed. To prevent accidental injuries, ensure that any tacks or nails used have their sharp points fully embedded in the wall or surface.

**Make sure the tacks or nails are securely anchored into the wall to prevent items from falling and causing potential harm.** Hang items out of the reach of young children to prevent them from pulling or playing with the objects.

**Consider the weight of the items being hung and use appropriate tacks or nails that can support the load securely.** Instead of using tacks or nails, consider using removable adhesive hooks or wall-mounted organizers specifically designed for kids' rooms, as these alternatives are less likely to damage the walls and can be easily re-positioned. If using tacks or nails on the walls, ensure that the wall coverings are childproof and do not pose any health risks if accidentally ingested. If you have older children who want to hang things themselves, supervise them to ensure they safely handle the tacks or nails.

**If possible, hang items on soft surfaces such as bulletin boards or fabric-covered walls, which are less likely to cause injuries if accidentally bumped.** Before using any hanging products, check for any safety recalls or warnings related to their use. Periodically inspect the items hung in the kids' bedroom to ensure that tacks or nails are still securely in place and that the objects are not damaged or worn.

---

<u>Children's Bedroom</u>
→ **Infant/Non-mobile: (Birth - 6 months)**
→ **Infant crawl/roll: (5 months - 1 year)**
→ **Toddler/Pre-school: (1 year - 4 years)**
→ **School-age: (5 years - 6+ years)**

# WHEN <u>NOT</u> TO SHARE

**Separating toys by age group is a great way to ensure that children have access to appropriate and safe toys for their developmental stage.** For infants from zero to 12 months, provide soft, plush toys without small parts that can be detached, rattles and teethers designed for young infants, high-contrast toys for visual stimulation, and activity mats and mobiles for sensory development.

**For toddlers from one to three years,** offer stacking toys and building blocks, shape sorters and puzzles with large pieces, push and pull toys for early walkers, play kitchen and food toys for pretend play, musical instruments designed for toddlers, and soft and safe ride-on toys. For preschoolers from three to five years, provide arts and crafts materials that are non-toxic and age-appropriate, playsets for imaginative play such as dollhouses and action figures, simple board games and puzzles with more pieces, sports equipment for gross motor development, and educational toys for learning numbers, letters, and basic concepts.

**For school-age children from six to 12 years,** offer more complex board games and strategy games, building sets with smaller pieces like LEGO sets, science kits and educational toys exploring STEM concepts, art supplies for more detailed artwork and creativity, and outdoor toys like bicycles, scooters, and sports gear. For teenagers 13 years and older, provide age-appropriate video games and gaming consoles, hobby-related items such as musical instruments or craft supplies, books and educational materials catering to their interests, and sports equipment or gear for more advanced sports activities.

**Keep in mind that children develop at different rates,** so the age groups provided here are general guidelines, as some children may show an interest in toys intended for older age groups while others may prefer toys designed for younger children. Always supervise playtime and ensure that toys are free from small parts or choking hazards, regardless of the child's age, and regularly inspect toys for wear and tear, replacing or repairing any damaged items to maintain a safe play environment for all age groups.

---



# Board game Concerns

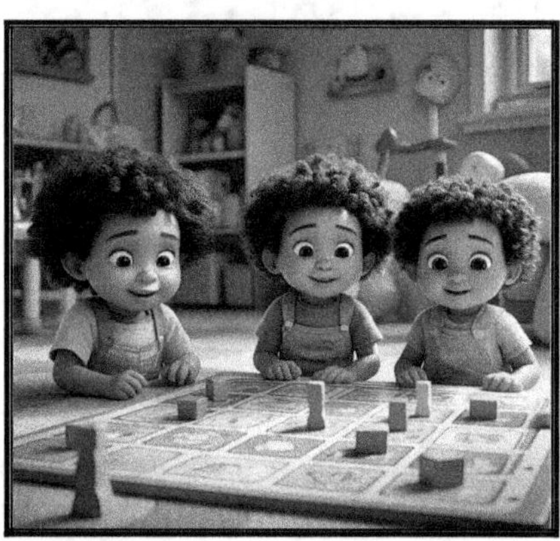

**Board games and other toys designed for older siblings can pose potential choking hazards for younger siblings**, so parents and caregivers need to be vigilant and take appropriate precautions when introducing toys or games with small parts into a household with children of different age groups.

**Always follow the age recommendations provided by the manufacturer on the toy's packaging**, as these recommendations are based on safety and developmental considerations. Ensure that younger children are supervised closely when older siblings are playing with toys that have small parts, and older siblings should be reminded to keep small game pieces away from younger siblings.

**Consider creating designated play areas for older and younger children**, where toys appropriate for their respective age groups are kept separate. Store small game pieces and other choking hazards out of the reach of younger children in storage containers with secure lids.

**Take the opportunity to educate older siblings** about the importance of keeping small parts and toys away from younger siblings to keep them safe. If possible, encourage older siblings to play with their small-piece toys during times when younger siblings are not present or are engaged in age-appropriate activities.

**Teach older siblings how to play responsibly and safely with their toys**, emphasizing the importance of keeping small parts and game pieces in designated play areas. Regularly inspect board games and toys for loose or broken parts that could pose a choking hazard, and repair or replace any damaged items promptly.

---

**Children's Bedroom**
→ **Infant/Non-mobile: (Birth - 6 months)**
→ **Infant crawl/roll: (5 months - 1 year)**
Toddler/Pre-school: (1 year - 4 years)
School-age: (5 years - 6+ years)

# NO STRINGS ON TOYS LONGER THAN 6 INCHES

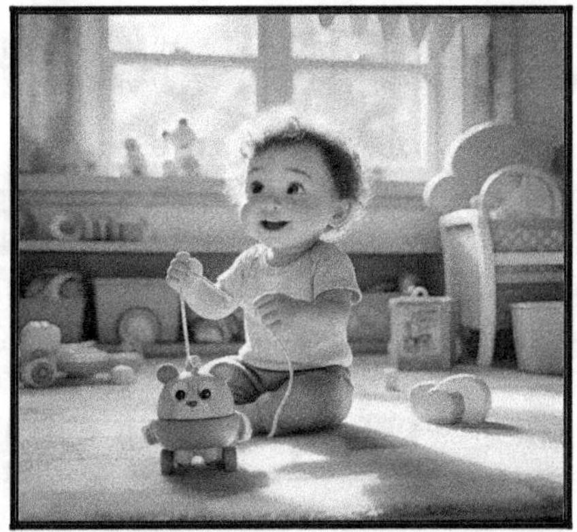

**Removing or avoiding strings longer than six inches on toys is an essential childproofing measure** to prevent potential strangulation hazards, as strings, cords, or ribbons that are too long can pose significant risks to young children, especially infants and toddlers, who may accidentally become entangled in them. Regularly inspect toys for any long strings or cords and trim them to a safe length if necessary. Be cautious of toys with pull cords, such as pull-along toys, and ensure they are kept out of reach when not in use. Ensure that any strings or cords attached to toys are securely fastened to prevent accidental detachment.

**For younger children who are at risk of entanglement**, choose age-appropriate toys that do not have long strings or cords. Unintentional suffocation causes around 1,200 child deaths each year, frequently due to unsafe sleep environments or household items like pillows and blankets.

**Avoid hanging toys with strings or cords on a crib or playpen, as they**

**can pose a strangulation hazard for infants.** Toys with long strings or cords should be kept away from areas where children sleep or play and avoided near cribs, beds, or playpens. Always supervise young children during playtime to ensure their safety and intervene if they encounter toys with long strings. Teach older siblings about the potential risks associated with toys that have long strings and encourage them to keep such toys away from younger siblings.

Consider using toys with short, safely attached strings, or opt for toys without strings altogether for added peace of mind.

---

**Children's Bedroom**
Infant/Non-mobile: (Birth - 6 months)
→ **Infant crawl/roll: (5 months - 1 year)**
→ **Toddler/Pre-school: (1 year - 4 years)**
→ **School-age: (5 years - 6+ years)**

# Never Lock a Child in a Bedroom

**Locking a child in their bedroom is not safe and should never be done under any circumstances, as it can be extremely dangerous** and poses severe risks to the child's safety and well-being. In the event of a fire or emergency, locking a child in their bedroom can prevent them from escaping quickly and safely, which could have tragic consequences. Locking the child's bedroom may hinder access for parents or caregivers in case the child needs assistance or medical attention urgently. Being locked in a room can cause anxiety, fear, and distress for the child, leading to emotional trauma that can have long-lasting effects. Locking a child in their bedroom can pose security risks, as they may be unable to leave the room if an intruder or dangerous situation arises.

**A child locked in their bedroom may try to escape by climbing out of a window or attempting other risky behaviors**, leading to potential injuries. Locking a child in their bedroom can be considered a violation of their rights and may be illegal in some jurisdictions. Instead, childproof the child's bedroom by securing furniture, covering electrical outlets, and removing any potential hazards. Always supervise young children to ensure their safety, especially during playtime or activities that may involve potential risks. Ensure that the child's bedroom has accessible exits and is not obstructed by furniture or other items. Use night lights to provide gentle illumination during the night, which can help alleviate the fear of the dark.

**Establish open communication with the child and address any fears or concerns** they may have about their bedroom or sleep environment.

Ensure that the child's crib or bed meets safety standards and is free from suffocation hazards.

---



# No Plastic Insulation Over Windows

**Plastic insulation or any plastic covering should not be used over windows in a child's bedroom or any living space**, especially if young children are present. Plastic insulation can pose a suffocation hazard for young children, who may accidentally come into contact with it and risk getting entangled or trapped. If not installed correctly, plastic insulation can interfere with proper air circulation and heating or cooling systems, leading to potential overheating in the room.

**Plastic is highly flammable,** and if it gets near heat sources like candles or heaters, it can quickly catch fire and spread throughout the room. Covering windows with plastic can obstruct visibility and make it difficult to see outside, potentially hindering escape in case of an emergency like a fire. Improperly installed plastic insulation may lead to condensation buildup, trapping moisture and potentially causing mold growth, which can be harmful to children's health. Instead, install curtains or drapes made of non-toxic, child-safe materials that can provide insulation and keep the room cozy.

**Use weather stripping around the window frames to prevent drafts and improve energy efficiency without obstructing visibility.** Apply caulk around the window frames to seal any gaps and prevent drafts from entering the room. Invest in thermal blinds or shades that provide insulation and help regulate the room's temperature without compromising safety.

**If necessary, window insulation kits should be specifically designed for safe indoor use, and the manufacturer's instructions should be followed carefully.** Install window safety locks to prevent young children from opening the window too wide and ensure childproofing.

---

# Closets Must Unlock from the Inside

**Ensuring that closets can be unlocked from the inside is an important safety measure, especially in children's bedrooms or playrooms where children might accidentally trap themselves.** If you use locks on closet doors, make sure to use childproof locks that can be easily opened from the inside, with these locks being accessible for a child's reach and simple to operate.

**Consider avoiding locks altogether on closet doors in children's rooms, as if privacy is not a significant concern, leaving the closet doors without locks** can provide easy access and prevent accidental entrapment. If the closet has a traditional doorknob with a keyhole, ensure the key can be removed from the outside when the closet is not in use, so children won't be able to accidentally lock themselves inside with the key left in the keyhole. If the closet has sliding or bi-folding doors, make sure they are easy to slide or open from the inside and avoid any mechanisms that could be difficult for a child to operate.

**Periodically test the closet door from the inside to ensure a child can easily unlock or open it.** Teach children how to unlock or open the closet door from the inside if they accidentally lock themselves in, as empowering them with this knowledge can help them stay calm and respond appropriately in such situations. Always supervise young children while they are in their bedrooms or playrooms to prevent accidental locking in closets.

---



# Remove Door Stoppers that Can be Disassembled

**Removing door stoppers that can be disassembled is an important childproofing measure, as door stoppers with small parts that can be taken apart pose a choking hazard for young children who may explore and put objects in their mouths.** Inspect all door stoppers in the house to identify if any of them have small parts that can be disassembled, looking for screws, nuts, bolts, or other removable components. If you find any door stoppers with small, removable parts, consider replacing them with childproof door stoppers that are designed to prevent accidental disassembly. If replacing the door stoppers is not immediately possible, secure the existing stoppers with solid adhesive or sealant to prevent small parts from coming loose.

**If you are unable to replace or secure the stoppers right away**, ensure that any small parts that might come loose are kept out of reach of young children. Always supervise young children to prevent them from accessing areas where door stoppers or small parts are present. Ensure that toys and other household objects are free from small parts or choking hazards. If you have older children, educate them about the importance of keeping small parts and potential hazards away from younger siblings.

---

**Children's Bedroom**
Infant/Non-mobile: (Birth - 6 months)
Infant crawl/roll: (5 months - 1 year)
→ **Toddler/Pre-school: (1 year - 4 years)**
→ **School-age: (5 years - 6+ years)**

# FINGER PINCH GUARDS

**A finger pinch guard, also called a door pinch guard, is designed to prevent fingers from getting caught or pinched in the gap between the door and the door frame when the door is being closed.** These devices are a valuable addition to childproofing measures and can help prevent painful finger injuries. A finger pinch guard is usually made of soft, flexible, and durable material, such as foam or rubber, and it comes in various shapes and designs, but the most common type is a long strip that attaches to the edge of the door. The finger pinch guard is installed on the edge of the door, either on the hinged side or the closing side, where fingers are most likely to get caught, and some models are designed to be easily adjustable or removable, making them convenient to use. When the door is being closed, the finger pinch guard acts as a cushion or barrier between the door and the frame, and if a child's fingers are accidentally in the way, the guard absorbs the pressure, preventing fingers from being pinched.

---

**Children's Bedroom**

Infant/Non-mobile: (Birth - 6 months)

Infant crawl/roll: (5 months - 1 year)

→ **Toddler/Pre-school: (1 year - 4 years)**

→ **School-age: (5 years - 6+ years)**

# WINDOW STOPPERS

Installing window stops is an effective childproofing measure to limit the opening of windows and prevent full access to children, as window stops are designed to restrict the movement of the window sash, reducing the risk of falls or other accidents. **Falls from windows result in over 500 fatalities and 10,000 non-fatal injuries among children annually in the United States**, frequently occurring in multi-story homes and apartments.

Choose window stops that are suitable for the type of window you have, as there are various types available, including sliding window locks, sash stops, and wedge-style stops. Measure the window's opening to determine the appropriate placement of the window stops, as the stops should be installed in a position that allows for proper ventilation while preventing full access.

**Read and follow the manufacturer's instructions** that come with the window stops, as different types of stops may have specific installation procedures. For windows that slide horizontally, install window stops on both sides of the window frame to prevent the sash from being opened too wide.

**Ensure that the window stops are securely attached to the window frame** and cannot be easily dislodged by a child. Periodically check the window stops to ensure they are still in place and functioning properly. While window stops are designed to prevent children from opening the window too wide, they should be easily accessible and operable by adults in case of an emergency or for regular cleaning and maintenance. Always supervise children around windows, even with window stops installed, as window stops are an added safety measure but do not replace the need for adult supervision. When appropriate, the window stops can be removed if they are no longer needed or if the child has outgrown the risk.

---

❦ *According to the CDC,* falls from windows result in **over 500 fatalities and 10,000 non-fatal injuries** among children annually in the U.S. frequently occurring in multi-story homes and apartments.

---

# PLACE GATES ON WINDOWS

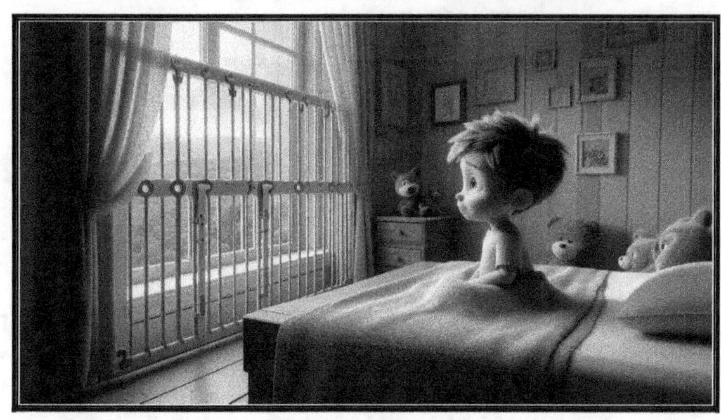

Placing gates on windows is an effective childproofing measure to enhance window safety and prevent young children from accessing or falling out of open windows, as window gates, also known as window guards, are designed to create a protective barrier over the window opening while still allowing for proper ventilation.

**Select window gates specifically designed for window safety and look for gates that meet safety standards and are appropriate for the size and type of windows in your home.** Accurately measure the dimensions of the window opening to ensure that the window gate fits securely, as the gate should cover the entire opening without any gaps that a child could slip through.

**Read and follow the manufacturer's instructions** that come with the window gates, as different types of window gates may have specific installation procedures. Properly install the window gate using the provided mounting hardware or brackets, and ensure that the gate is securely attached to the window frame or wall to prevent it from being dislodged by a child.

**Window gates should be easily operable by adults in case of emergency** or for regular cleaning and maintenance, and some gates come with quick-release mechanisms or swing-open features for easy adult access. Periodically inspect the window gates to ensure they are still in place and functioning properly. Check that the gaps between the window gate's bars are small enough to prevent a child from squeezing through. Always supervise children around windows, even with window gates installed, as window gates are an added safety measure but do not replace the need for adult supervision. Ensure that window gates do not impede emergency escape routes in case of a fire or other emergencies, and make sure that adults can quickly remove the gates if needed. When appropriate, the window gates can be removed if they are no longer needed or if the child has outgrown the risk.

---

**Children's Bedroom**
Infant/Non-mobile: (Birth - 6 months)
Infant crawl/roll: (5 months - 1 year)
→ **Toddler/Pre-school: (1 year - 4 years)o**
→ **School-age: (5 years - 6+ years)**

# Teach Children How to Call 911

**Teaching a child how to call 911 is a crucial life skill that can help them in emergencies and potentially save lives.** Start by explaining to your child what 911 is and why it is essential, emphasizing that 911 is a special number to call for help during emergencies, such as when someone is hurt, there's a fire, or a dangerous situation.

**Assess the child's age, maturity level, and ability to comprehend the concept of an emergency, as generally children around age four or five can start learning about 911, but remember that each child is different.** Role-play various emergency scenarios with your child, for example, pretending that there is a fire, someone is injured, or a stranger is causing trouble, and practice what they should say to the 911 operator in each situation.

**Teach your child essential information they should share with the 911 operator,** such as their full name, home address, and phone number, ensuring they know how to spell their name and address correctly. Show your child how to use a phone and dial 911, and explain that they should stay calm and speak clearly when talking to the operator.

**Make sure your child understands that 911 is only for real emergencies**, not for playing or non-urgent situations, and give them examples of when to call and when not to call. Teach your child to stay on the line until the 911 operator tells them it's okay to hang up, and explain that the operator may need additional information or instructions. Continually reinforce safety messages, such as not talking to strangers or playing with matches, and emphasize that calling 911 is for serious situations. Always supervise the child when practicing calling 911 and repeat the process occasionally to reinforce their understanding.

---

# SMALL PETS: GERBILS, RABBITS, ETC.

**To create a safe and harmonious environment for children and small pets like gerbils, rats, and rabbits, follow these comprehensive guidelines**. Before acquiring a pet, research to find a suitable match considering the animal's temperament and care requirements to ensure compatibility with your family. Always supervise children during their interactions with pets, teaching them gentle handling and avoiding loud noises to prevent startling the animals.

**Ensure cages are secure, escape-proof, and free of sharp edges, with safe bedding materials that won't cause respiratory issues.** Emphasize hand washing before and after handling pets and instruct children on proper food handling to avoid sharing human food with pets, which can make them sick.

**Schedule regular vet checkups and adhere to vaccination guidelines to keep pets healthy.** Set up a designated play area for supervised interactions and teach children empathy and respect for the animals, assigning them age-appropriate responsibilities for pet care. Though these bites make up less than one percent of all pediatric animal bites, they can nonetheless cause painful punctures and carry infection risks, and in rare documented instances, rabbits have transmitted Pasteurella infections, so even minor bites may require stitches or medical care.

---

❦ According to the CDC, small mammals including gerbils and rabbits can carry a range of transmissible diseases .Among them Salmonella, ringworm, rat-bite fever, and Leptospirosis. And can spread these germs even when they look perfectly clean and healthy. CDC. The risk falls hardest on the youngest children: Salmonella infection can cause serious disease especially in children younger than 5 years of age. King County **And here's the part most parents miss.** You don't even have to touch the animal to get sick. Pet food, equipment, and habitats can all be contaminated with Salmonella and other germs. CDC. Gerbils will bite or scratch when startled, and since they are nocturnal, a child waking one from sleep may trigger a defensive bite without warning. Hutch and Cage -*CDC Healthy Pets / Small Mammals page, cdc.gov; King County Public Health / CDC disease reference; Hutch and Cage gerbil safety guide*

# |Ch. 7| Children's Bathroom

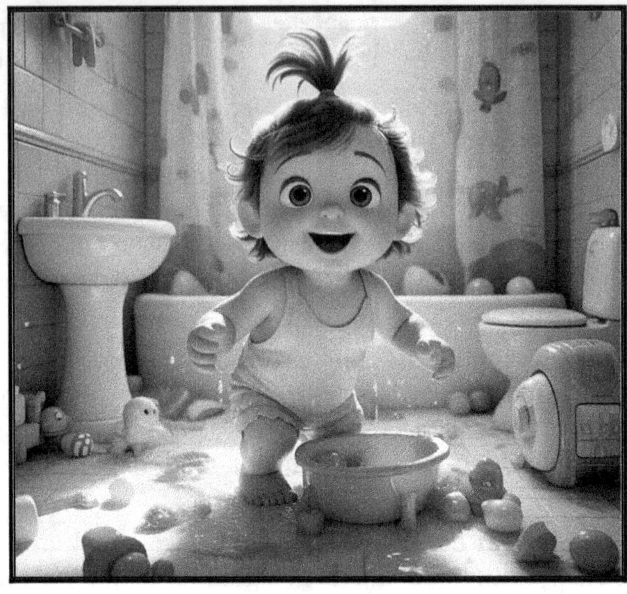

**Introduction**: In the bustling journey of parenthood, the bathroom can often be overlooked as a potential danger zone for young explorers. Yet, this space, brimming with slippery surfaces, sharp corners, and an array of chemicals and cosmetics, harbors numerous hazards for little ones. As we venture into this critical chapter, we will guide you through comprehensive strategies to transform your child's bathroom into a haven of safety. From securing potentially harmful products to installing preventative measures against slips and falls. We aim to equip you with the knowledge and tools to create a bathroom environment where your child can safely grow and learn. Let's embark on this essential step in childproofing, ensuring peace of mind each time your child enters the bathroom.

---

**Children's Bathroom**
→ Infant/Non-mobile: (Birth - 6 months)
→ Infant crawl/roll: (5 months - 1 year)
→ Toddler/Pre-school: (1 year - 4 years)
→ School-age: (5 years - 6+ years)

# BATHING A CHILD

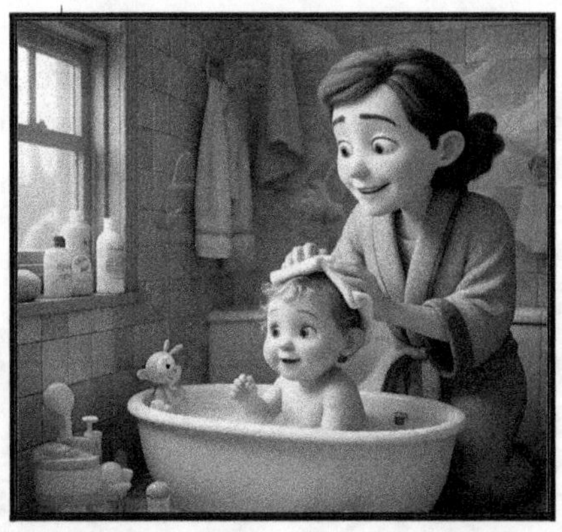

**Each year, approximately 5,000 children are injured by falls or drownings in overfilled bathtubs, stressing the importance of bath supervision and water level control.** Bath time is an important part of a child's day, and while splashing and playing in the water can be fun and enjoyable for your child, it is essential to keep the slippery tub a safe spot for your child to get clean and have fun. The most significant concern during bath time is drowning, as even a small amount of water can pose a significant risk to a young child.

**Never leave a child unattended in the bath, even for a moment, and always stay within arm's reach of the child during bath time. If you need to leave the bathroom for any reason, take your child with you or wrap them in a towel and bring them along rather than leaving them alone even briefly.**

The bathroom floor can be slippery, leading to slips and falls during bath time, so use non-slip bathmats both inside and outside the bathtub to provide secure footing. Consider placing non-slip stickers on the bathtub floor to reduce slipping further, and install grab bars in the bathroom to provide additional support and stability for both children and adults.

**Hot water can cause severe burns to a child's delicate skin, so set your water heater temperature to 120 degrees Fahrenheit or below to prevent scalding.** Always test the water temperature with your wrist or elbow before placing the child in the bath, as these areas are more sensitive to temperature than your hands. Consider using a bathtub spout cover to prevent accidental contact with hot faucets. To effectively prevent burns or other injuries, it's imperative to choose a cover that is durable and compatible with your specific valve, and frequently checking the integrity of the cover ensures that it remains a reliable safety feature in your home.

**Keep electrical appliances like hairdryers, curling irons, and electric**

**razors away from the bathtub to avoid the risk of electrocution.** Use electrical appliances in a different area of the bathroom, away from water sources, and unplug electrical devices after use, storing them out of the child's reach. Be cautious of cords from devices like radios, phones, or other electronic gadgets in the bathroom, keeping cords away from the water and out of the child's reach, and store electronic devices outside the bathroom or in a secure location.

**To prevent accidental ingestion, store toiletries and medications out of the child's reach in a high cabinet away from the child's reach, and lock all medications away in a secure medicine cabinet.** To prevent overflowing water in the bathtub, never leave the water running without supervision, and be mindful of the water level while filling the tub. Use child-friendly bath products that are free from harmful chemicals, and choose mild and hypoallergenic bath products designed for children's sensitive skin. Ensure that the bathtub drains properly to avoid standing water and reduce the risk of slips, and clean the bathtub drain regularly to prevent clogs. If you have older siblings, educate them about the importance of keeping the bathroom safe during bath time.

**For infants and younger babies, consider using a bathtub or seat that provides additional support and stability during bath time.** Install toilet seat locks to prevent young children from accessing the toilet during bath time, as children can be curious and might try to play with the water or objects inside the toilet, which can be hazardous. When the bathroom is not in use, keep the doors closed and secure with childproof doorknob covers, which prevents children from entering the bathroom without supervision. If your child enjoys playing with toys during bath time, ensure the toys are safe, free from small parts, and non-toxic, and supervise water play closely to avoid any potential choking or ingestion risks. Be cautious about using slippery bathrobes or towels, as they can make it challenging for a child to stay stable when stepping out of the bathtub. To reduce the risk of slips and falls, encourage children to sit in the bathtub instead of standing. Throughout the bath, continue to check the water temperature to ensure it remains comfortable for the child, as water can cool down or heat up over time.

**Always have emergency numbers, including poison control, readily available in the bathroom or nearby in case of accidents.** As children grow older, teach them water safety rules, such as not diving or running near water and how to call for help in case of an emergency. After bath time, ensure the bathtub is empty and the drain is closed, and remove toys or bath accessories that could pose a hazard when not used. Make bath time a positive and enjoyable experience for your child by staying calm, patient, and reassuring, which will help build their confidence and make them feel safe during baths.

---

**Children's Bathroom**
Infant/Non-mobile: (Birth - 6 months)
Infant crawl/roll: (5 months - 1 year)
→ **Toddler/Pre-school: (1 year - 4 years)**
→ **School-age: (5 years - 6+ years)**

# SHOWER CURTAIN

**Shower curtains seem harmless, but they can pose risks of strangulation or entanglement that parents need to address.** Opt for shower curtains with weighted hems, which reduces the likelihood of your child grabbing and pulling the curtain down or getting tangled. Attach magnets to the bottom corners of the shower curtain and tub to keep them closed and less accessible. If you're in full childproofing mode, replace the curtain with a glass shower door for zero curtain access. Ensure shower hooks are not within reach, as they can be a choking hazard, and use hidden or snap-on hooks for a cleaner, safer look. Shower curtains and rods may seem harmless, but they can present surprising dangers to toddlers, as plastic liners can wrap around little ones, leading to suffocation or strangulation, and loose tension rods are equally risky, with real cases where a collapsing rod fell onto a child's face, leaving a deep tear, showing that even everyday bathroom fixtures need secure installation and careful oversight.

---

🌱 Shower curtains and rods may seem harmless, but they can present surprising dangers to toddlers. **Plastic liners can wrap around little ones, leading to suffocation or strangulation.** Loose tension rods are equally risky. There have been real cases where a collapsing rod fell onto a child's face, leaving a deep tear. It shows that even everyday bathroom fixtures need secure installation and careful oversight.

---

**Children's Bathroom**
→ **Infant/Non-mobile: (Birth - 6 months)**
→ **Infant crawl/roll: (5 months - 1 year)**
→ **Toddler/Pre-school: (1 year - 4 years)**
→ **School-age: (5 years - 6+ years)**

# ANTIBACTERIAL SOAP CONCERNS

**There are several concerns about children using antibacterial soaps,** even after the FDA banned chemicals like triclosan and triclocarban, as some remaining antibacterial agents, such as benzalkonium chloride, may still pose risks. These chemicals can be harsh on a child's sensitive skin, causing irritation or allergic reactions. **Frequent use of antibacterial products may also disrupt the skin's natural microbiome, which plays a key role in immune system development.** Overuse of antibacterial soaps can strip the skin of natural oils and beneficial bacteria, weakening the skin's protective barrier and making it more susceptible to dryness and infections. Additionally, there is concern about how antibacterial soaps contribute to antimicrobial resistance, as overuse may promote the growth of bacteria that are resistant to antibiotics, making infections harder to treat in the future, which is especially concerning for children who are more vulnerable to infections. **Some antibacterial agents may also be absorbed through the skin, potentially impacting a child's developing immune system.** Environmental concerns also exist, as some antibacterial chemicals do not fully break down and may enter water systems, affecting wildlife and ecosystems. Given these risks, healthcare professionals often recommend using regular soap and water for children, which is both effective in reducing germs and safer than antibacterial alternatives.

---

**Children's Bathroom**
Infant/Non-mobile: (Birth - 6 months)
Infant crawl/roll: (5 months - 1 year)
→ **Toddler/Pre-school: (1 year - 4 years)**
→ **School-age: (5 years - 6+ years)**

# Bathroom Garbage Can

**Garbage cans can be an irresistible treasure trove for curious little hands in the bathroom.** Choose a garbage can with a pedal-operated, locking lid, as the lock will prevent tiny fingers from accessing whatever's inside, whether it's bathroom waste or more dangerous items like razors. Store the garbage can in a locked cabinet or under the sink with childproof cabinet locks if possible. While it sounds futuristic, some cans have motion sensors that close before your child can dive in, providing an extra layer of protection. If you cannot keep the garbage can out of reach, use adhesive strips or anti-tip devices to prevent your toddler from tipping it over in a moment of playful curiosity.

---

# No In-toilet Cleaning Supplies

Childproofing bathroom cleaning supplies is crucial to prevent accidental poisoning or harm to young children who may be curious and explore their surroundings. **Keep all cleaning supplies, including toilet bowl cleaners, disinfectants, bleach, and other chemicals, in a locked cabinet or high out of the child's reach, and choose a storage location that is not easily accessible to young children.** Install childproof cabinet locks on bathroom cabinets that contain cleaning supplies to prevent curious children from opening them. Store cleaning supplies separately from personal care items and food items, which reduces the risk of accidental ingestion if a child mistakes cleaning products for something else. Use childproof bottles for cleaning supplies whenever possible, as these bottles require a specific action like pressing and turning to open, making it difficult for young children to access the contents. Label all cleaning supplies clearly with their contents and warning labels, which helps adults identify the products easily and reminds them of potential hazards. Dispose of empty cleaning supply containers safely and promptly, rinsing them thoroughly before recycling or discarding them to eliminate any residual product. Consider using non-toxic and eco-friendly cleaning products that are safer for both children and the environment. Avoid transferring cleaning supplies into other containers, as this can lead to confusion and accidental misuse. Keep children out of the bathroom or in a separate room when cleaning is in progress, which reduces the risk of accidental exposure to cleaning products. Use cleaning supplies carefully, following instructions and safety guidelines, and always close containers tightly after use. **If you have older siblings, educate them about the importance of keeping cleaning supplies out of reach of younger siblings.** Use childproof trash bins with secure lids to prevent children from accessing discarded cleaning supply containers. If you use cleaning tools like scrub brushes or sponges with cleaning products, store them out of the of children.

---

# TOILET SEAT CLOSED AND SECURED

**Keeping the toilet seat closed and installing safety measures are essential steps in childproofing the bathroom effectively.** Always keep the toilet seat and lid closed when not in use, which prevents young children from accessing toilet water, which can be hazardous and unhygienic. Install toilet locks or latches to secure the toilet seat and lid, as these locks prevent young children from lifting the seat and accessing the toilet bowl. A toilet paper dispenser is essential to prevent young kids from creating a mess or potentially clogging the toilet, so opt for dispensers with covers or controlled dispensing mechanisms to limit access and waste. Consider mounting the dispenser higher on the wall or using childproof locks to keep it out of children's reach, or alternatively, a freestanding dispenser placed in a less accessible spot can also help. Store extra rolls out of reach and always supervise young children in the bathroom.

**If you have older children, teach them the importance of keeping the toilet seat closed and using the toilet locks to prevent accidents.** Always supervise young children in the bathroom to ensure they don't access the toilet or play with toilet paper. Use toilet cleaners that are safe, non-toxic, and labeled as child friendly, and store these cleaning products securely out of your child's reach. Use childproof trash bins in the bathroom to prevent children from accessing and handling discarded toilet paper or other bathroom waste. As children grow older, explain the rules about toilet safety, such as not playing in or near the toilet and not flushing toys or objects down the toilet. To prevent unsupervised access to the bathroom, consider using childproof doorknob covers or installing locks on the doors.

**Teach children proper handwashing techniques** after using the toilet to maintain good hygiene. Keep the bathroom free from clutter to reduce the risk of accidents and provide a safe space for children.

---

# TOILET PAPER

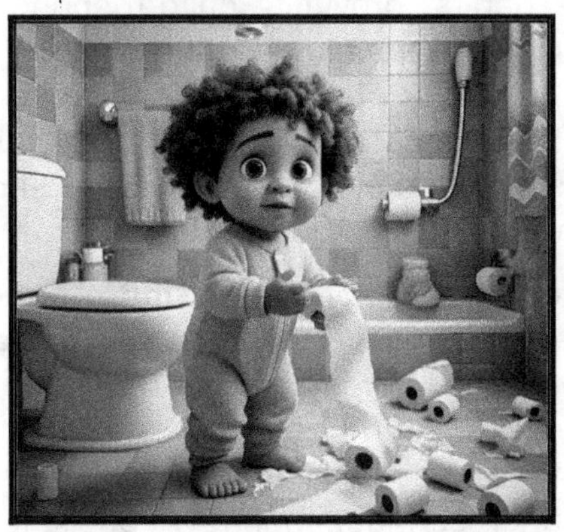

**Childproofing toilet paper in a child's bathroom is important to prevent waste, clogged toilets, and unnecessary messes.** One of the simplest solutions is using a toilet paper guard or dispenser with a controlled-release mechanism to limit how much paper can be pulled at once. Placing the toilet paper holder slightly higher or reversing the roll so it unravels from the back can also make it more challenging for little hands to unroll large amounts. Teaching your child the proper amount to use and explaining that too much can clog the toilet helps reinforce good habits. For younger children, replacing the roll with a tissue box can provide better control over usage. Additionally, securing the roll with a Velcro strap or a simple latch can slow down excessive unrolling. Until your child fully understands how to use toilet paper properly, supervising their bathroom habits can prevent unnecessary waste and ensure they develop good practices.

---

**Children's Bathroom**
Infant/Non-mobile: (Birth - 6 months)
Infant crawl/roll: (5 months - 1 year)
→ **Toddler/Pre-school: (1 year - 4 years)**
School-age: (5 years - 6+ years)

# POTTY TRAINING SAFETY

Potty crucial for success. **Always supervise your child during potty training, as accidents can happen, and being nearby ensures you can**

**provide immediate assistance.** Childproof the bathroom to minimize potential hazards by keeping cleaning supplies, medications, and other hazardous items out of the child's reach in locked cabinets or on high shelves. Use a stable and sturdy step stool to help your child reach the potty or the sink for hand washing, making sure the step stool has a non-slip surface. Encourage proper hand washing after using the potty to instill good hygiene habits, providing child-friendly soap and teaching them how to thoroughly lather and rinse their hands. If using a standalone potty chair, choose one with a stable base and secure handles to help the child feel comfortable and safe while using it. If you're using a regular toilet with a potty seat or training seat, always keep your child within arm's reach near water to prevent accidents or falls.

**To prevent pinched fingers, consider using a soft-close toilet seat, which slowly lowers the seat and lid without slamming.** Use slip-resistant bathmats or rugs in the bathroom to reduce the risk of slipping and falling. Dress your child in clothing that is easy to remove quickly during potty training, as elastic waistbands or pull-up pants can make it easier for them to undress independently. For nighttime potty training, use a nightlight in the bathroom and along the path from the child's bedroom to the bathroom to help them navigate safely in the dark. Use positive reinforcement and praise when your child successfully uses the potty, as this positive reinforcement helps build confidence and encourages them in the process. Potty training can be a challenging time for both the child and the parent, so be patient, understanding, and supportive during this learning phase

---

<u>Children's Bathroom</u>
→ **Infant/Non-mobile: (Birth - 6 months)**
→ **Infant crawl/roll: (5 months - 1 year)**
→ **Toddler/Pre-school: (1 year - 4 years)**
School-age: (5 years - 6+ years)

# KEEP BABY OIL OUT OF REACH

**Baby oil, while a common household item for skin care, can pose a significant safety risk to young children due to its slippery texture and potential for accidental spills.** Store baby oil in a locked cabinet or shelf that is well out of reach of children, which prevents them from accessing the bottle and reduces the risk of accidental ingestion or spills. Always ensure the bottle is tightly closed before placing it away, as a loose lid can allow the oil to leak out, making it more accessible to children. When using baby oil during massage or skincare routines, dispense only the necessary amount and keep the bottle away from the baby's reach, which prevents the baby from grabbing the bottle and potentially spilling or ingesting the oil. Educate all caregivers, including babysitters and nannies, about the potential hazards of baby oil and the importance of storing it securely, ensuring they are aware of the proper handling and storage procedures.

---

<u>**Children's Bathroom**</u>
→ **Infant/Non-mobile: (Birth - 6 months)**
→ **Infant crawl/roll: (5 months - 1 year)**
→ **Toddler/Pre-school: (1 year - 4 years)**
School-age: (5 years - 6+ years)

# Baby Powder Concerns

**Baby powder is talcum powder which is often used to keep babies' skin dry and prevent diaper rash, however, there are some dangers associated with baby powder.** Talcum powder is mined from the ground, and there is a risk that it can be contaminated with asbestos, which is a known carcinogen, and exposure to asbestos can increase the risk of developing lung cancer, mesothelioma, and other respiratory diseases. Talcum powder can be inhaled, and this can irritate the lungs, and in some cases, inhalation of talcum powder can lead to a condition called Talcosis, which is a type of lung scarring. Talcum powder can irritate the skin, especially in sensitive babies, and in some cases, skin irritation from talcum powder can lead to a condition called contact dermatitis. Because of these dangers, the

**FDA has advised consumers to avoid using talcum powder on babies and to use alternatives.** Cornstarch is a natural powder that is often used as an alternative to talcum powder, and while cornstarch is not as absorbent as talcum powder, it is still effective at keeping skin dry. Arrowroot powder is another natural powder that can be used as an alternative to talcum powder, and arrowroot powder is just as absorbent as cornstarch and is also gentle on the skin. Baby oil is a liquid that can be used to keep skin dry, and while baby oil is not as absorbent as talcum powder, it can help to prevent chafing and irritation. Petroleum jelly is a thick, oily substance that can be used to keep skin dry, and while petroleum jelly is not as absorbent as talcum powder, it can help to prevent chafing and irritation. If you are looking for an alternative to baby powder, talk to your doctor or a pharmacist, as they can help you choose a product that is safe and effective for your needs.

---

# CHILDREN'S TOOTHPASTE CONCERNS

**Fluoride is a mineral that helps to strengthen teeth and prevent cavities, however, too much fluoride can be harmful, especially for young children**, and the American Dental Association recommends that children under the age of six use toothpaste that contains no more than 500 parts per million of fluoride. Some children's toothpaste contains artificial sweeteners like xylitol and sorbitol, and while these sweeteners can be beneficial for oral health, they may cause digestive issues, such as stomach upset or diarrhea, in some children. Many children's toothpastes feature artificial flavors like bubble gum or fruit, and these flavors can make brushing more enjoyable for kids but can also be irritating to the mouth, especially if used excessively.

**Artificial colorings are often added to children's toothpaste to make it visually appealing, however, these colorings can be irritating to the mouth and may contribute to allergies** or sensitivities in some children. If you are concerned about the safety of children's toothpaste, talk to your dentist, as they can recommend a toothpaste that is safe and effective for your child. Choose a toothpaste that is specifically designed for children, as these toothpastes typically contain less fluoride and artificial sweeteners than adult toothpastes. Look for a toothpaste that is labeled as kid-friendly, as these toothpastes are typically free of artificial flavors and colors. Read the label carefully and make sure that the toothpaste you choose does not contain any ingredients that your child is allergic to.

**Start with a pea-sized amount of toothpaste**, as this is enough to clean your child's teeth without too much fluoride. Rinse your child's mouth thoroughly after brushing, which will help to remove any toothpaste that may have been swallowed.

---

# NEVER CALL MEDICINE "CANDY"

**One rule that should be non-negotiable is to never refer to medicine as candy, as children, especially at a very young age, can easily be confused by this and may seek out medicine unsupervised, thinking it's a treat.** This miscommunication can lead to dangerous and potentially life-threatening situations. Therefore, always store medicine in a secure place and educate children about the potential dangers of consuming it without adult supervision. Over seven million patients in the US are impacted by medication errors annually, and more than 100,000 reports of medication errors are received by the FDA each year. **Medication errors injure over 1.3 million people annually in the US. As many as 30% of medication errors reported to US Poison Control Centers involve pediatric patients, and dosage errors are common, with 7.8% of caregivers reporting insufficient doses and 6.6% reporting overdoses. Over 50% of parents have given incorrect acetaminophen doses to their children, making proper medication education and storage absolutely critical.**

---

🌰 **Medication Error Statistics:** Over 7 million patients in the US are impacted by medication errors annually. **More than 100,000 reports of medication errors are received by the FDA each year.** Medication errors injure over 1.3 million people annually in the US. **Pediatric Medication Errors:** As many as 30% of medication errors reported to US Poison Control Centers involve pediatric patients. Dosage errors are common, with 7.8% of caregivers reporting insufficient doses and 6.6% reporting overdoses. Over 50% of parents have given incorrect acetaminophen doses to their children.

---

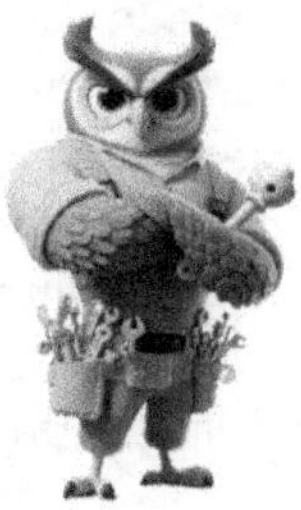

 # Parents/Guest Bedrooms

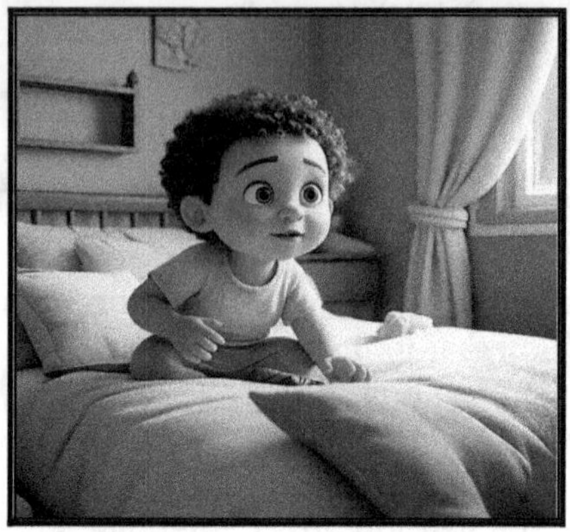

**Introduction:** In the sanctuary where parents retreat for relaxation, the nuances of childproofing often go overlooked. Yet, the parents' bedroom harbors a myriad of potential hazards for little explorers. From securing heavy furniture to ensuring that small, swallowable items are out of reach, this chapter guides you through creating a safe haven that doesn't compromise on its comforting appeal. As we delve deeper, we'll explore innovative and simple strategies to childproof your bedroom, ensuring that curious little hands and nimble little feet navigate a space that is as safe as it is serene. Let's embark on this journey to foster a home where safety meets tranquility, beginning with the cornerstone of adult sanctuaries, the parents' bedroom.

---

**Parent's and Guest Bedroom**
→ **Infant/Non-mobile: (Birth - 6 months)**
→ **Infant crawl/roll: (5 months - 1 year)**
→ **Toddler/Pre-school: (1 year - 4 years)**
School-age: (5 years - 6+ years)

# Never Allow Children Under 2 Years to Sleep in an Adult Bed

Adult beds lack safety features of cribs and pose serious risks including falls, suffocation from soft mattresses and pillows, and entrapment in gaps between mattress and frame. Always provide age-appropriate sleeping environments with firm mattresses free from blankets, pillows, and stuffed animals. Place infants on their backs to sleep and keep sleep areas clutter-free. If co-sleeping is preferred, use co-sleeper bassinets that provide separate space while keeping baby close.

<u>**Parent's and Guest Bedroom**</u>
Infant/Non-mobile: (Birth - 6 months)
Infant crawl/roll: (5 months - 1 year)
→ **Toddler/Pre-school: (1 year - 4 years)**
→ **School-age: (5 years - 6+ years)**

# INSTALL SAFETY NETTING ON BALCONIES AND DECKS

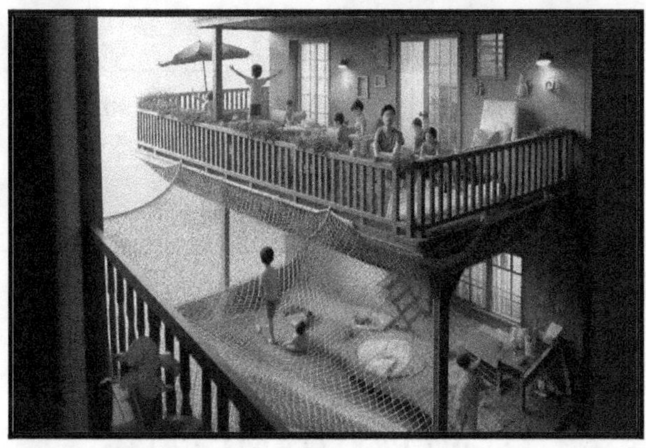

**Installing safety netting on balconies and decks prevents falls, manages children's curiosity, and fills gaps in railings.** Use durable, weather-resistant, see-through materials for easy installation. While netting provides protection, it doesn't replace adult supervision. Ensure compliance with local building codes and inspect regularly for wear.

---

<u>**Parent's and Guest Bedroom**</u>
Infant/Non-mobile: (Birth - 6 months)
Infant crawl/roll: (5 months - 1 year)
→ **Toddler/Pre-school: (1 year - 4 years)**
→ **School-age: (5 years - 6+ years)**

# GUN SAFETY

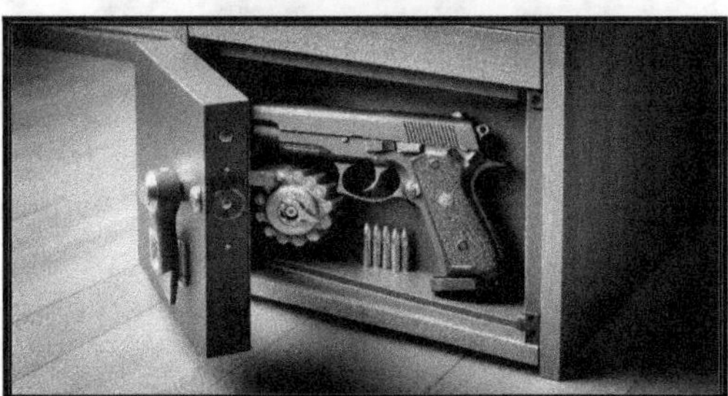

**Each year, firearm accidents cause serious injuries to children.** Store firearms in securely locked gun safes inaccessible to children, keeping keys away from their reach. Use cable or trigger locks if a safe isn't available. Store ammunition separately in locked containers.

**Educate children early that guns are dangerous and should never be touched,** establishing strict zero-tolerance policies. Always supervise when firearms are present, unload guns when not in use, and double-check they're unloaded before storing. Teach older children proper handling under adult supervision only. Enroll in reputable gun safety courses and discuss storage practices with other parents whose homes your children visit.

---

🐝 *Research cited by the* ***American Academy of Pediatrics (AAP)*** has found that children as young as **3 years old** have the physical hand strength required to pull the trigger on most standard handguns.

---

<u>**Parent's and Guest Bedroom**</u>
Infant/Non-mobile: (Birth - 6 months)
Infant crawl/roll: (5 months - 1 year)
→ **Toddler/Pre-school: (1 year - 4 years)**
→ **School-age: (5 years - 6+ years)**

# JEWELRY DANGERS

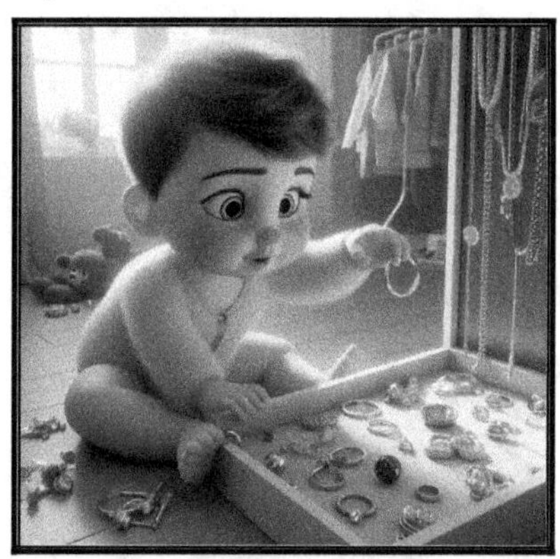

**Small jewelry poses choking hazards for children under three. Prevent ingestion of beads and gemstones.** Be aware of allergic reactions to metals like nickel, strangulation risks from long necklaces, and dangers of swallowing magnetic components. Avoid sharp edges and lead content. Choose age-appropriate jewelry, supervise usage, avoid magnetic pieces for young children, use hypoallergenic options, ensure secure closures, check safety certifications, remove during play, and inspect regularly for damage.

---

<u>**Parent's and Guest Bedroom**</u>
Infant/Non-mobile: (Birth - 6 months)
Infant crawl/roll: (5 months - 1 year)
→ **Toddler/Pre-school: (1 year - 4 years)**
→ **School-age: (5 years - 6+ years)**

# Keep All Sleep Medication Out of Reach

**Critical statistics show 65,000-75,000 young children (ages 0-6) visit emergency rooms annually after accessing medications, with melatonin alone involved in 11,000 yearly poisoning visits.** Store all medications in locked cabinets with childproof locks, keep in original containers with child-resistant caps, label clearly, use childproof bottles, never call medicine "candy," keep out of sight, use time-lock dispensers if needed, dispose of expired medications safely, separate from vitamins, and save emergency contact numbers including Poison Control.

---

<u>**Parent's and Guest Bedroom**</u>
Infant/Non-mobile: (Birth - 6 months)
Infant crawl/roll: (5 months - 1 year)
→ **Toddler/Pre-school: (1 year - 4 years)**
→ **School-age: (5 years - 6+ years)**

# Walk-in Closet Safety

**Control access with childproof locks or knob covers.** Keep items off floors to reduce tripping hazards. Store heavy or dangerous items on high shelves. Secure shelving units to walls with anchors. Use childproof containers for small items like jewelry and buttons. Organize cables with ties or covers. Place hanging rods at heights inaccessible to children. Pad sharp furniture corners and install drawer latches. Use LED lighting that doesn't heat up. Never store cleaning supplies or chemicals unless in locked childproof cabinets. Place laundry baskets in elevated areas. Conduct regular inspections as children grow and mobility increases.

---

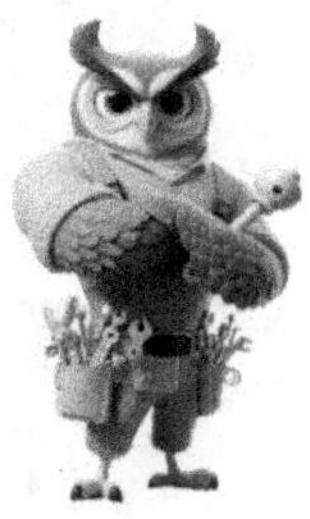

# |Ch. 9| Parents Bathroom

**Introduction:** In this chapter, we delve into the critical task of childproofing the parent's bathroom, a place often laden with potential hazards for your little ones. As parents, we must transform this space into a safe space where the risk of accidents is minimized. From securing potentially harmful substances found in cabinets to ensuring the safe use of electrical appliances, we will guide you step-by-step to create a bathroom environment that combines safety with functionality. As we navigate through this chapter, you will be equipped with practical tips and insights to foster a secure and child-friendly bathroom without compromising its adult-oriented utilities. Let's embark on this journey to safeguard our children while preserving the sanctity of our personal retreat.

---

**Parents Bathroom**
→ Infant/Non-mobile: (Birth - 6 months)
→ Infant crawl/roll: (5 months - 1 year)
→ Toddler/Pre-school: (1 year - 4 years)
→ School-age: (5 years - 6+ years)

## Tips on How to Use the Bathroom Alone

Communicate your whereabouts, set expectations with older children about privacy, lock the door if possible, engage children with distractions, time bathroom trips strategically, use visual cues like timers for younger children, practice independence, prepare essentials beforehand, childproof the bathroom, and plan ahead for longer trips. Keep visits relatively short since young children may need occasional supervision.

---

🐞 Every parent knows the feeling. You need 90 seconds alone in the bathroom, and suddenly it feels like a national emergency. Turns out, the anxiety is warranted. Childproofing experts note that toddlerhood is the stage where parents learn they need to take bathroom trips with lightning speed. Because in their absence, however brief, a child will either find a way around existing safeguards or turn their attention to something less protected. Thewildwest3. The solution most safety professionals recommend isn't willpower. It's a designated safe zone. A freestanding play yard or corral gives parents a baby-proof area to leave their child in while they use the bathroom, answer the phone, or cook nearby. Berkeley Parents Network And according to the CPSC, no safety device is completely childproof. Determined toddlers have been known to overcome or disable them._So the goal is buying yourself enough time, not achieving perfection. The practical tip: child development experts recommend establishing independent playtime from early on, working toward a child being content playing alone for 10–20 minutes. With safety being the key issue, placing them somewhere safe and within earshot. *BabyWise Mom The Wild Wild West Parenting Blog; Berkeley Parents Network; BabywiseMom.com; U.S. CPSC*

---

**Parents Bathroom**
Infant/Non-mobile: (Birth - 6 months)
Infant crawl/roll: (5 months - 1 year)
→ **Toddler/Pre-school: (1 year - 4 years)**
→ **School-age: (5 years - 6+ years)**

# Secure Razors, Nail Clippers, Tweezers, Makeup...

**Approximately 2,500 children are injured yearly by hair accessories, while over 15,000 sustain burns from styling tools.** Switch to electric razors when possible for built-in safety features. Store traditional razors in locked drawers or high cabinets with guards or covers. Keep nailclippers in childproof containers with safety features. Store tweezers out of reach, preferably child-friendly versions with rounded edges. Store makeup in locked cases, never leave unattended, and use childproof containers. Always supervise when using these items, keep out of reach when not in use, and inspect storage regularly.

---

❦ That pretty makeup bag on the bathroom counter is practically an invitation to a toddler. A study by researchers at Nationwide Children's Hospital found that 64,686 children younger than five were treated in U.S. emergency departments for injuries related to personal care products over a 14-year period. The equivalent of one child every two hours. Nationwide Children's Hospital

The most dangerous items aren't the ones parents expect. Nail care products caused the most injuries at 28%, followed by hair care at 27% and skin care at 25%. And about 60% of those injured were under age 2. UPI The reason? Young children can't read labels, so a bottle of nail polish remover looks just like juice, and lotion smells exactly like something edible. *-Nationwide Children's Hospital*

And it gets more alarming: hair relaxers and permanent solutions contain sodium hydroxide. The same ingredient found in drain cleaner. And children exposed to these products are over three times more likely to be hospitalized than those exposed to other personal care products. UPI Even a small bottle of perfume, mixed in 100% alcohol, can cause intoxication in a small child. UPI

As for razors, nail clippers, and tweezers. Childproofing experts specifically call_these out as items that are frequently left out and unattended, posing a sharp object threat to curious children, and recommend keeping them organized in a locked cabinet. Tundraland. *Nationwide Children's Hospital / Clinical Pediatrics study; UPI health reporting on the same study; Tundraland childproofing guide*

---

<u>**Parents Bathroom**</u>
Infant non-mobile: (Birth-6 mo.)
Infant crawl/roll: (5 mo.-2 yrs.)
→ **Toddler/Pre-School: (1 yr.-4 yrs.)**
→ **School-age: (5 yrs.-6 yrs.)**

# MOUTHWASH CONCERNS

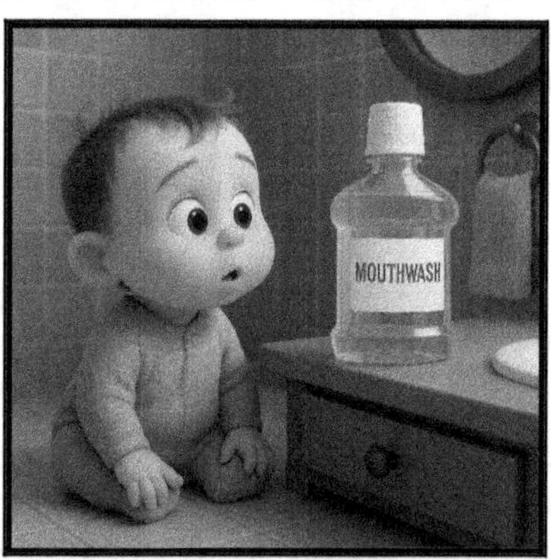


**Each year around 3,000 preschoolers under six are reported to poison control after ingesting mouthwash, with nearly 170 cases per 100,000 kids. Between 1987-1993,** three toddlers died from swallowing alcohol-rich rinses. Swallowing mouthwash can cause gastrointestinal distress, nausea, vomiting, and alcohol poisoning. Many mouthwashes contain alcohol that children's smaller bodies can't process safely. Excessive swallowing of fluoride-containing mouthwash can lead to dental fluorosis or other health issues. Some children may have sensitivities to ingredients causing irritation. Don't give mouthwash to children under the recommended age, always supervise older children, use sparingly, educate about proper use and spitting out, store out of reach, and consult pediatric dentists before introducing to oral care routines.

---



# DON'T STORE MEDICINE IN THE MEDICINE CABINET

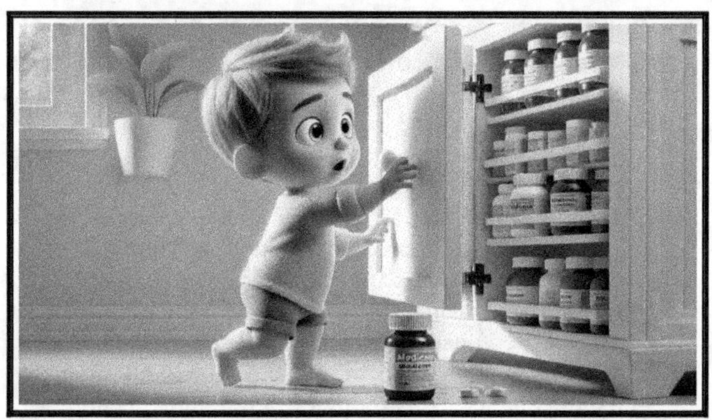

**Each year around 3,000 preschoolers under six are reported to poison control after ingesting mouthwash, with nearly 170 cases per 100,000 kids.** Between 1987-1993, three toddlers died from swallowing alcohol-rich rinses. Swallowing mouthwash can cause gastrointestinal distress, nausea, vomiting, and alcohol poisoning. Many mouthwashes contain alcohol that children's smaller bodies can't process safely. Excessive swallowing of fluoride-containing mouthwash can lead to dental fluorosis or other health issues. Some children may have sensitivities to ingredients causing irritation. Don't give mouthwash to children under the recommended age, always supervise older children, use sparingly, educate about proper use and spitting out, store out of reach, and consult pediatric dentists before introducing to oral care routines.

---

<u>**Parents Bathroom**</u>
Infant/Non-mobile: (Birth - 6 months)
→ **Infant crawl/roll: (5 months - 1 year)**
→ **Toddler/Pre-school: (1 year - 4 years)**
→ **School-age: (5 years - 6+ years)**

# Talk to Guests About Their Contents

Warmly welcome guests and mention your childproofing practices. When appropriate, inquire if guests carry medication. Offer secure, childproof storage locations like lockable drawers. Share safety tips about keeping medications out of reach and secured. Politely remind guests of their role in ensuring children's safety. Share emergency contact numbers including Poison Control. Approach conversations with understanding without judgment. Demonstrate childproofing measures in your home. Thank guests for cooperation in maintaining child safety.

---

🐝 The most dangerous object in a walk-in closet is often sitting on the floor or a low shelf: a visitor's bag. Nearly **70% of medication ingestions** in children involve a child taking someone else's medicine—not their parents'. Guests often leave purses or toiletry kits on the floor of a walk-in closet. These bags are "treasure chests" for toddlers, containing "candy-lookalike" pills (ibuprofen, heart meds), colorful hand sanitizers (high alcohol content), and loose coins (choking/lithium batteries). One child is treated in an emergency department for accidental medicine poisoning **every 8 minutes**. A guest's "overnight bag" in an unlocked closet is a primary -*Safe Kids Worldwide / American Association of Poison Control Centers (AAPCC).*

---

**Notes:**

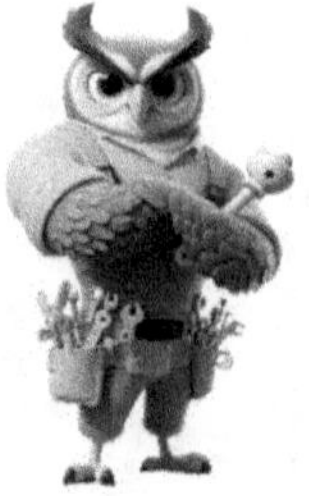

# |Ch. 10| Nursery

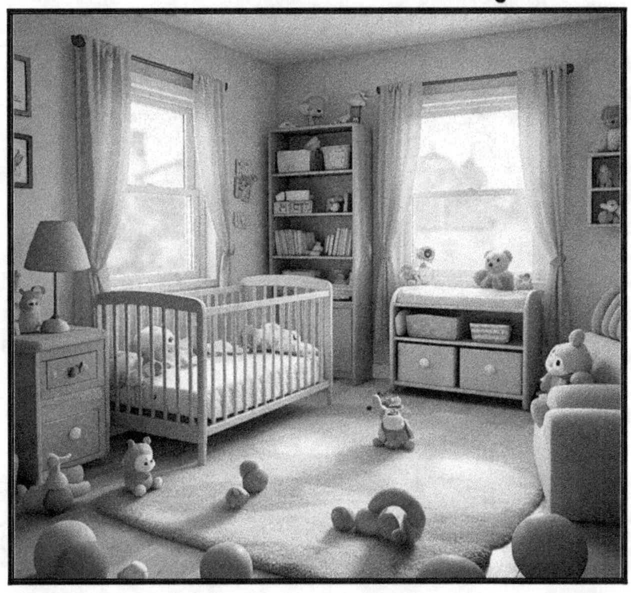

**Introduction:** As the nursery is undoubtedly the most important room in your house, we will dedicate significant time to ensuring that the space where your baby spends most of their early life is exceptionally safe. We understand that you might have already taken some safety measures when setting up the nursery, such as reading safety manuals and choosing appropriate window treatments. However, that won't deter us from meticulously detailing every aspect of this room to maximize its safety and security from top to bottom. Your baby's well-being is our top priority, and we want to create a nurturing environment where they can thrive and explore with confidence. Let's go through the nursery step by step to implement the best safety practices and give you peace of mind knowing that your little one is protected in every possible way.

**Notes:**

→ **Infant/Non-mobile: (Birth - 6 months)**
→ **Infant crawl/roll: (5 months - 1 year)**
Toddler/Pre-school: (1 year - 4 years)
School-age: (5 years - 6+ years)

# CRIB INFORMATION

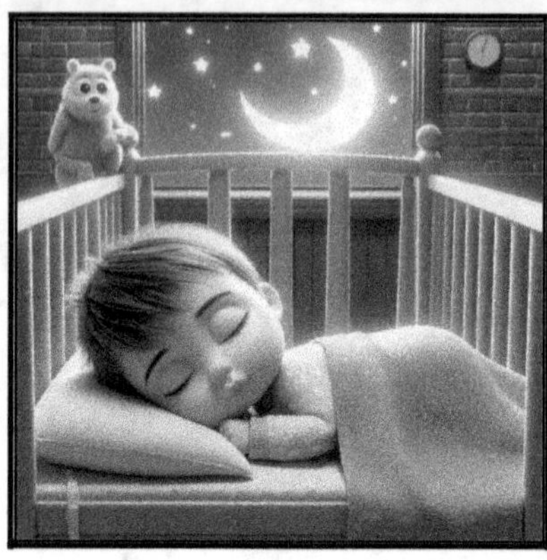

_According to the Consumer Product Safety Commission_
_and the American Academy of Pediatrics_

**Approximately 9,561 children under two are injured in crib-related accidents annually.** Ensure slats are spaced no more than 2.375 inches apart with no decorative cutouts. Check for rough or sharp edges. Ensure sturdy construction with no wobbling, tightening all screws securely. Place away from outlets, cords, heating sources, and windows. Ensure mattress fits snugly with no gaps. Use fitted sheets only, avoiding soft bedding, pillows, comforters, and stuffed animals. Unintentional suffocation from bedding causes approximately 500 child deaths annually. Remove mobiles once baby can sit up. Monitor baby's development and adjust mattress height. Always place baby on back to sleep. Follow manufacturer's guidelines and conduct regular maintenance.

---

🐞 _According to Pediatrics Journal, Nationwide Children's Hospital,_ **approximately 9,561 children under 2 years old are injured in crib-related accidents annually in the US.**

---

<u>**Nursery**</u>
→ **Infant/Non-mobile: (Birth - 6 months)**
→ **Infant crawl/roll: (5 months - 1 year)**
Toddler/Pre-school: (1 year - 4 years)
School-age: (5 years - 6+ years)

# MESH-SIDED CRIB

**Choose sturdy, tightly woven mesh meeting safety standards, free from tears or holes.** Mesh provides excellent visibility and breathability for better air circulation. Ensure mattress fits snugly with no gaps. Use fitted sheets only, avoiding additional bedding. Regularly inspect mesh for secure attachment and adjust sagging areas promptly. Follow weight limits and transition to toddler bed when exceeded or when baby can climb out. Ensure no gaps between mattress and mesh sides. Check corner fasteners are secure. Always supervise baby and transition when showing climbing signs.

---

<u>**Nursery**</u>
→ **Infant/Non-mobile: (Birth - 6 months)**
Infant crawl/roll: (5 months - 1 year)
Toddler/Pre-school: (1 year - 4 years)
School-age: (5 years - 6+ years)

# BASSINET SAFETY

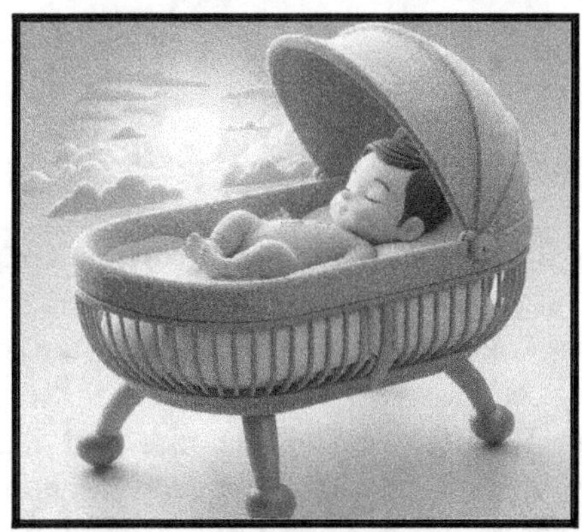

**Choose sturdy, stable frames unlikely to tip over with all components securely attached.** Use firm, flat mattresses fitting snugly within frames. Follow age and weight limitations, transitioning to crib when exceeded or when baby can roll over. Ensure sufficient ventilation in sides. Use fitted sheets only, avoiding additional bedding. Place away from cords, curtains, and heating sources. If equipped with wheels, ensure locking mechanisms work. Meet safety standards with JPMA or ASTM certification. Always supervise during sleep. Inspect regularly for wear or damage. Avoid additional accessories like toys or mobiles. If equipped with canopy, ensure secure attachment without suffocation risks.

---



# Location, Location, Location (Crib location)

**Place in your bedroom for first six months to year for easier nighttime care.** Keep away from windows, curtains, cords, blinds, heaters, radiators, and air vents. Position at safe distance from furniture to prevent items falling into crib. Don't place under wall hangings or heavy pictures. Ensure easy accessibility for comfortable care. Use bassinet or co-sleeper if preferring baby near bed initially. Avoid high-traffic areas. Keep away from cords to prevent entanglement. Place safely from pets. Follow manufacturer's recommendations. Ensure baby monitor accessibility.

---



# Teething

**Use crib rail covers with non-toxic materials to prevent chewing.** Provide safe teething toys to redirect behavior. Remove items encouraging chewing like loose bumpers or blankets. Offer positive reinforcement when not chewing. Address teething discomfort with chilled teething rings. Ensure crib paint is safe and non-toxic, addressing peeling immediately with rail covers. Always supervise crib time. Distract with age-appropriate activities. Consult pediatrician if chewing persists.

---

# PREVENT OVERHEATING

**Maintain room temperature between 68-72°F using a thermometer.** Dress baby in light, breathable sleepwear suitable for temperature. Use breathable bedding like cotton sheets, avoiding heavy comforters or quilts. Layer clothing for easy adjustment. Avoid overburdening or swaddling beyond first few months or when baby starts rolling. Use fan or ensure proper air circulation. Keep room dark with blackout curtains on hot days. Regularly check baby's skin for heat, sweating, flushed skin, or rapid breathing. Monitor regularly during sleep. Follow safe sleep guidelines with back sleeping and firm mattress. Avoid sleep positioners and loose bedding.

---



# CRIB TENTS

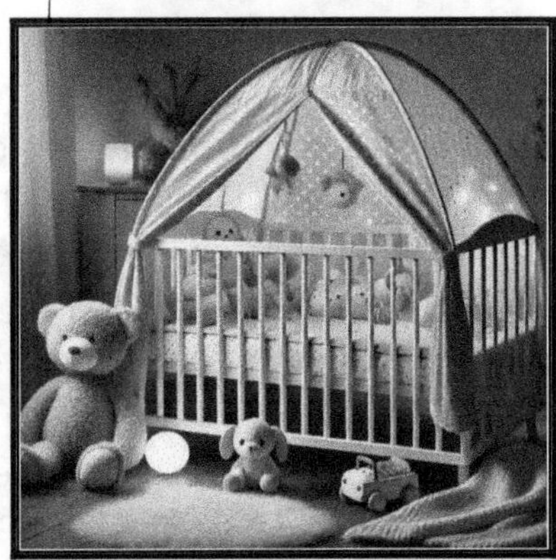

**Crib tents create mesh canopy preventing climbing or falling from crib.** Follow manufacturer's age and weight recommendations. Install properly and securely with close attention to fasteners. Continue supervising even with tent in place. Regularly check for wear, tears, or loose parts. Consider alternatives and evaluate overall sleep environment. Ensure crib meets safety standards with firm mattress and properly fitting sheets. Transition to toddler bed when appropriate age or showing climbing attempts.

---

**Nursery**
→ **Infant/Non-mobile: (Birth - 6 months)**
→ **Infant crawl/roll: (5 months - 1 year)**
→ **Toddler/Pre-school: (1 year - 4 years)**
School-age: (5 years - 6+ years)

# Crib Mounting Attachments

While mounting crib attachments on the wall side to prevent climbing may seem logical, consider safety guidelines and manufacturer instructions carefully. Not all attachments are designed for wall mounting, and improper installation poses safety risks.

**Follow Manufacturer's Instructions:** Always follow guidelines for crib attachments. Manufacturers design and test products based on specific safety standards; proper usage is crucial for your child's safety.

**Crib Attachment Compatibility:** Ensure any attachments are compatible with your crib model and installed correctly. Some cribs include specific attachments designed to prevent climbing.

**Wall Mounting Safety:** If mounting anything on the wall side, ensure it's securely anchored and doesn't risk falling or tipping onto the crib.

**Crib Slats and Design:** Check spacing between slats meets safety standards to prevent entrapment or climbing.

**Correct Mattress Height:** Keep mattress at appropriate height based on child's age and developmental stage. Lower it as the child grows and becomes more mobile to prevent climbing out.

**Supervision:** Always supervise your child in the crib, especially as they reach the age where climbing attempts are more likely.

**Transition to Toddler Bed:** Once your child shows signs of attempting to climb out or reaches the recommended age, consider transitioning to a toddler bed for safety and comfort.

The primary goal is creating a safe sleep environment. While crib attachments can offer additional safety features, they must be used correctly according to manufacturer guidelines. If you have doubts or questions about crib attachments or safety, consult with a pediatrician or child safety expert to ensure appropriate measures for your child's well-being!

**Nursery**
→ **Infant/Non-mobile: (Birth - 6 months)**
→ **Infant crawl/roll: (5 months - 1 year)**
→ **Toddler/Pre-school: (1 year - 4 years)**
School-age: (5 years - 6+ years)

# CRIB SLEEP SAFETY

**Over 1,500 children are injured annually by electrical heating pads.** Choose safe cribs meeting standards with no missing or broken parts. Avoid drop-sides and used cribs. Remove all soft bedding, pillows, toys, and loose blankets. Use firm mattress fitting snugly without gaps. Always place baby on back to sleep. Once baby can roll both ways independently, they can choose position. Dress appropriately in light sleepwear for room temperature. Avoid overcrowding crib with items. Keep away from windows, blinds, cords, and strangulation hazards. Monitor room temperature, avoiding electric blankets or heating pads. Never smoke around baby. Place crib in your room for first six months to year. Regularly inspect crib for loose screws or sharp edges.

---

**Nursery**
→ **Infant/Non-mobile: (Birth - 6 months)**
→ **Infant crawl/roll: (5 months - 1 year)**
→ **Toddler/Pre-school: (1 year - 4 years)**
School-age: (5 years - 6+ years)

# INSTALL CRIB SHEET SECURITY CLIPS

**Installing crib sheet security clips can provide an added layer of safety to keep the fitted sheet securely in place on the crib mattress.** These clips, also known as sheet savers or sheet fasteners, help prevent the fitted sheet from coming loose, bunching up, or slipping off the mattress, which can reduce the risk of suffocation or entanglement for your baby.

**Secure Fit:** Babies are active sleepers and can move around a lot during the night. Crib sheet clips keep the fitted sheet snugly fitted to the mattress, reducing the chances of it getting loose and creating potential hazards.

**Prevent Suffocation Risks:** A loose sheet can accidentally cover the baby's face during sleep, increasing the risk of suffocation. Security clips help keep the sheet taut and properly positioned.

**Ease of Use:** Crib sheet clips are easy to install and remove when it's time to change the sheets. They typically come in sets and can be attached to the corners of the fitted sheet.

**Peace of Mind:** For parents or caregivers, using crib sheet security clips offers peace of mind, knowing that the baby's sleep environment is safer and more secure.

When using crib sheet security clips, it's essential to follow the manufacturer's instructions for proper installation. Additionally, always ensure that the clips are placed in a way that doesn't create any additional hazards or discomfort for the baby.

Remember that while crib sheet security clips can be helpful, they are not a substitute for maintaining a safe sleep environment. Always follow safe sleep guidelines, keep the crib free from loose bedding, and place the baby on their back to sleep. Regularly check the crib and sheets for wear and tear and replace them if needed.

As with baby-related products, if you have any doubts or concerns about using crib sheet security clips, consult your pediatrician or a childproofing expert for guidance. Safety should always be the top priority when it comes to your little one's sleeping environment.

---

<u>**Nursery**</u>
→ **Infant/Non-mobile: (Birth - 6 months)**
→ **Infant crawl/roll: (5 months - 1 year)**
→ **Toddler/Pre-school: (1 year - 4 years)**
School-age: (5 years - 6+ years)

# Sleep Positioning Pads are Not Recommended

The American Academy of Pediatrics strongly advises against sleep positioning pads due to suffocation and SIDS risks. These products can restrict baby's movement, cause overheating, and create entrapment hazards. Always place baby on back to sleep until they can roll independently. Use firm, flat sleep surface like crib mattress fitting snugly. Clear crib of soft bedding, toys, pillows, and bumpers. Room-share for first six to twelve months. Keep home smoke-free. Breastfeed if possible as it reduces SIDS risk.

---

<u>**Nursery**</u>
→ **Infant/Non-mobile: (Birth - 6 months)**
→ **Infant crawl/roll: (5 months - 1 year)**
→ **Toddler/Pre-school: (1 year - 4 years)**
School-age: (5 years - 6+ years)

# REMOVE CRIB BUMPER PADS

The CPSC recommends against bumper pads due to suffocation and entrapment risks where babies can get faces pressed against pads or bodies caught between pad and slats. Bumpers contribute to overheating (SIDS risk factor), reduce airflow, and provide climbing footholds as babies grow. Use bare, empty crib with firm mattress and fitted sheet only. Always place baby on back to sleep. Use properly fitted sheet without bunching or sagging. Keep crib empty of soft bedding, bumpers, stuffed animals, and pillows. Room-share for first six to twelve months.

---

<u>**Nursery**</u>
→ **Infant/Non-mobile: (Birth - 6 months)**
→ **Infant crawl/roll: (5 months - 1 year)**
Toddler/Pre-school: (1 year - 4 years)
School-age: (5 years - 6+ years)

# IF YOUR CHILD IS UNDER 12 MONTHS:
# BE AWARE OF SIDS
# (SUDDEN INFANT DEATH SYNDROME)

**Sudden Infant Death Syndrome is unexplained death of healthy baby during sleep, typically under one year with highest risk between 1-4 months.** Always place baby on back for naps and nighttime. Use firm, flat sleep surface with fitted sheet. Room-share for at least six months, ideally up to one year. Keep crib bare without soft bedding, blankets, pillows, bumpers, or stuffed animals. Dress baby in light sleepwear to prevent overheating. Keep home and car smoke-free. Consider breastfeeding as it reduces SIDS risk. Attend regular check-ups and vaccinations. Encourage supervised tummy time when awake. Consider offering pacifier at nap and bedtime (wait until breastfeeding established).

---

# Hanging Toy Concerns

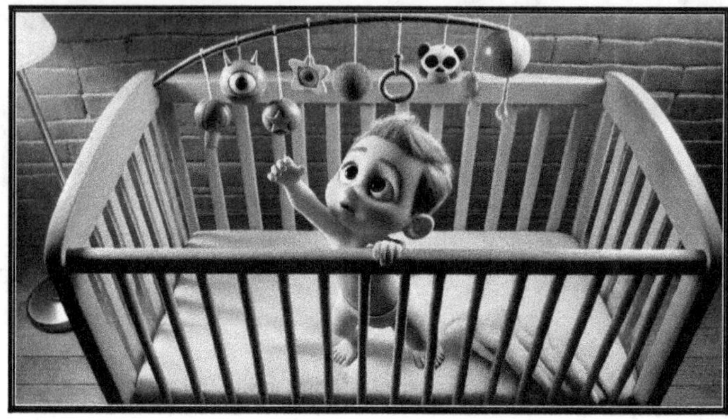

**Do not hang toys, mobiles, or objects over crib due to strangulation hazards from strings, cords, or ribbons. Small parts can detach and become choking hazards.** As babies become mobile, they may reach for items increasing fall risk. Remove all hanging items, keeping crib bare. Follow safe sleep practices with back sleeping on firm surface. Avoid wall hangings above crib. If providing crib toys, choose ones designed for cribs, securely attached to rails, and out of reach when lying down.

---



# Pillow Concerns

**A recent CDC report analyzing Georgia data found nursing pillows present in 5% of 1,685 Sudden Unexpected Infant Deaths, most under 4 months old.** Children don't need pillows until at least one year old. Pillows pose suffocation risk for babies with limited movement control. Infants' undeveloped neck muscles can be pushed forward by pillows, interfering with breathing. Pillows contribute to overheating (SIDS risk factor). For mobile children, pillows can become climbing obstacles. After one year when transitioning to toddler bed, consider small, firm pillow designed for toddlers. Always place baby on back to sleep. Use firm mattress with fitted sheet. Keep crib bare. Room-share for at least six months. Use appropriate sleepwear for room temperature.

---

🍼 *A recent CDC report (May 2025)* analyzing Georgia data from 2013-2022 found that **nursing pillows were present in the sleep space of 84 (5%) of 1,685 Sudden Unexpected Infant Deaths (SUIDs)**. Most of these infants were under 4 months old.

---

**Nursery**
→ **Infant/Non-mobile: (Birth - 6 months)**
Infant crawl/roll: (5 months - 1 year)
Toddler/Pre-school: (1 year - 4 years)
School-age: (5 years - 6+ years)

# Changing Table Guards

Install guards correctly following manufacturer instructions. Never leave baby unattended even briefly. Check age and weight limits ensuring product suits child's size. Regularly inspect for secure attachment and wear. **Avoid distractions during changes.** Use safety straps designed to secure baby. Ensure table is in safe location away from hazards. Use comfortable height for caregiver. Consider non-slip pad to prevent sliding.

---

**Nursery**
→ **Infant non-mobile: (Birth-6 mo.)**
→ **Infant crawl/roll: (5 mo.-2 yrs.)**
Toddler/Pre-School: (1 yr.-4 yrs.)
School-age: (5 yrs.-6 yrs.)

# Breast Milk Safety

**Wash hands before expressing. Use clean containers, labeling with date and time.** Refrigerate up to four days or freeze for extended periods. Never microwave to prevent nutrient loss and uneven heating. Don't shake vigorously. Don't add fresh milk to frozen batch. Check temperature before feeding. Use within two hours at room temperature. Maintain hygiene with breast pumps. Be cautious about alcohol and medication as they transfer through milk. Consult healthcare provider if ill.

---

# Baby Bottle Tooth Decay

**Baby Bottle Tooth Decay (ECC)** Early Childhood Caries results from prolonged exposure to sugary liquids during sleep. Avoid letting child fall asleep with bottle. Limit juice consumption. Regularly clean gums and teeth. Schedule regular dental visits. Encourage healthy eating habits. Lead by example with good oral hygiene. Discuss fluoride supplements with healthcare provider. Avoid sharing utensils or cleaning pacifiers with your mouth to prevent bacteria transfer.

---

<u>**Nursery**</u>
→ **Infant/Non-mobile: (Birth - 6 months)**
→ **Infant crawl/roll: (5 months - 1 year)**
→ **Toddler/Pre-school: (1 year - 4 years)**
School-age: (5 years - 6+ years)

# Baby Wipes and Lotions Safety

**Wipes can contain harsh chemicals causing skin irritation, trigger allergic reactions, clog pores, harbor bacteria increasing infection risk, and ingredients may cause choking if ingested.** Lotions may cause similar issues plus create moist environments increasing infection risk. Store out of reach. Choose fragrance-free, dye-free, alcohol-free products. Apply lotion sparingly. Clean wipes thoroughly after use. Use water and washcloth when possible. Avoid wipes on face. Stop use if irritation occurs.

---

<u>**Nursery**</u>
→ **Infant/Non-mobile: (Birth - 6 months)**
→ **Infant crawl/roll: (5 months - 1 year)**
Toddler/Pre-school: (1 year - 4 years)
School-age: (5 years - 6+ years)

# No Bibs in Crib

Always supervise when wearing bibs. **Choose properly fitting bibs appropriate for age without long strings or ties.** Never let baby wear bib while sleeping or napping as it could cover face or become entangled. Use breathable materials like cotton. Ensure fastening is safe but not too tight. Avoid loops or drawstrings around neck. Remove immediately after feeding or when wet. Never leave in crib.

<u>**Nursery**</u>
→ **Infant/Non-mobile: (Birth - 6 months)**
Infant crawl/roll: (5 months - 1 year)
Toddler/Pre-school: (1 year - 4 years)
School-age: (5 years - 6+ years)

# TOY RATTLE CONCERNS

**Rattles should have no small detachable parts posing choking hazards.** Ensure secure assembly before giving to baby.

Choose non-toxic, BPA-free materials meeting safety standards. Follow age recommendations. Ensure appropriate size and shape for baby's development. Always supervise during play. Avoid strings, cords, or ribbons. Clean and inspect regularly. Use for playtime only, not as sleep aids. Rotate toys for engagement. Plush toys pose suffocation hazards if covering baby's face, overheating risks, choking from small detachable parts, entanglement risks as babies become mobile, and create uneven sleep surfaces. Keep crib bare without plush toys, blankets, or pillows. Use sleep sacks instead of loose blankets. Separate playtime from sleep time. Room-share for first six to twelve months. Offer toys during supervised playtime only.

---

<u>**Nursery**</u>
→ **Infant/Non-mobile: (Birth - 6 months)**
→ **Infant crawl/roll: (5 months - 1 year)**
→ **Toddler/Pre-school: (1 year - 4 years)**
School-age: (5 years - 6+ years)

# PLUSH TOY CONCERNS

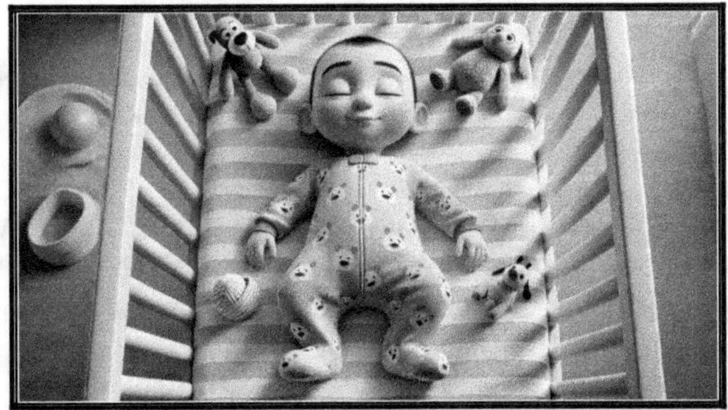

Plush toys, also known as stuffed animals or soft toys, can pose several dangers when placed in a crib with a baby. It's essential to prioritize safety and create a safe sleep environment.

**Suffocation Hazard:** Plush toys have soft, fluffy surfaces that can accidentally cover a baby's face during sleep. This poses a suffocation risk if the baby is unable to move the toy away.

**Risk of Overheating:** Plush toys can trap heat, leading to overheating, which is a risk factor for sudden infant death syndrome (SIDS).

**Choking Hazard:** Some plush toys may have small parts, loose threads, or accessories like buttons or eyes that can become detached. If the baby puts them in their mouth, these items pose a choking hazard.

**Crib Clutter:** Placing plush toys in the crib adds to the clutter and increases the risk of entanglement, especially when the baby becomes more mobile.

**Interference with Sleep Surfaces:** Plush toys can create uneven surfaces in the crib, making providing a firm and safe sleep environment challenging.

### Create a Safe Sleep Environment for Your Baby

**Bare is Best:** Keep the crib free from plush toys, blankets, pillows, and other soft items. A firm, flat sleep surface is the safest for your baby.

**Use Sleep Sacks:** To keep your baby warm during sleep, consider using sleep sacks or wearable blankets instead of loose blankets.

**Separate Playtime from Sleep Time:** Keep playtime and sleep time separate. Remove all toys and distractions from the crib when it's time for sleep.

**Room-sharing:** Consider room-sharing with your baby for the first six to twelve months. Room-sharing allows you to monitor your baby easily while they sleep.

**Offer Toys for Playtime:** Instead of placing plush toys in the crib, give them to your baby during supervised playtime when they can interact with them safely.

Always consult with your pediatrician or a child safety expert if you have any questions or concerns about creating a safe sleep environment for your baby. By prioritizing safety and following these guidelines, you can reduce the risk of sleep-related incidents and make a secure space for your little one to rest and grow.

**Nursery**
→ **Infant/Non-mobile: (Birth - 6 months)**
→ **Infant crawl/roll: (5 months - 1 year)**
→ **Toddler/Pre-school: (1 year - 4 years)**
School-age: (5 years - 6+ years)

# SHOWER/WASH YOUR HANDS FIRST (HYGIENE IMPORTANCE)

**Shower or wash before handling children, especially newborns, to prevent germ spread.** Wash hands thoroughly before and after diaper changes and feeding. Clean hands provide comfortable, hygienic environment promoting bonding. Prevents skin irritation from substances. Postpone handling if unwell or have someone else care for child. Wash hands for at least 20 seconds, especially after bathroom, diaper changes, or handling food. Use alcohol-based sanitizer with 60% alcohol if soap unavailable. Avoid smoking or strong odors before handling baby. Regularly clean and sanitize frequently touched surfaces and baby equipment.

---

**Nursery**
→ **Infant/Non-mobile: (Birth - 6 months)**
→ **Infant crawl/roll: (5 months - 1 year)**
→ **Toddler/Pre-school: (1 year - 4 years)**
School-age: (5 years - 6+ years)

# BABY MONITORS

**Approximately 200 children are injured yearly by baby monitors including electrical shocks and choking from small parts.** Choose reputable brands with good reviews and safety features. Use monitors with secure, encrypted connections. Avoid sharing sensitive information through monitor features. Regularly update firmware for latest security patches. Test range within home. Position at safe distance from baby's sleep area without direct contact. Use as supplemental tool, not replacement for direct supervision. Follow manufacturer's setup and usage guidelines. (Source: U.S. Consumer Product Safety Commission (CPSC) - Baby Monitor Safety) use.

---

**Nursery**
**Infant/Non-mobile: (Birth - 6 months)**
**Infant crawl/roll: (5 months - 1 year)**
**Toddler/Pre-school: (1 year - 4 years)**
School-age: (5 years - 6+ years)

# NURSERY CARE KIT SHOULD AT LEAST CONTAIN:

A Nursery Care Kit is a handy collection of essential items to help parents and caregivers care for their baby's basic needs. While the specific contents may vary depending on the brand and type of kit, a comprehensive Nursery Care Kit typically includes the following items:

☐ **Digital Thermometer:** A digital thermometer to measure the baby's temperature accurately. Opt for a rectal or forehead thermometer explicitly designed for infants.

☐ **Nasal Aspirator or Bulb Syringe:** Used to clear a baby's nasal passages from mucus and congestion, helping them breathe more comfortably.

☐ **Nail Clippers or Scissors:** These are specially designed to trim babies' tiny nails safely and prevent scratching.

☐ **Baby Brush and Comb:** Soft-bristled brush and comb to gently groom and style the baby's hair.

☐ **Medicine Dispenser:** A device to administer liquid medication in precise doses to the baby.

☐ **Medicine Spoon or Dropper:** This is used to give oral medication accurately to the baby.

☐ **Emery Boards:** Gentle emery boards can be used to file baby's nails, offering an alternative to nail clippers or scissors.

☐ **Gauze Pads or Cotton Balls:** These are used for various cleaning purposes, such as applying ointments or wiping sensitive areas.

☐ **Baby Lotion:** A mild, hypoallergenic baby lotion for moisturizing the baby's skin.

☐ **Petroleum Jelly:** Protects baby's sensitive skin from moisture and prevents diaper rash.

☐ **Diaper Cream or Ointment:** To soothe and protect the baby's skin from diaper rash.

☐ **Alcohol Swabs:** These are used to clean items like thermometers before use.

☐ **Safety Nail File:** A gentle nail file as an alternative to nail clippers or scissors.

☐ **Teething Toy or Gel:** An item to soothe the baby's gums during teething.

☐ **Baby Pacifier:** A pacifier can help soothe a fussy baby and promote self-soothing.

☐       **Organizing Case:** A convenient case to keep all the items neatly organized and easily accessible.

Remember that every baby is different, and some items in the Nursery Care Kit may be more useful than others, depending on your baby's needs.

---

**Nursery**
→ **Infant/Non-mobile: (Birth - 6 months)**
→ **Infant crawl/roll: (5 months - 1 year)**
Toddler/Pre-school: (1 year - 4 years)
School-age: (5 years - 6+ years)

# Infant Carrier Safety

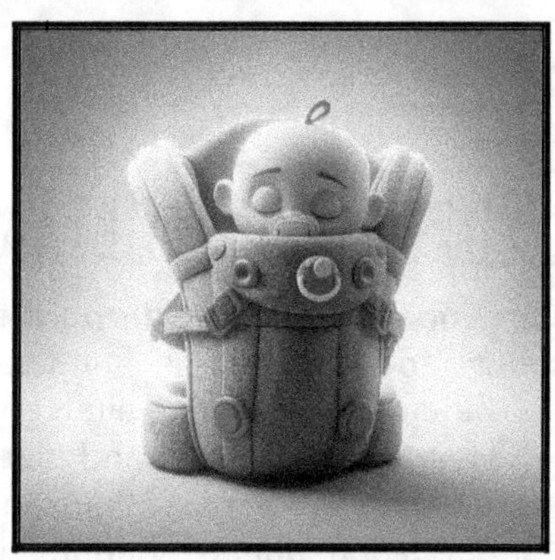

**The U.S. Consumer Product Safety Commission (CPSC) provides important guidelines and recommendations for the safe use of infant carriers, also known as baby carriers or baby slings.**

Follow manufacturer instructions for specific carrier. Choose age-appropriate carriers for baby's size. Position baby upright with face visible and clear of fabric. Keep chin away from chest to maintain airway. Keep nose and mouth free from fabric. Support head and neck for young infants. Ensure snug but not tight fabric and straps. Stay alert and supervise frequently. Take breaks for position changes. Avoid overheating by keeping face and head uncovered. Dress appropriately for weather. Inspect regularly for wear and tear. Use on stable ground, supporting baby's weight when bending. Avoid additional accessories posing strangulation or choking hazards.

---

**Nursery**
→ **Infant/Non-mobile: (Birth - 6 months)**
→ **Infant crawl/roll: (5 months - 1 year)**
Toddler/Pre-school: (1 year - 4 years)
School-age: (5 years - 6+ years)

# Diaper Pail Concerns

Choose pails with good odor control reviews. Clean regularly per manufacturer instructions. Consider eco-friendly liners or reusable cloth liners. Place safely away from children's reach. Empty regularly to prevent buildup. Ensure proper ventilation. Use locks if accessible to older children. Place at safe distance from baby's sleeping area.

---

**Nursery**
→ **Infant/Non-mobile: (Birth - 6 months)**
→ **Infant crawl/roll: (5 months - 1 year)**
→ **Toddler/Pre-school: (1 year - 4 years)**
→ **School-age: (5 years - 6+ years)**

# Air Purifier Importance

**Over 1,200 children are injured yearly by air purifiers and humidifiers from electrical shocks and burns.** Air purifiers benefit children's developing respiratory systems by removing allergens, dust, pet dander, pollen, mold spores. Help with asthma and allergy relief. Capture bacteria and viruses reducing infection risk. Minimize secondhand smoke exposure. Promote better sleep quality. Reduce indoor air pollution effects. Enhance concentration. Particularly useful in nurseries. Help manage pet allergies. Remove harmful VOCs from cleaning products and paints. Reduce airborne disease transmission. Choose appropriate filtration system and room size coverage. Replace filters regularly. Secure properly to prevent tipping. (Source: U.S. Consumer Product Safety Commission (CPSC) - Appliance Safety)

---

**Nursery**
→ **Infant/Non-mobile: (Birth - 6 months)**
→ **Infant crawl/roll: (5 months - 1 year)**
→ **Toddler/Pre-school: (1 year - 4 years)**
→ **School-age: (5 years - 6+ years)**

# Mist Humidifiers

**Safer than vaporizers as they don't produce hot steam.** Provide cool or room temperature mist. Add moisture soothing dry nasal passages and throats. Help reduce airborne allergens. Prevent dry, itchy skin. Promote restful sleep. Don't significantly affect room temperature. Many have built-in features preventing bacterial growth. Clean regularly per instructions. Use distilled or demineralized water. Place safely out of children's reach. Monitor humidity levels, maintaining 30-50%. Use in moderation.

---

<u>**Nursery**</u>
→ **Infant/Non-mobile: (Birth - 6 months)**
→ **Infant crawl/roll: (5 months - 1 year)**
→ **Toddler/Pre-school: (1 year - 4 years)**
→ **School-age: (5 years - 6+ years)**

# EAR PIERCING SAFETY

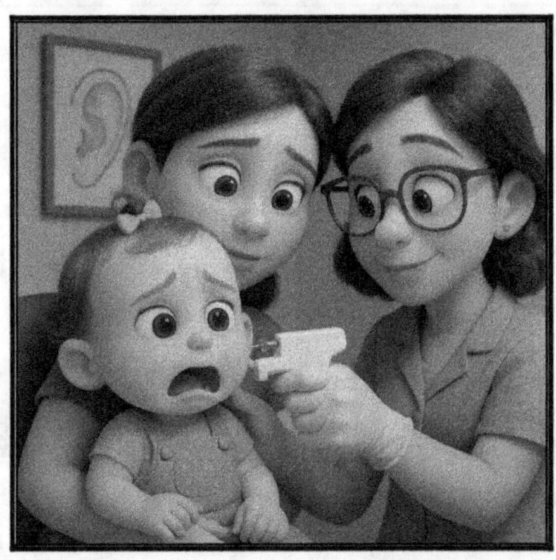

**Up to 35% of ear piercings result in complications including infections (20-30% of cases), allergic reactions, keloid scarring, and embedded earrings.** Higher infection rates with piercing guns and inadequate aseptic technique. Nickel allergy and permanent ear deformities well-documented, particularly in children pierced before age 11. About 13% of piercing-associated ED visits involve infections, with 3% requiring hospitalization. Consider child's age and ability to provide informed consent. Understand pain and discomfort involved. Follow proper aftercare to prevent infection. Choose hypoallergenic materials. Allow adequate healing time. Consider impact on activities. Avoid DIY piercing kits. Choose reputable, experienced piercer using sterile equipment. Consider potential future regret. Respect cultural and family traditions.

---

# |Ch. 11| Children with Diverse Needs

Childproofing a home is like crafting the ultimate safety zone, especially when it comes to children with special needs. These kids are superheroes in their own right, and just like superheroes, they need a space that caters to their unique abilities and challenges. Your home should be their safe space, whether it's mobility issues, sensory sensitivities, behavioral tendencies, or medical conditions. This chapter is your guide to making sure you've got every angle covered, with a sprinkle of humor to keep things light!

---

**Children with Diverse Needs**
→ Infant/Non-mobile: (Birth - 6 months)
→ Infant crawl/roll: (5 months - 1 year)
→ Toddler/Pre-school: (1 year - 4 years)
→ School-age: (5 years - 6+ years)

# UNDERSTANDING CHILDREN WITH DIVERSE NEEDS

**Every child is unique requiring tailored childproofing approaches.** Physical mobility challenges require ramps, wider doorways, trip-hazard removal, non-slip mats, and padding. Sensory processing disorders need balanced environments - hypo-sensitive children need safe excitement zones, hypersensitive children need calm, low-stimulation spaces. Behavioral and cognitive delays require extra supervision and multiple safety layers, especially for children with autism, ADHD, or severe cognitive delays who may not grasp danger concepts. Medical needs require secure storage of equipment like feeding tubes and oxygen tanks, keeping them accessible for adults but away from siblings.

---

**Children with Diverse Needs**
→ Infant/Non-mobile: (Birth - 6 months)
→ Infant crawl/roll: (5 months - 1 year)
→ Toddler/Pre-school: (1 year - 4 years)
→ School-age: (5 years - 6+ years)

# GENERAL SAFETY MEASURES

**Anchor all furniture to walls.** Use extra-wide, reinforced gates at stairs. Pad sharp corners. Use sliding outlet covers. Keep cords hidden and secured. Install smoke detectors with vibrating or visual alarms for noise-sensitive children. Create sensory retreats with soft pillows, weighted blankets, dimmable lights, minimal clutter. Add padded walls if needed for head-banging behaviors.

---

<u>**Children with Diverse Needs**</u>
→ **Infant/Non-mobile: (Birth - 6 months)**
→ **Infant crawl/roll: (5 months - 1 year)**
→ **Toddler/Pre-school: (1 year - 4 years)**
→ **School-age: (5 years - 6+ years)**

# Childproofing for Sensory Processing Issues

**Use dimmable lighting and blackout curtains for light sensitivity.** Add acoustic panels and plush rugs for noise dampening. Have noise-canceling headphones available. Offer safe sensory materials like soft blankets, smooth toys, textured walls (all non-toxic). Avoid irritating materials like shag rugs or rough upholstery.

---

<u>**Children with Diverse Needs**</u>
Infant/Non-mobile: (Birth - 6 months)
Infant crawl/roll: (5 months - 1 year)
→ **Toddler/Pre-school: (1 year - 4 years)**
→ **School-age: (5 years - 6+ years)**

# Behavioral Safety Concerns

**Install high locks or deadbolts out of reach but easy for adults. Use alarms or motion sensors for doors and windows.** Add soft padding to walls, floors, and furniture in frequently used rooms. Offer sensory gloves or chewable jewelry for children who bite or scratch. Use tamper-proof locks on medication and hazardous substance cabinets.

---

<u>**Children with Diverse Needs**</u>
→ **Infant/Non-mobile: (Birth - 6 months)**
→ **Infant crawl/roll: (5 months - 1 year)**
→ **Toddler/Pre-school: (1 year - 4 years)**
→ **School-age: (5 years - 6+ years)**

# Mobility and Accessibility Adjustments

**Remove tripping hazards like rugs and cords.** Ensure doorways and hallways accommodate wheelchairs and walkers. Install grab bars in bathrooms, near beds, and along hallways. Consider stairlifts or home elevators for multiple floors. Ensure lifts have safety features like seatbelts and secure footrests. Use tamper-proof locks on medication and hazardous substance cabinets.

---

# |Ch. 12| Laundry Room

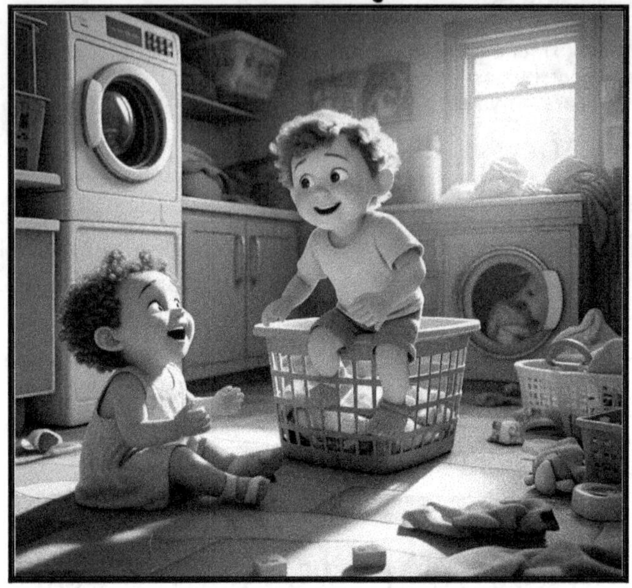

**Introduction:** In the bustling heart of every home lies a room often overlooked in the childproofing process - the laundry room. This seemingly innocuous space, brimming with the fragrance of fresh linen and fabric softener, holds a myriad of hidden dangers for our little explorers. As we venture into this chapter, we will unearth the secrets to transforming this bustling hub into a safe haven devoid of the perils that lurk in laundry baskets and behind laundry cupboard doors. From securing hazardous cleaning agents to ensuring the washing machine remains an appliance rather than a playground, we will guide you step-by-step to foster a safe and secure environment. Let's embark on this journey to create a laundry room where little dreams can't be dampened, and tiny adventurers play safely under the watchful eyes of their guardians.

---

**<u>Laundry Room</u>**
Infant non-mobile: (Birth-6 mo.)
Infant crawl/roll: (5 mo.-2 yrs.)
→ **Toddler/Pre-School: (1 yr.-4 yrs.)**
→ **School-age: (5 yrs.-6 yrs.)**

# LAUNDRY ROOM SAFETY

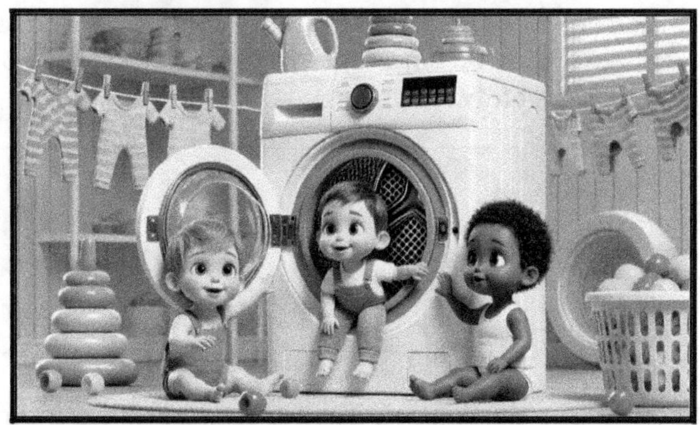

**Approximately 2,000 children are injured yearly by laundry machines.** Install childproof locks on washer and dryer doors. Elevate machines if possible. Store detergents, fabric softeners, and supplies in locked cabinets. Secure power cords. Educate older children about risks. Supervise laundry time. Teach safe operation. Unplug when not in use. Keep area tidy to prevent tripping.

---

**<u>Laundry Room</u>**
Infant/Non-mobile: (Birth - 6 months)
Infant crawl/roll: (5 months - 1 year)
→ **Toddler/Pre-school: (1 year - 4 years)**
→ **School-age: (5 years - 6+ years)**

# IRON AND IRONING BOARD SAFETY

**Over 50,000 children sustain burns yearly from hot surfaces including irons.** Store ironing board in locked closet, fully collapsed. Choose sturdy design with secure locking. Elevate storage. Designate child-free zone. Supervise usage. Avoid overloading. Use safety cover with childproof fastener. Store iron on high shelf or locked cabinet. Use cord holder. Educate older children. Designate cooling area with heat-resistant pad. Always unplug after use. Avoid leaving water inside steam irons. Inspect regularly.

---

# CLOTHING STEAMERS

**Store in locked cabinet or high shelf when not in use.** Unplug immediately after use with cord out of reach. Choose models with automatic shutoff and safety lock.

---



# DRYING RACK SAFETY

**Place in elevated position out of reach or use wall-mounted version.** Ensure sturdy, stable design. Secure wall mounting with appropriate hardware. Avoid sharp edges. Supervise usage. Avoid overloading. Designate child-free zone. Secure folding legs when in use. Store safely when not in use. Educate older children. Avoid hanging heavy or sharp items. Keep area tidy.

---



# DETERGENT AND BLEACH SAFETY

**Detergent pods are dangerous despite convenience. Ensure containers have childproof tops and store high or locked.** Read and follow label instructions. Use in well-ventilated areas. Wear protective gear for concentrated bleach. Store in locked cabinets out of reach. Store separately, never mix together. Never mix bleach with ammonia or acids. Use recommended amounts. Clean spills promptly with proper precautions. Keep in original labeled containers. Dispose properly. Childproof laundry area. Teach children about dangers.

---

**Laundry Room**
Infant/Non-mobile: (Birth - 6 months)
Infant crawl/roll: (5 months - 1 year)
→ **Toddler/Pre-school: (1 year - 4 years)**
→ **School-age: (5 years - 6+ years)**

# STANDING WATER CONCERNS

**Standing water creates slip and fall hazards, electrical hazards when contacting outlets or appliances, damage to flooring and property, appliance damage, health hazards from bacterial growth and mold, water contamination risks, and structural damage.** Address leaks immediately. Ensure proper drainage. Regularly inspect for water damage. Promptly address plumbing issues. Use water-resistant flooring. Install leak detectors or flood sensors.

---

**Laundry Room**
Infant/Non-mobile: (Birth - 6 months)
Infant crawl/roll: (5 months - 1 year)
→ **Toddler/Pre-school: (1 year - 4 years)**
→ **School-age: (5 years - 6+ years)**

# LAUNDRY BASKET CONCERNS

**Choose child-safe design with rounded edges, lightweight material.** If equipped with lid, ensure childproof safety lock. Store out of reach in locked closet or high shelf. Avoid overloading. Always supervise usage. Teach proper use. Remove tripping hazards from laundry area. Educate about risks.

---

❦ While it seems impossible in a "dry" closet, laundry baskets are a leading contributor to non-pool-related infant injuries. Large, solid-wall plastic laundry baskets are essentially portable bathtubs. If left in a walk-in closet near a bathroom or a "lifestyle sink," they can collect water from a leak or an overflowing basin. Because of their high walls, a baby who crawls into a basket containing as little as **2 inches of water** cannot right themselves if they flip over. The "ribbed" sides of many baskets actually make it harder for a slippery infant to find purchase to push themselves up.

*-Consumer Product Safety Commission (CPSC) reports on "Submersion in Household Containers."*

---

# |Ch. 13| Home Office/Den

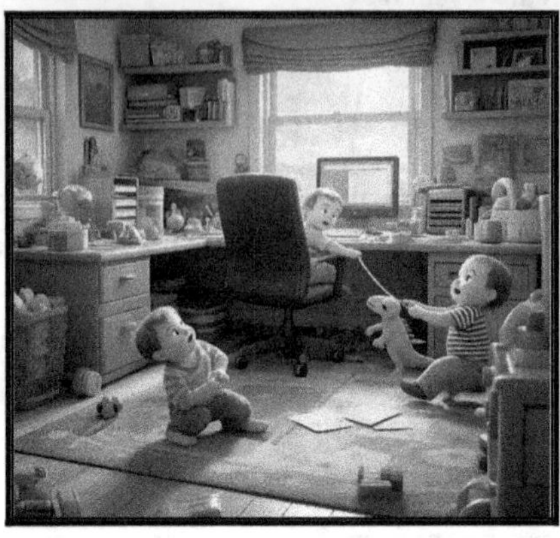

**Introduction:** In the modern home, the home office often stands as a sanctuary of productivity and creativity, a place where great ideas come to life. However, to the curious eyes of a child, it transforms into a wonderland of intriguing gadgets, colorful stationery, and mysterious nooks. As we delve into this chapter, we will guide you in crafting a space that nurtures both your professional aspirations and your child's safety. From securing heavy furniture to organizing cords and electrical outlets, we will explore comprehensive strategies to foster a child-friendly environment without compromising your workspace aesthetics. Join us in sculpting a home office that harmoniously blends safety and functionality, allowing peace of mind to fuel your productivity while nurturing the budding curiosity of the little ones.

---

**Home Office/Den**
Infant/Non-mobile: (Birth - 6 months)
Infant crawl/roll: (5 months - 1 year)
→ **Toddler/Pre-school: (1 year - 4 years)**
→ **School-age: (5 years - 6+ years)**

## HOME OFFICE DOORKNOBS

Childproofing doorknobs prevents young children from accessing certain areas or leaving rooms unsupervised.

**Doorknob Covers:** Use doorknob covers or childproof locks designed to fit over existing doorknobs. These covers are typically made of durable materials difficult for young children to manipulate.

**Door Lever Locks:** If doors have lever-style handles, install door lever locks specifically designed to prevent children from operating them.

**Height Adjustment:** Adjust the height of doorknob covers or locks to ensure they're out of your child's reach. Higher placement makes them more challenging to access.

**Secure External Doors:** Install childproof locks on external doors to prevent young children from wandering outside unsupervised.

**Educate Older Children:** If you have older children who can open doors, educate them about the importance of securing doorknob covers or locks.

**Consistent Use:** Always use the doorknob cover or lock whenever you leave a room.

**Keep Keys Out of Reach:** If your door has a key lock, keep keys out of children's reach to prevent unlocking.

**Regular Maintenance:** Inspect doorknob covers or locks regularly for signs of wear or damage. Replace promptly if needed.

Creating a safer environment gives peace of mind knowing certain areas are securely off-limits. As with all childproofing efforts, vigilance and consistency are key to maintaining a safe home for little ones.

---

**Home Office/Den**
Infant/Non-mobile: (Birth - 6 months)
→ **Infant crawl/roll: (5 months - 1 year)**
→ **Toddler/Pre-school: (1 year - 4 years)**
→ **School-age: (5 years - 6+ years)**

# OFFICE SUPPLIES

Everyday office items like scissors, staples, and paper clips frequently cause eye injuries and punctures. Office furniture accounts for 70% of tip-over injuries, happening every 46 minutes in ERs. Store supplies in locked cabinets or drawers. Use childproof containers for small items. Secure cords with organizers and clips. Bundle cables to avoid tangles. Keep sharp objects in secure drawers with childproof features. Childproof electronics placement. Secure heavy equipment to prevent tipping. Educate older children. Keep chemicals separate in locked cabinet. Maintain organized, tidy workspace.

---

*According to Nationwide Children's Hospital, everyday items like scissors, staples, and paper clips frequently lead to eye injuries and puncture wounds in young children. And with office desks or shelves toppling over, youngsters account for 70% of furniture-tip-over injuries, happening as often as* **one child every 46 minutes in**

**ERs.** Together, these risks show that even quiet office areas need childproofing.

---

**Home Office/Den**
Infant/Non-mobile: **(Birth - 6 months)**
Infant crawl/roll: **(5 months - 1 year)**
→ **Toddler/Pre-school: (1 year - 4 years)**
→ **School-age: (5 years - 6+ years)**

# Paper Shredder Safety

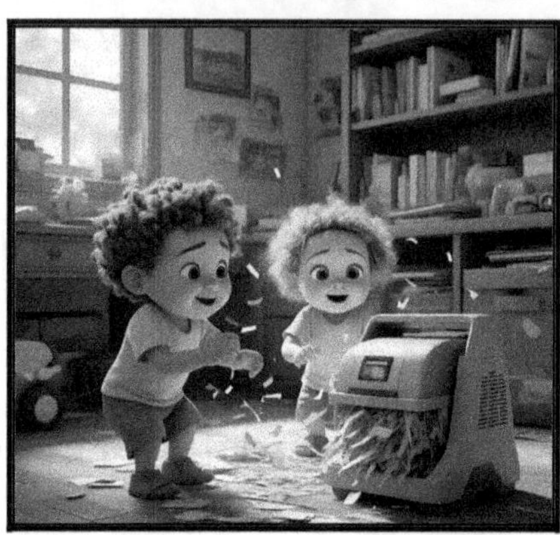

**Always unplug when not in use with cord out of reach.** Engage safety lock feature when not in use. Store in locked cabinet or inaccessible room. Educate older children about dangers, supervising usage. Keep hands and objects away from opening. Use sensors that automatically shut off if hands get close. Secure waste bin to shredder. Always monitor during operation. Inspect regularly, replacing damaged parts promptly.

---

**Home Office/Den**
Infant/Non-mobile: (Birth - 6 months)
Infant crawl/roll: (5 months - 1 year)
→ **Toddler/Pre-school: (1 year - 4 years)**
→ **School-age: (5 years - 6+ years)**

# Ink and Toner Concerns

**Store in childproof containers with secure lids and proper labels.** Use elevated storage on high shelves or locked cabinets. Educate older children. Clean spills immediately, keeping children away. Monitor usage. Avoid transferring to other containers. Follow proper disposal guidelines. Keep caps secure after use. Store away from food and drink. Lock printer trays if possible.

---

# COPIER AND PRINTER SAFETY

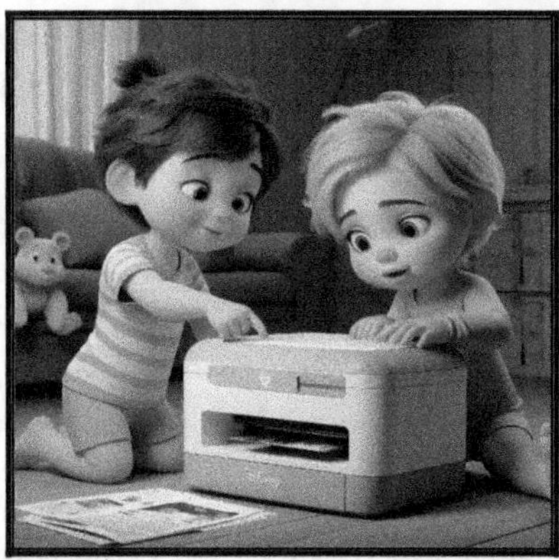

**Place on stable surfaces out of reach, avoiding low furniture. Secure cables with organizers.** Use childproof covers for removable parts. Activate child lock features in settings. Educate older children. Supervise usage. Store supplies in locked cabinets. Secure or lock paper trays. Inspect regularly. Follow proper disposal guidelines.

---

**Home Office/Den**
Infant/Non-mobile: (Birth - 6 months)
Infant crawl/roll: (5 months - 1 year)
→ **Toddler/Pre-school: (1 year - 4 years)**
→ **School-age: (5 years - 6+ years)**

# COMPUTER EQUIPMENT

**Over 5,000 children injured yearly by computers and laptops. Place on sturdy desk out of reach. Secure cords with organizers.** Use childproof covers for removable parts. Store accessories in locked cabinets. Use childproof power strips. Educate older children. Implement parental controls and limit screen time. Monitor usage. Install child-friendly software. Inspect regularly. Lock screen when unattended. Empty bathtub after use.

---

# Stapler Safety

**Store manual staplers in locked drawers. Educate older children. Supervise usage.** Teach safe usage. Use safety guards. For electric staplers, unplug when not in use. Store safely in locked areas. Use safety features like automatic shut-off. Monitor usage. Keep hands clear. Inspect regularly.

---



# Laser Pointer Concerns

**Laser light can damage retina causing vision problems including blindness.** Children's developing eyes are more vulnerable. Keep out of reach. Teach about dangers. Never point at eyes. Direct beam away from audience during presentations. Check local laws on laser pointer regulations. Take child to doctor immediately if injured.

---



# Door Security

**Childproofing every door in your home is vital in safeguarding young children from potential hazards.** This involves securing various types of doors, including front and back doors, by installing high-placed deadbolts and door alarms and using safety glass to prevent breakage. Interior doors, such as those in bedrooms and bathrooms, should have knob covers, finger pinch guards, and door stoppers to prevent injuries and accidental lock-ins. Sliding doors, often leading to patios, require top locks, window films, and safety bars to deter children from opening them and to prevent shattering. Garage doors should have remote controls stored safely, safety sensors installed, and childproofing straps on emergency levers to avoid unauthorized access. Closet doors need special attention, with bi-fold door locks and magnetic locks to prevent children from getting trapped or accessing unsafe items. Educating children about the potential dangers and supervising them closely are general safety practices that should be adopted. These measures help in fostering a safe and secure home environment for children to explore without risks.

---

**Home Office/Den**
Infant/Non-mobile: (Birth - 6 months)
Infant crawl/roll: (5 months - 1 year)
→ **Toddler/Pre-school: (1 year - 4 years)**
→ **School-age: (5 years - 6+ years)**

# EMERGENCY DISTRACTION KIT

Coloring books and washable crayons, sticker sheets, age-appropriate puzzle books, favorite storybooks, Play-Doh or modeling clay, small quiet toys, activity cards, healthy non-messy snacks, travel games, educational flashcards, water wow books, headphones and audiobooks (if comfortable with screen time), pipe cleaners and beads for older kids, scavenger hunt lists, notebooks and gel pens. Customize based on age and interests, rotating items regularly.

---

**Notes:**

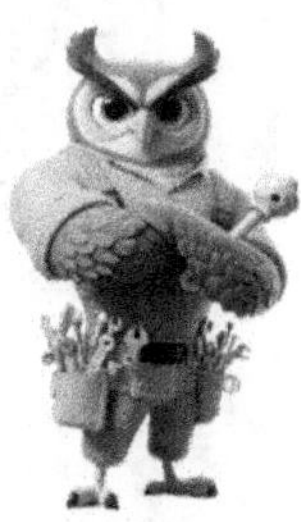

 # Sunroom/Patio

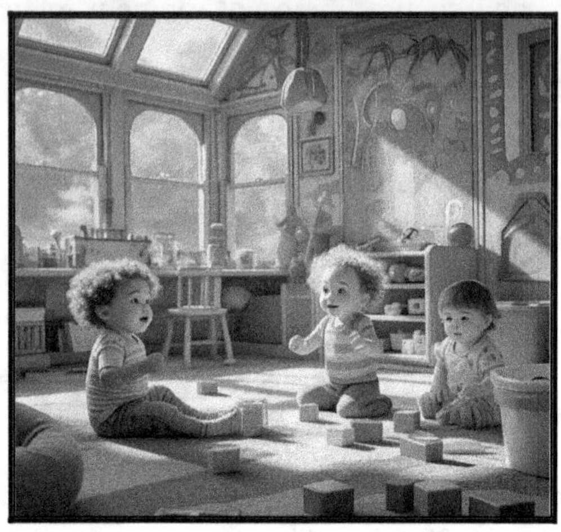

**Introduction:** In the blissful embrace of your home's sunroom or patio, where sunlight filters through, and laughter echoes, the safety of your little ones remains paramount. This chapter is dedicated to transforming your sunroom or deck into a haven where curiosity meets safety, allowing your children to explore without encountering hazards. From securing railings to ensuring the safety of outdoor furniture, we will guide you through comprehensive strategies to childproof these spaces. Let's embark on this journey of creating a sunroom or patio that harmonizes the joyous melodies of childhood with the comforting embrace of safety, fostering a space where memories are made with peace of mind.

---

**Sunroom/Patio**
Infant/Non-mobile: **(Birth - 6 months)**
→ **Infant crawl/roll: (5 months - 1 year)**
→ **Toddler/Pre-school: (1 year - 4 years)**
→ **School-age: (5 years - 6+ years)**

## REMOVE CHAIRS WITH RUBBER-STRIPED SEATS AND BACKS

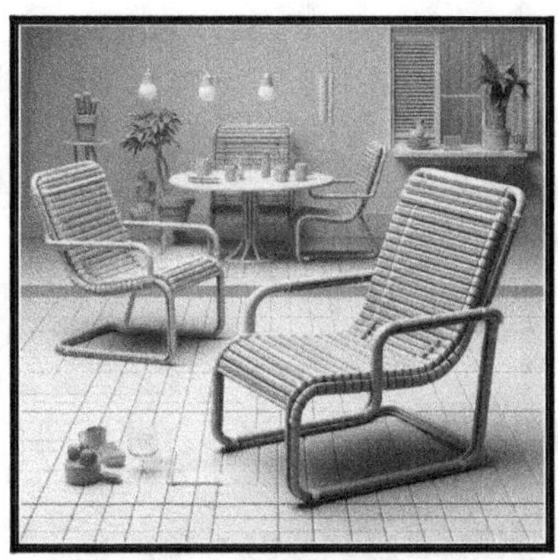

**These pose significant choking hazards, particularly for toddlers.**

Inspect thoroughly for loose or detachable rubber strips. Conduct regular checks for wear and tear. Remove chairs entirely from accessible areas or store in locked rooms. Replace with safer alternatives having solid backs and seats without detachable elements. Extend safety approach to other areas - anchor furniture, check sharp edges, educate family and visitors. Consider first aid course for choking incidents. Keep emergency numbers accessible.

---

**Sunroom/Patio**
Infant/Non-mobile: (Birth - 6 months)
Infant crawl/roll: (5 months - 1 year)
→ **Toddler/Pre-school: (1 year - 4 years)**
→ **School-age: (5 years - 6+ years)**

# WICKER SAFETY

**Inspect for loose fibers and stability.** Sand sharp edges smooth. Secure loose fibers by weaving back or trimming. Add padding to cover gaps. Schedule regular maintenance. Clean regularly. Position away from windows and hazardous areas. Install corner protectors. Educate family members. Be prepared with first aid kit and emergency training.

---

**Sunroom/Patio**
Infant/Non-mobile: (Birth - 6 months)
Infant crawl/roll: (5 months - 1 year)
→ **Toddler/Pre-school: (1 year - 4 years)**
→ **School-age: (5 years - 6+ years)**

# INSTALL SECURITY WINDOW LOCKS

**Conduct comprehensive window assessment. Select high-quality, child-resistant locks designed to withstand force. Install at height out**

**of children's reach.** Consider integrating alarms for opening attempts. Ensure quick-release mechanism for emergencies. Educate household about functioning and benefits.

---

**Sunroom/Patio**

Infant/Non-mobile: (Birth - 6 months)
Infant crawl/roll: (5 months - 1 year)
→ **Toddler/Pre-school: (1 year - 4 years)**
→ **School-age: (5 years - 6+ years)**

# Beware of Exposed Metal

**(Heat Concerns)**

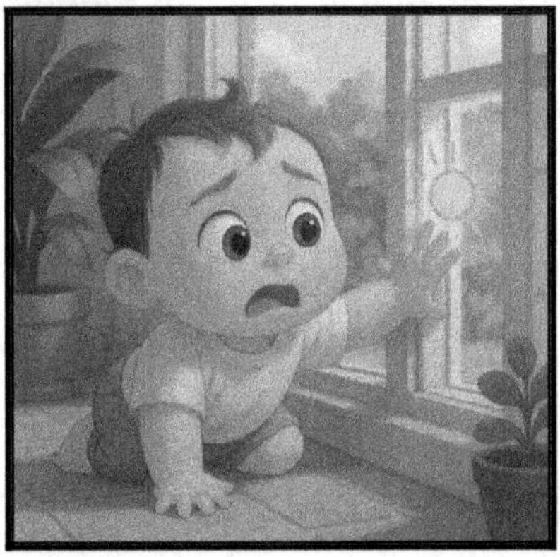

**A 2012-2017 study documented 58 children (median age 17 months) suffering contact burns from sun-heated surfaces.** Identify metal areas that heat significantly. Install shades to control sunlight. Consider replacing with non-conductive materials. Cover exposed metal with heat-resistant materials like insulating foam or silicone. Establish child-friendly zone away from these areas. Educate children about touching hot surfaces. Keep first-aid kit equipped for burns readily available. Supervision is key.

---

❦ A study from *Children's Hospital Colorado* (2012–2017) documented 58 children (median age 17 months) who suffered contact burns from sun-heated surfaces around the home, think metal thresholds, toilet lids, or other surfaces heated by sunlight.

---

# |Ch. 15| Attic

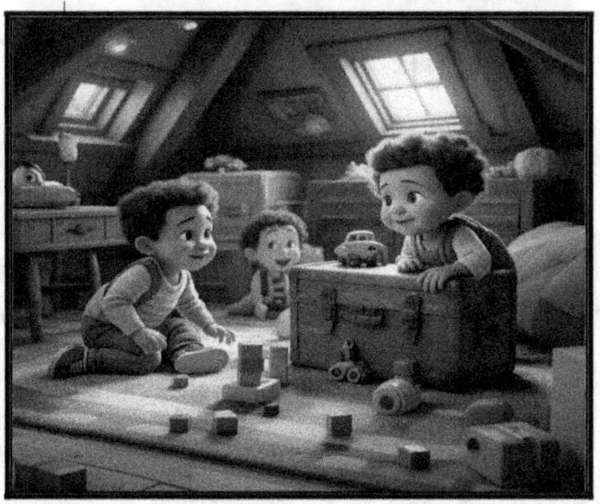

**Introduction:** Due to its specific characteristics, childproofing an attic requires a combination of traditional techniques and unique considerations.

---

**Attic**
Infant/Non-mobile: (Birth - 6 months)
Infant crawl/roll: (5 months - 1 year)
→ **Toddler/Pre-school: (1 year - 4 years)**
→ **School-age: (5 years - 6+ years)**

## Attic Access Control

**Install childproof lock or gate at entrance.** If accessed via stairs, install safety gates at top and bottom. Add non-slip pads to steps. Install childproof window locks. Add window guards for low or large windows.

---

**Attic**
Infant/Non-mobile: (Birth - 6 months)
→ **Infant crawl/roll: (5 months - 1 year)**
→ **Toddler/Pre-school: (1 year - 4 years)**
→ **School-age: (5 years - 6+ years)**

## Floor Security

**Inspect floor for weak or rotten spots, repairing immediately.** Ensure no protruding nails or screws. Cover rough material with carpeting or rugs. Remove clutter and tripping hazards. Secure rugs properly. Create designated play area with safe toys away from stairs or windows. Add padding to play area. Ensure no loose cords. Cover floor-level outlets. Lock harmful substances away. Always supervise.

# Childproofing Electricity in the Attic

**Install tamper-resistant outlet covers**. Use cord organizers to hide electrical cords. Fasten loose cords with clips. Replace standard outlets with GFCI outlets. Secure light bulbs, using safety cages. Choose LED bulbs. Install lockable cover on electrical panels. Educate children on electrical safety. Supervise constantly. Conduct routine safety inspections.

---

**Attic**
→ **Infant/Non-mobile: (Birth - 6 months)**
→ **Infant crawl/roll: (5 months - 1 year)**
→ **Toddler/Pre-school: (1 year - 4 years)**
→ **School-age: (5 years - 6+ years)**

# Insects and Pests

**Natural Repellents:** Use natural repellents like peppermint oil or cedarwood to deter pests without introducing harmful chemicals.

**Check for Pests:** Regularly inspect the attic for signs of pests like rodents or insects and address any infestations promptly.

---

**Attic**
→ **Infant/Non-mobile: (Birth - 6 months)**
→ **Infant crawl/roll: (5 months - 1 year)**
→ **Toddler/Pre-school: (1 year - 4 years)**
→ **School-age: (5 years - 6+ years)**

# Temperature

**Ensure well-insulated attic with insulated windows.** Install efficient ventilation system with roof vents. Set up safe heating and cooling systems with safeguarded elements. Install temperature monitoring system. Use thermal curtains. Designate temperature-regulated play area with neutral-temperature flooring. Educate children. Ensure supervision. Conduct regular maintenance and professional inspections.

---

# Attic Play Zone

**Studies show falls from elevated spots like attics are nearly seven times more likely to cause skull fractures or brain injuries. Over 10,000 preschoolers hospitalized yearly from falls.** Inspect floor for splinters and uneven surfaces. Use soft flooring like plush carpets or play mats. Install soft wall coverings. Establish temperature control with insulation and heating/cooling. Use child-friendly furniture with rounded edges, securing heavy pieces to walls. Install sufficient lighting with nightlights. Add window locks and guards. Cover outlets and manage cords. Keep tidy with secure storage. Ensure clear exit access. Stock first-aid kit. Maintain vigilant supervision. Educate about safety rules. Conduct regular maintenance.

---

**Notes:**

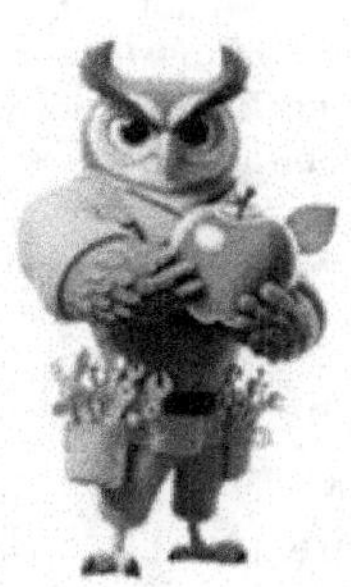

 # Panic/Safe Room

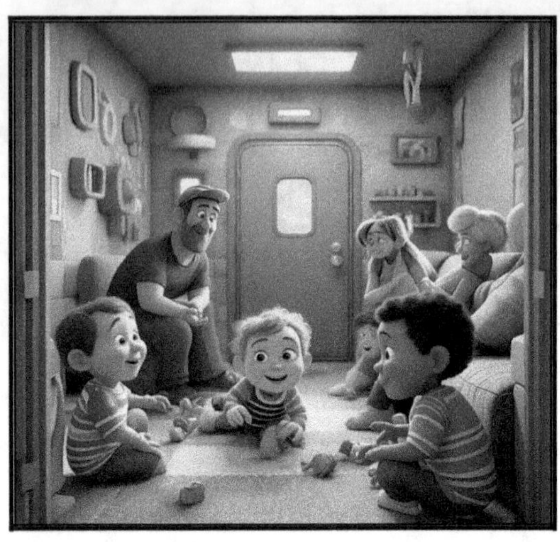

**Introduction:** In the modern home, a panic room stands as a fortress of safety, a haven designed to shield its occupants from unforeseen dangers and emergencies. Yet, in the eyes of a child, this secure space can morph into a realm of mystery and adventure, beckoning them with the lure of the unknown. As we venture into this chapter, we delve deep into the essential strategies to transform your panic room into a zone that safeguards not only against external threats but also the curious and ever-adventurous spirits of little ones. From installing child-resistant locks to securing potential tripping hazards, we will guide you step-by-step to ensure that your fortress of safety remains impenetrable to young explorers, keeping them safe from both external dangers and the bumps and bruises of unintended adventures.

---

**Panic/Safe Room**
Infant/Non-mobile: (Birth - 6 months)
Infant crawl/roll: (5 months - 1 year)
→ **Toddler/Pre-school: (1 year - 4 years)**
→ **School-age: (5 years - 6+ years)**

## CONTROL ACCESS

**Install biometric locks** (fingerprint or retina scan) recognizing only adults. Include secondary manual lock for electronic failures that children can't manipulate.

---

**Panic/Safe Room**
Infant/Non-mobile: (Birth - 6 months)
Infant crawl/roll: (5 months - 1 year)
→ **Toddler/Pre-school: (1 year - 4 years)**
→ **School-age: (5 years - 6+ years)**

# FLOOR AND WALL CONCERNS

**Use non-slip flooring mats or tiles.** Add padded walls for soundproofing and injury prevention.

___________________________________________

<u>**Panic/Safe Room**</u>
Infant/Non-mobile: (Birth - 6 months)
Infant crawl/roll: (5 months - 1 year)
→ **Toddler/Pre-school: (1 year - 4 years)**
→ **School-age: (5 years - 6+ years)**

# FURNITURE PREFERENCES

**Blend safety with functionality using rounded corners and securing heavy pieces to walls.** Choose soft materials, avoid glass. Include lockable storage for emergency supplies, comfortable padded seating, foldable cot, small desk with communication devices. Use carpeted or rubber-matted flooring. Designate play area with soft, non-toxic toys. Include air purifier or ventilation for extended stays.

___________________________________________

<u>**Panic/Safe Room**</u>
→ **Infant/Non-mobile: (Birth - 6 months)**
→ **Infant crawl/roll: (5 months - 1 year)**
→ **Toddler/Pre-school: (1 year - 4 years)**
→ **School-age: (5 years - 6+ years)**

# INTERCOM COMMUNICATION

**Essential for emergency communication with outside world and household members.** Select easy-to-use system with large, clear buttons operable by children. Install at height accessible to both adults and children. Consider video display to monitor surroundings before opening door. Ensure child operability if adults incapacitated.

___________________________________________

**Panic/Safe Room**
→ Infant/Non-mobile: (Birth - 6 months)
→ Infant crawl/roll: (5 months - 1 year)
→ Toddler/Pre-school: (1 year - 4 years)
→ School-age: (5 years - 6+ years)

# Separate Air Source

**Independent sealed air source ensures clean, uncontaminated air during fires or chemical hazards.** System should filter smoke, chemicals, hazardous substances. Design to be easily activated, even by children. Display clear instructions. Include safety features preventing tampering during non-emergencies. Consider oxygen supply unit for sufficient levels, especially with infants.

---

**Panic/Safe Room**
→ Infant/Non-mobile: (Birth - 6 months)
→ Infant crawl/roll: (5 months - 1 year)
→ Toddler/Pre-school: (1 year - 4 years)
→ School-age: (5 years - 6+ years)

# Needed Supplies

**Food and water:** non-perishable variety, baby food/formula if needed, bottled water, child-friendly utensils.

**Health and hygiene:** first aid kit with child-specific medications, baby wipes, hygiene items, diapers.

**Comfort:** bedding like sleeping bags, spare clothes including warm options. Entertainment: toys, books, board games, activity kits.

**Communication:** intercom system, charging station.

**Special supplies:** separate air source, masks, air purifiers, emergency lighting, essential documents. Regular maintenance and updates crucial.

---

**Panic/Safe Room**
→ Infant/Non-mobile: (Birth - 6 months)
→ Infant crawl/roll: (5 months - 1 year)
→ Toddler/Pre-school: (1 year - 4 years)
→ School-age: (5 years - 6+ years)

# Surveillance

**Install cameras strategically mounted high with infrared capabilities.** Conceal and secure wiring. Mount monitoring screens at adult-accessible height with password protection. Use simple interface older children can navigate under supervision. Install silent alarms and panic buttons at various heights. Educate children about system importance. Use safety covers on outlets. Conduct regular emergency drills. Maintain emergency contact access.

---

**Panic/Safe Room**
Infant/Non-mobile: (Birth - 6 months)
Infant crawl/roll: (5 months - 1 year)
→ **Toddler/Pre-school: (1 year - 4 years)**
→ **School-age: (5 years - 6+ years)**

# PROPER LIGHTING

**Use soft LED lights with dimmable features.** Securely install recessed fixtures. Use diffused lighting to prevent harsh glares. Include battery-powered emergency lights and night lights. Integrate remote-controlled systems. Use childproof switches at unreachable heights with safety covers. Ensure no exposed wires. Employ heat-resistant covers on fixtures.

---

**Panic/Safe Room**
Infant/Non-mobile: (Birth - 6 months)
Infant crawl/roll: (5 months - 1 year)
→ **Toddler/Pre-school: (1 year - 4 years)**
→ **School-age: (5 years - 6+ years)**

# EDUCATE AND SUPPORT CHILDREN

**Panic Rooms:** Prepare children with age-appropriate conversations about the room's purpose. Conduct regular drills. Teach basic safety (intercom use, panic buttons, staying quiet). Let them choose comfort items. During emergencies: stay calm, offer physical comfort, engage in quiet activities, maintain open communication. After: debrief gently, seek professional support if needed.

Panic rooms can feel like cages to toddlers, triggering fear or dissociation. Young children may trip over supplies or trap fingers. Safe rooms need simple exits, soft edges, and comforting caregiver presence.

---

# PRACTICE

**Drills:** Regularly conduct drills with all family members, including children, so they know how to behave in the safe room during emergencies.

**Escape Plan:** Even in a safe room, there should be a way out in case of unforeseen circumstances. Ensure this escape route is childproofed to prevent unsupervised access but can be used with guidance during emergencies.

**By combining security measures with childproofing techniques, a panic or safe room can be both a fortress against external threats and a safe haven for the family's youngest members. Regular reviews and updates to the safety protocols are essential.**

---

🐦 Panic or safe rooms are designed to protect, but for toddlers they can feel more like cages. Enclosed spaces with reinforced doors can cause acute fear and anxiety. Sometimes triggering panic or dissociation. Young children may trip over emergency supplies, head-butt reinforced walls, or trap their fingers in door hinges. In the chaos of an actual crisis, a locked door can be terrifying if they can't quickly release it themselves. That's why safe rooms meant for families must be intentionally child-safe, equipped with simple exits, soft edges, and comforting input from caregivers.

---

**Notes:**

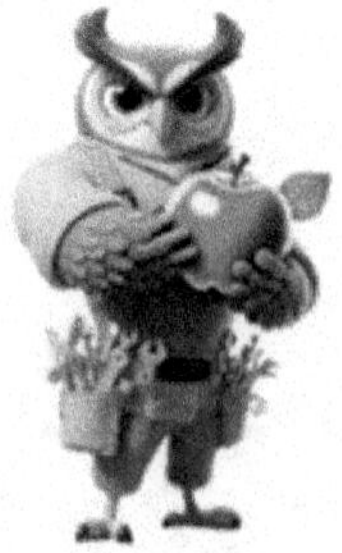

 # Prayer/Meditation Room

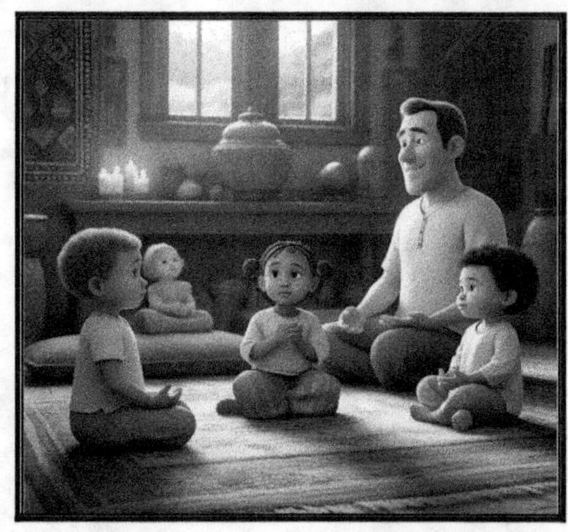

**Introduction:** In the journey of spiritual growth, a prayer and meditation room serves as a sanctuary, a place of solace and introspection. As we invite the younger members of our family into this sacred space, it becomes imperative to ensure their safety without compromising the room's spiritual essence. Childproofing such a room requires a delicate balance, ensuring that the space remains conducive to spiritual practices and safe for curious little souls.

---

**Prayer/Meditation Room**
Infant/Non-mobile: (Birth - 6 months)
Infant crawl/roll: (5 months - 1 year)
→ **Toddler/Pre-school: (1 year - 4 years)**
→ **School-age: (5 years - 6+ years)**

# YOUR SPIRITUAL HAVEN

Keep candles/incense out of reach. Use battery-operated alternatives. Use soft furnishings without sharp edges. Secure small items (beads, statues) on high shelves or locked cabinets. Non-slip flooring, secure rugs. Install window guards and gentle lighting with protective covers. Store materials safely and avoid high stacks. Educate children on the room's importance. Even peaceful spaces hide dangers. Candles, incense, beaded decor, hanging fabrics, and diffusers can cause choking, burns, or strangulation. Most home injuries happen within five minutes of unsupervised play.

---

# |Ch. 18| Game/Recreation/ Fitness Room

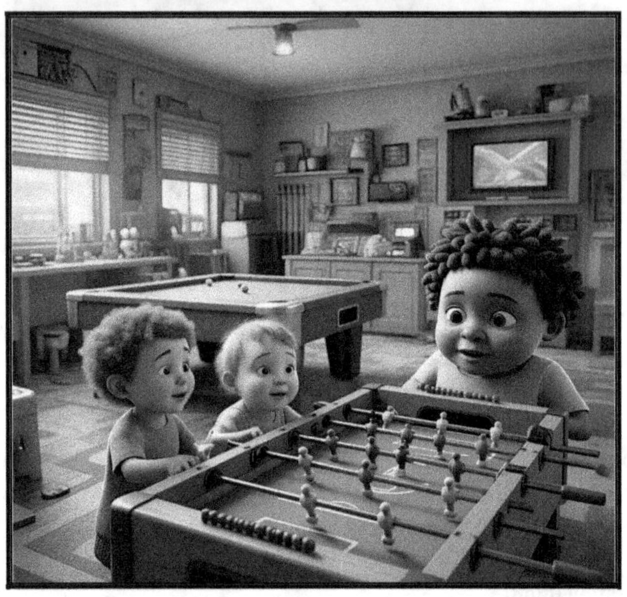

**Introduction:** In the heart of every home, the game, recreation, or fitness room pulsates with laughter, energy, and the spirit of family bonding. It's a sanctuary where fun meets fitness, children cultivate a love for physical activity, and cherished memories are created. However, amidst the joyous chaos, our guardians must weave a safety net that guards the youthful zest yet shields the tender limbs from potential hazards. This chapter is dedicated to helping you foster a space that nurtures both fun and safety in equal measure. From securing heavy equipment to creating zones that encourage safe play, we guide you in crafting a stimulating and secure environment. Let us embark on this mission to create a haven where little feet can run, little hands can explore, and little hearts can enjoy, all under the watchful eyes of safety and precaution.

# GAME CONSOLE

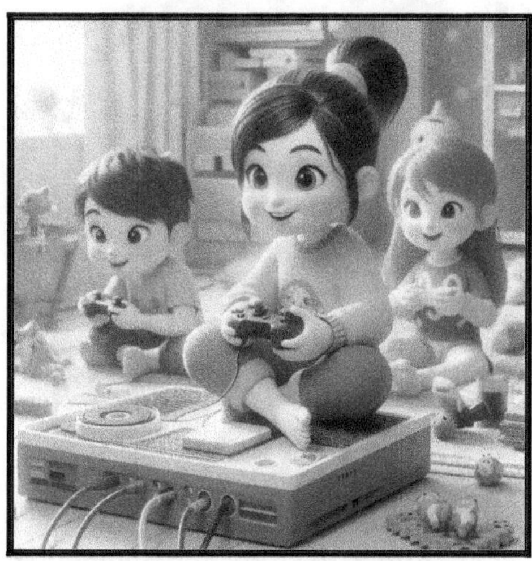

**Game Console:** Activate parental controls. Set time limits. Place in family room for monitoring. Password-protect settings. Choose age-appropriate games. Store safely. Secure wired cords. Monitor online interactions. Teach responsible gaming. Data shows roughly 6,800 gaming-related injuries yearly in kids under 10. Mostly fingers, hands, wrists from repetitive play.

---

🌱 Game consoles may seem harmless, but they can cause real injuries even in preschoolers. Anecdotal cases of 'Nintendo thumb' (tendonitis and swelling) have appeared in young children after repetitive play. *NEISS data* shows **roughly 6,800 gaming-related injuries yearly in kids under 10**. Mostly to fingers, hands, and wrists, including strains and sprains. These findings highlight the need for younger gamers to take breaks, use proper posture, and limit extended play.

---

# POOL TABLE

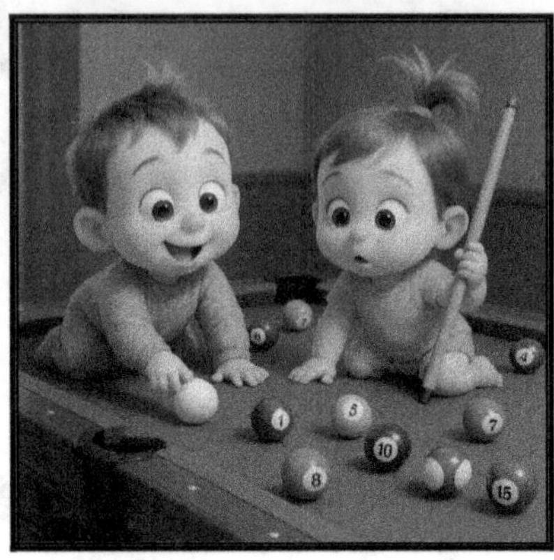

Install corner cushions and edge guards. Store balls in locked cabinet (heavy, can hurt). Lock cues away or offer foam alternatives. Create child-friendly zone nearby. According to Library of Medicine, from 2000 to 2020, U.S. emergency departments treated an **estimated 78,500 billiards-related injuries, including cuts, bruises, and strikes from pool cues.**

---

**Game/Recreation/ Fitness Room**
Infant/Non-mobile: (Birth - 6 months)
Infant crawl/roll: (5 months - 1 year)
→ **Toddler/Pre-school: (1 year - 4 years)**
→ **School-age: (5 years - 6+ years)**

# PING-PONG TABLE

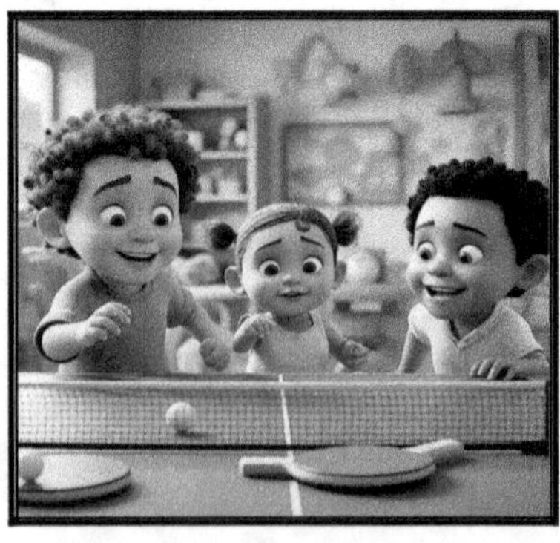

Ping-Pong: Install corner protectors, ensure stable setup. Store balls securely (choking hazard). Lock paddles; offer foam alternatives. Non-slip flooring, clear surrounding area.

**Note:** Unstable tables have collapsed causing injuries. Tiny balls are swallowing hazards (Rethink Childhood).

---

🍎 Ping-pong tables and accessories may look harmless, but they hide risks for toddlers. Even a quick game can cause repetitive strains in wrists and shoulders, while unstable folding tables have collapsed under light pressure, resulting in falls and bruises. Tiny ping-pong balls are also swallowing hazards for little ones. **In one U.S. recall, a table's sudden collapse injured four people.** That's why young children need close supervision, use age-appropriate gear, and safe, stabilized table setups, even for fun backyard rallies."

*-Rethink Childhood*

---

<u>**Game/Recreation/ Fitness Room**</u>
Infant/Non-mobile: **(Birth - 6 months)**
Infant crawl/roll: **(5 months - 1 year)**
→ **Toddler/Pre-school: (1 year - 4 years)**
→ **School-age: (5 years - 6+ years)**

# FOOSBALL SAFETY

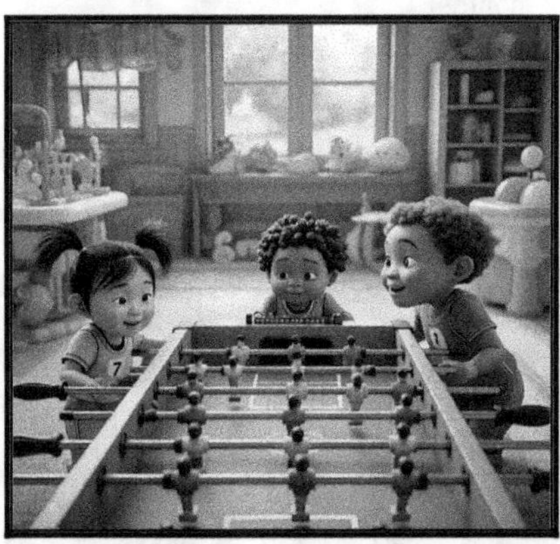

Install corner protectors, edge guards, rod bumpers, handle grips, rod locks. Store balls securely. Supervise play. Spacious area with non-slip flooring.

---

**Game/Recreation/ Fitness Room**
Infant/Non-mobile: (Birth - 6 months)
Infant crawl/roll: (5 months - 1 year)
→ **Toddler/Pre-school: (1 year - 4 years)**
→ **School-age: (5 years - 6+ years)**

# DARTBOARD SAFETY

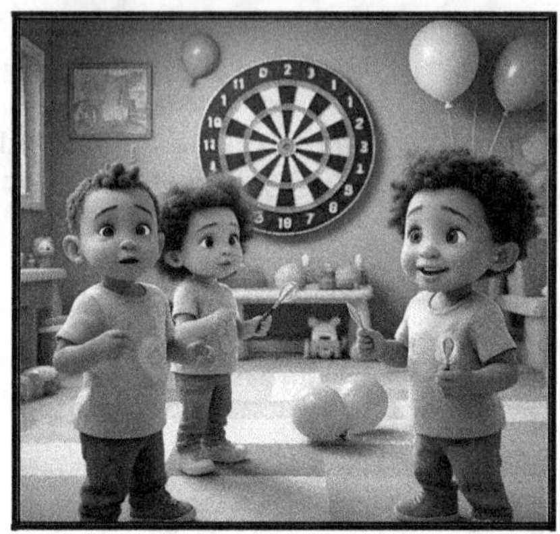

Install high, in isolated area. Use magnetic or rubber-tipped darts. Store in locked containers. Always supervise.

**Note:** UK study found 31.4% of sharp implement-related eye injuries occurred at home, often involving darts.

---

**Game/Recreation/ Fitness Room**
Infant/Non-mobile: (Birth - 6 months)
→ **Infant crawl/roll: (5 months - 1 year)**
→ **Toddler/Pre-school: (1 year - 4 years)**
→ **School-age: (5 years - 6+ years)**

# SLOT MACHINES

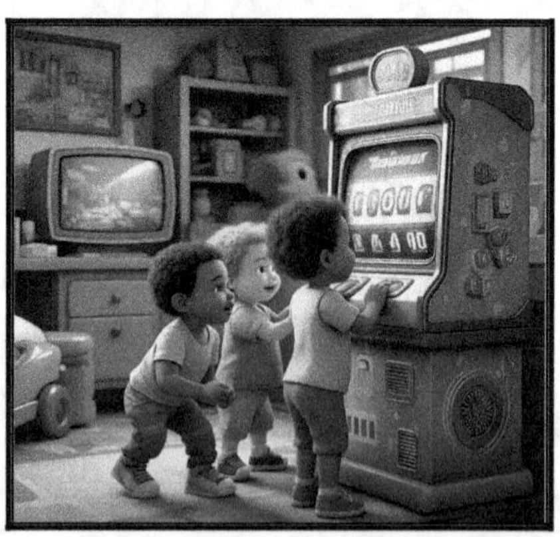

Childproofing slot machines requires meticulous attention given electronic components, movable parts, and coin or token systems.

**Physical Components:** The exterior and interior components fascinate children. Secure the machine to the wall or stable base to prevent tipping. Use corner protectors to cover sharp edges or corners.

**Coin/Token Slot:** The slot can be a curious spot for children. Block the slot with a cover to prevent children from inserting foreign objects or fingers. If possible, make the slot lockable to prevent access.

**Buttons and Levers:** Often the most attractive components for children. Disable buttons when the machine is not in use to prevent tampering. If the machine has a lever, consider installing one that can be removed when not in use.

**Electrical Safety:** Slot machines are electrical devices requiring safeguarding from hazards. Ensure cords are appropriately managed with no exposed wires that might pose electrical shock risks. Use a surge protector to prevent electrical mishaps and protect the machine.

---

**Game/Recreation/ Fitness Room**
Infant/Non-mobile: (Birth - 6 months)
Infant crawl/roll: (5 months - 1 year)
→ **Toddler/Pre-school: (1 year - 4 years)**
→ **School-age: (5 years - 6+ years)**

# BOARDGAMES

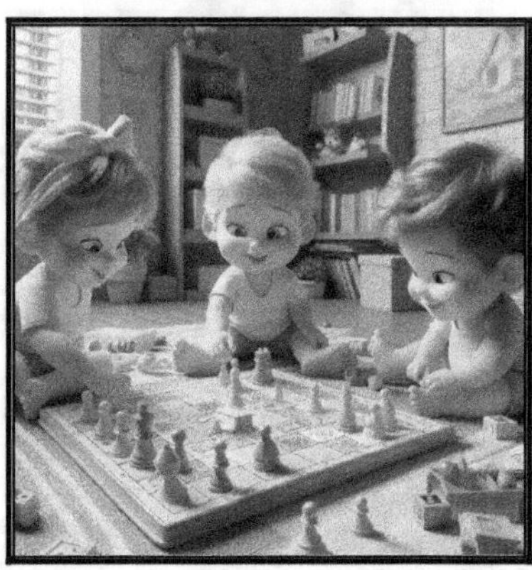

Various elements must be addressed when childproofing board games to ensure safe and enjoyable playtime for children.

**<u>Game Pieces and Accessories:</u>** Most board games contain small pieces that could pose choking hazards.

**Organized Storage:** Store small pieces in containers with secure lids, which prevents young children from accessing them unsupervised.

**Age-Appropriate Alternatives:** Consider purchasing or creating age-appropriate versions of the game with larger, non-choke hazard pieces for young children to use.

**Board and Game Surfaces** The board itself can have some areas of concern, primarily related to its corners and potential pinching points.

**Corner Cushions:** Apply corner cushions to board game corners to prevent injuries from sharp points.

**Smooth Edges:** Ensure that the board's edges are smooth and free of splinters or rough areas that could cause injuries.

**Card Safety**

**Card Protectors:** Use card protectors to prevent young children from bending, tearing, or attempting to ingest parts of the cards.

**Teaching Careful Handling:** Educate older children on carefully handling cards to prevent damage and potential hazards.

---

**Game/Recreation/ Fitness Room**
Infant/Non-mobile: (Birth - 6 months)
Infant crawl/roll: (5 months - 1 year)
→ **Toddler/Pre-school: (1 year - 4 years)**
→ **School-age: (5 years - 6+ years)**

# Popcorn Maker

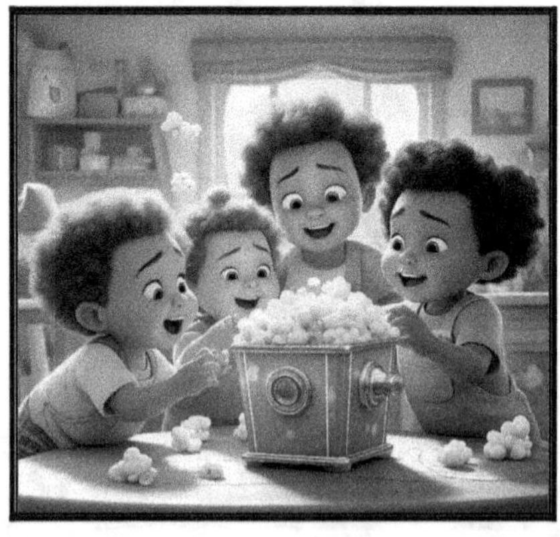

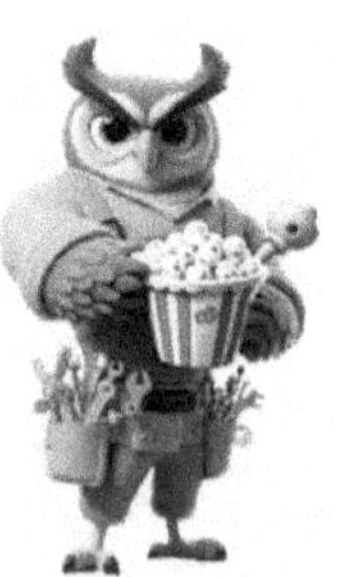

## Hot Surfaces

Large popcorn makers often have surfaces that can get quite hot. To prevent burns:

**Safety Gates:** Install safety gates to keep children at a safe distance from the popcorn maker.

**Heat-Resistant Covers:** Use heat-resistant covers on handles and other parts that may become hot to the touch.

## Electrical Concerns

Electrical components can be hazardous for children.

**Safety Plugs:** Use safety plugs to cover any unused electrical outlets on the popcorn maker.

**Cord Management:** Ensure cords are properly managed, avoiding any hanging parts that children could pull or get tangled in.

## Moving Parts

Moving parts in a popcorn maker can pose a risk of injury.

**Guard Rails:** Install guard rails or screens around the moving parts to prevent children from sticking their hands or fingers in them.

**Locking Mechanisms:** Use locking mechanisms to prevent children from being able to open doors or lids where there are moving parts.

**Cleaning Agents** used to clean popcorn makers can be toxic.

**Non-Toxic Cleaners:** Use only non-toxic cleaners to clean the popcorn maker, avoiding any potential poisoning hazards.

**Secure Storage:** Ensure cleaning agents are stored in a secure location that is out of reach of children.

---

**Game/Recreation/ Fitness Room**
Infant/Non-mobile: (Birth - 6 months)
Infant crawl/roll: (5 months - 1 year)
→ **Toddler/Pre-school: (1 year - 4 years)**
→ **School-age: (5 years - 6+ years)**

# BAR OR WET BAR

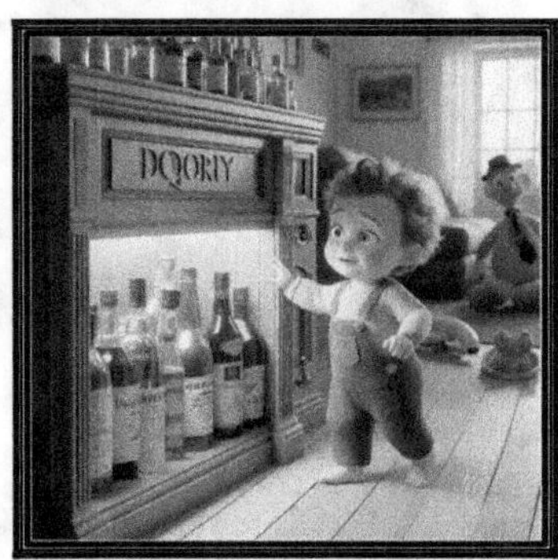

Lock alcoholic beverages. Use plastic alternatives to glassware. Non-slip mats, prompt cleanup. Safety covers on outlets, appliance locks.

---

**Game/Recreation/ Fitness Room**
Infant/Non-mobile: (Birth - 6 months)
Infant crawl/roll: (5 months - 1 year)
→ **Toddler/Pre-school: (1 year - 4 years)**
→ **School-age: (5 years - 6+ years)**

# Fitness Room Safety

**Install safety locks on machines.** Position equipment against walls. Store accessories (dumbbells, bands, balls) in locked cabinets or high locations. Soft flooring. Safety outlet covers.

**Average 12,714** annual injuries to children involving exercise equipment. 71% in kids under 10 (NEISS 1990–2008). CPSC reports 8,700 children under 5 and 16,500 aged 5–14 treated yearly.

---

**Game/Recreation/ Fitness Room**
Infant/Non-mobile: (Birth - 6 months)
Infant crawl/roll: (5 months - 1 year)
→ **Toddler/Pre-school: (1 year - 4 years)**
→ **School-age: (5 years - 6+ years)**

# Fitness Room Flooring and Electrical

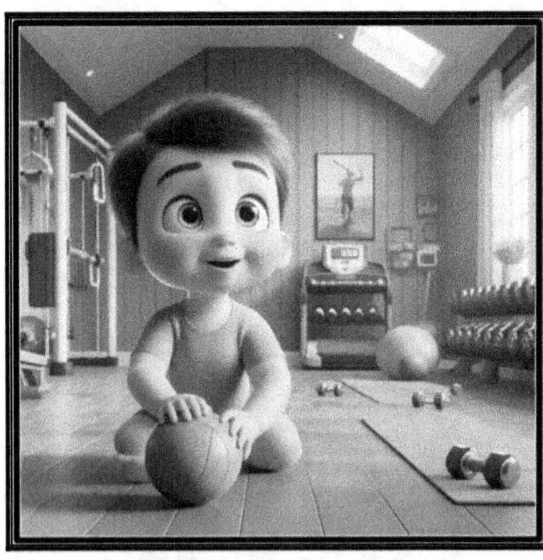

The flooring and electrical components in a fitness room must also be secured.

**Soft Flooring:** Install soft flooring such as foam mats to prevent injuries from falls.

**Outlet Covers:** Use safety outlet covers to prevent children from inserting objects or fingers    into electrical outlets.

Childproofing a home fitness room involves a detailed strategy that encompasses various aspects. One critical area to address is the presence of heavy equipment, such as treadmills and weight machines, which could pose a significant danger to children.

**Installing safety locks on these machines will prevent children from being able to operate them,** thus averting potential accidents. Moreover, positioning such heavy equipment against the wall will deter children from going behind them, minimizing the risk of injury.

Furthermore, loose accessories common in fitness rooms, like dumbbells and resistance bands, can be hazardous to children. Establishing secure storage systems for these accessories is essential.

**Cabinets equipped with childproof locks** can effectively prevent children from accessing these potentially dangerous items. Additionally, maintaining a high degree of organization by storing smaller accessories in bins or baskets, preferably out of children's reach, can be another safety layer.

The safety of flooring and electrical components within the fitness room is also a pivotal concern. **Installing soft flooring options such as foam mats** can be instrumental in preventing injuries resulting from falls. Also, the use of safety outlet covers can prevent curious children from inserting objects or their fingers into electrical outlets, thus averting potential electrocution hazards.

Implementing these detail-oriented strategies can transform your home fitness room into a space that is safe for children and conducive for adults to focus on their fitness goals, fostering a safe and healthy environment for the entire family.

---

# |Ch. 19| Theater/ Entertainment Room

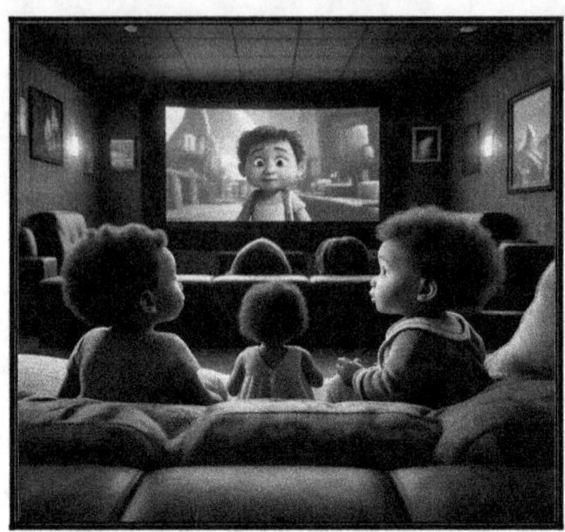

**Introduction:** Childproofing a home theater or entertainment room is essential to keep little ones safe while allowing the family to enjoy movies, music, and other entertainment without worry. From securing heavy furniture and electronics to managing cords and small components, here's a detail-oriented plan to make your entertainment room child-friendly.

---

**Theater/Entertainment Room**
Infant/Non-mobile: (Birth - 6 months)
Infant crawl/roll: (5 months - 1 year)
→ **Toddler/Pre-school: (1 year - 4 years)**
→ **School-age: (5 years - 6+ years)**

## GENERAL SAFETY

**Use furniture anchor**s. Secure TVs with anti-tip straps. Install corner protectors. Cord management systems. Safety outlet covers. Hide power strips. Store remotes and media in closed cabinets. For **projectors:** mount high, secure cables, protect lenses.

> **Note:** 11,500 ER visits yearly for furniture/TV tip-overs—70% kids under 6. Child treated every 46 minutes. One child dies every 2–3 weeks from TV tip-over (Consumer Report, ABC News).

---

 # Hobby/Scrapbooking/Sewing Room

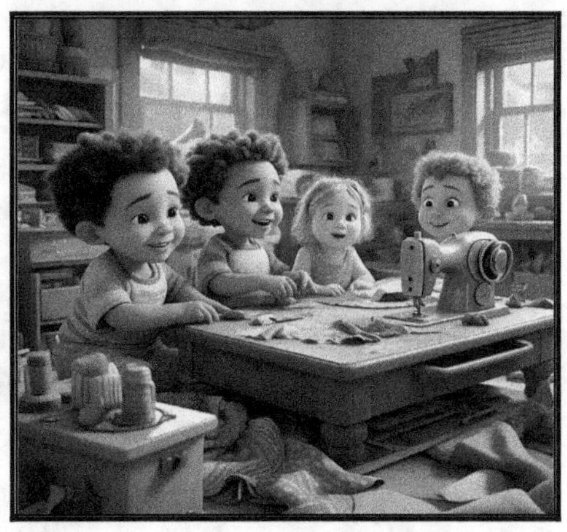

**Introduction:** In the vibrant world of hobby rooms, where creativity knows no bounds, and every corner is a treasure trove of artistic potential, safeguarding our little artists becomes paramount. This chapter is dedicated to transforming your hobby, scrap booking, or sewing room into a haven where creativity and safety coexist harmoniously. From organizing an enticing yet secure space for children to explore their artistic inclinations to selecting child-friendly tools and materials, we will guide you through comprehensive strategies to foster their creativity while keeping those precious fingers and curious minds safe. Dive into this chapter to craft a nurturing environment where your child's imagination can soar, free from the worries of potential mishaps, allowing the seeds of creativity to blossom safely and splendidly.

---

**Hobby/Scrap booking/Sewing Room**
Infant/Non-mobile: (Birth - 6 months)
Infant crawl/roll: (5 months - 1 year)
→ **Toddler/Pre-school: (1 year - 4 years)**
→ **School-age: (5 years - 6+ years)**

# GENERAL SAFETY

Store sharp tools (scissors, needles, cutters) in locked drawers. Use safety caps. Corner protectors on tables. Store small items (beads, buttons, pins) in secure containers on high shelves. Proper ventilation. Lock harmful chemicals. Soft flooring. **Over 50,000 children treated yearly for arts/crafts injuries** (NEISS-CDC).

---

 # Unfinished Basement Furnace/Water Heater

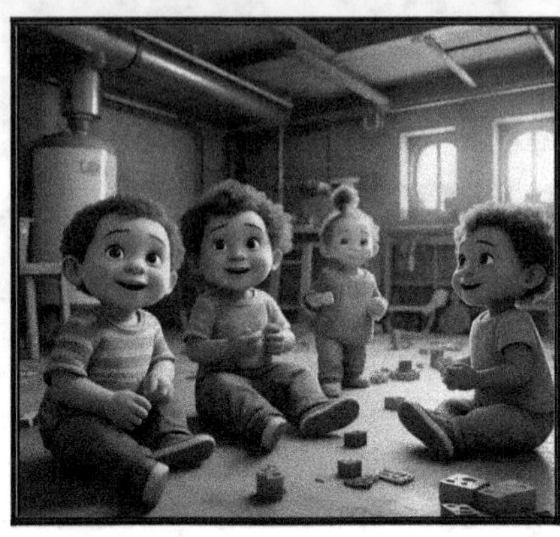

**Introduction**: In the hidden corners of our homes, where the furnace hums and the water heater stands sentinel, lies an area often overlooked in the childproofing process, the unfinished basement. This chapter is your guiding light in transforming this space, often brimming with potential hazards, into a secure zone that keeps the little adventurers at bay. From securing heavy appliances and shielding hot surfaces to creating barriers around potentially dangerous zones, we will walk you through meticulous steps to ensure safety without compromising the functionality of these vital home systems. As you turn the pages, you'll find insightful tips and innovative solutions that will help you foster a home where curiosity can flourish without fear and where every nook and cranny echoes with the laughter of safe and happy children.

---

**Unfinished Basement/Furnace/Water Heater**
Infant/Non-mobile: (Birth - 6 months)
Infant crawl/roll: (5 months - 1 year)
Toddler/Pre-school: (1 year - 4 years)
→ **School-age: (5 years - 6+ years)**

# WINDOW FIRE ESCAPES

**Install window guards (quick-release for adults).** Child-safe locks. Window alarms. Educate children. Regular drills. Store escape ladder nearby. Emergency toolkit.

---

# Uncovered Doors and Vents

Keeping the doors and vents in an unfinished basement uncovered can indeed have some benefits, especially when considering ventilation, moisture control, and easy access to various utilities.

## Ventilation and Air Circulation

**Improved Airflow:** Leaving vents uncovered can facilitate better airflow, which can help reduce the buildup of stale or moist air, which is often a problem in basements.

**Preventing Mold:** Increased airflow can also help prevent mold and mildew growth, which thrive in damp, stagnant environments.

## Easy Access to Utilities

**Quick Access:** Not having door covers allows for fast and easy access to utilities and storage areas, which is often necessary in a basement where many home utilities are located.

**Safety:** In case of emergencies, such as gas or water leaks, having uncovered doors can facilitate a quicker response time as you can easily spot and address the issue.

## Cost Effectiveness

**Saving Money:** Leaving the basement unfinished, including not adding door or vent covers, can save a considerable amount of money, which might be preferable if the basement is primarily used for storage or utilities.

**Flexibility:** Without permanent fixtures, you retain the flexibility to make changes or upgrades to the basement layout without the additional cost of removing and replacing doors and vents.

---

🍎 Unfinished basements with exposed furnaces and water heaters can hide serious burn hazards. In the U.S. alone, **nearly 3,800 scald injuries from hot water are treated annually.** Often near water heater systems, with **over 30 deaths**. Altogether, **about 435 children per day end up in emergency rooms** due to burns from hot equipment, making supervision and protective barriers around utility zones essential. *(The American Burn Association (ameriburn.org) and the CDC)*

---

<u>**Unfinished Basement/Furnace/Water Heater**</u>
Infant/Non-mobile: (Birth - 6 months)
Infant crawl/roll: (5 months - 1 year)
→ **Toddler/Pre-school: (1 year - 4 years)**
→ **School-age: (5 years - 6+ years)**

# Water Heater Area

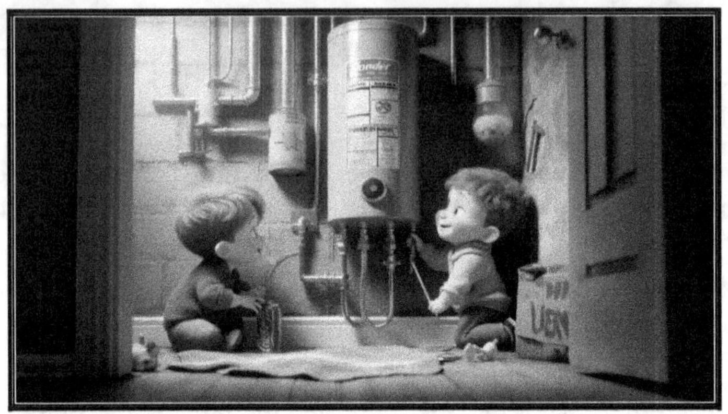

Each year, 1,000+ children injured by hot water heaters (CPSC). Install safety gates. Lower temperature below 120°F. Thermal insulation. Anchor to wall. Cover pipes. Secure gas lines. Install smoke/CO detectors. First-aid kit nearby.

**Nearly 3,800 scald injuries from hot water treated annually, 30+ deaths. About 435 children daily in ERs for burns from hot equipment** (American Burn Association, CDC).

---

<u>**Unfinished Basement/Furnace/ Water Heater**</u>
→ **Infant/Non-mobile: (Birth - 6 months)**
→ **Infant crawl/roll: (5 months - 1 year)**
→ **Toddler/Pre-school: (1 year - 4 years)**
→ **School-age: (5 years - 6+ years)**

# Furnace Concerns

**Sturdy gates around furnace.** Locked doors or plexiglass barriers. Heat-resistant guards on hot surfaces. Insulate pipes. Keep flammables away. Regular maintenance. Secure gas lines. Bundle cords. CO detectors. Proper ventilation. Educate children.

---

# PROVIDE GOOD VENTILATION

Childproofing an unfinished basement while ensuring good ventilation is a meticulous process that aims to create a safe and healthy environment for children.

## Install Quality Ventilation Systems

**Air Purifiers:** Set up air purifiers to remove impurities and allergens.

**Dehumidifiers:** Utilize dehumidifiers to control humidity levels and prevent mold growth.

**Exhaust Fans:** Install exhaust fans to eliminate stale air and bring in fresh air.

---

## Open Windows

**Window Guards:** Install window guards to prevent children from falling or climbing out.

**Window Screens:** Incorporate window screens to keep insects and debris out.

## Natural Ventilation

**Vented Doors:** Use vented doors to facilitate air circulation.

**Ventilation Grills:** Install ventilation grills at strategic points to enhance airflow.

## Chemical and Fume Control

**Chemical Storage:** Store any chemicals, paints, or solvents in a secured cabinet, inaccessible to children.

**Safety Latches:** Install safety latches on storage cabinets to prevent children from accessing potentially harmful substances.

## Heating and Cooling Systems

**HVAC Maintenance:** Regular maintenance of heating and cooling systems to ensure they function properly and do not emit harmful substances.

**Carbon Monoxide Detectors:** Install carbon monoxide detectors to alert in case of gas leaks or harmful emissions.

---

 # Rooftop Terrace

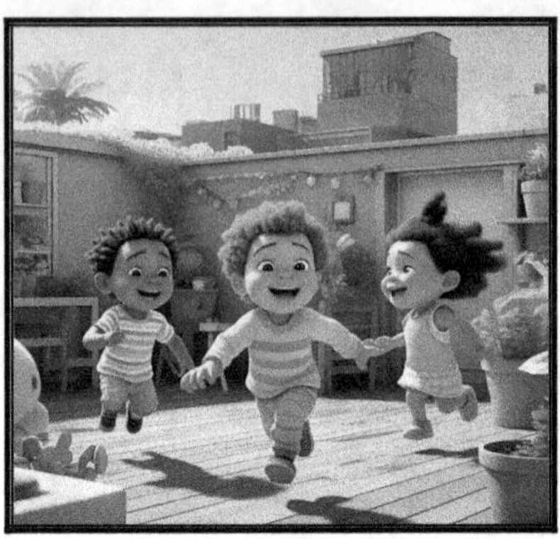

**Introduction:** In the bustling embrace of urban living, a rooftop terrace stands as a serene oasis, offering a breath of fresh air and a slice of the sky amidst concrete jungles. Yet, as parents, we must remember that this elevated paradise comes with its own set of challenges when it comes to ensuring the safety of our little explorers. This chapter delves deep into the nuances of childproofing your rooftop terrace, transforming it into a haven where your children can play and explore without any looming dangers. From securing the railings to creating a safe play zone, we guide you in crafting a space that combines safety with the joyous freedom a rooftop terrace can provide. Let's embark on this journey of creating a secure yet enchanting kingdom in the sky for our little ones, where adventures await at every corner, sans the perils

---

**Rooftop Terrace**
Infant/Non-mobile: (Birth - 6 months)
Infant crawl/roll: (5 months - 1 year)
→ **Toddler/Pre-school: (1 year - 4 years)**
→ **School-age: (5 years - 6+ years)**

# RAILING CONCERNS

**Railings at least 4 feet high, spaces less than 4 inches.** Reinforced materials. Smooth vertical railings. No footholds. Position furniture away from edges. Non-slip flooring. Cushioned areas. Remove splinters/nails.

---

<u>**Rooftop Terrace**</u>
Infant/Non-mobile: (Birth - 6 months)
Infant crawl/roll: (5 months - 1 year)
→ **Toddler/Pre-school: (1 year - 4 years)**
→ **School-age: (5 years - 6+ years)**

# Anti-Climbing

**Smooth Railings:** Railings should be vertical and smooth, with no horizontal bars or decorative elements that can act as footholds.

**Furniture Positioning:** Place furniture, especially the climbable types, centrally and away from the edges. This reduces the temptation for children to climb and reach the railings.

---

<u>**Rooftop Terrace**</u>
Infant/Non-mobile: (Birth - 6 months)
Infant crawl/roll: (5 months - 1 year)
→ **Toddler/Pre-school: (1 year - 4 years)**
→ **School-age: (5 years - 6+ years**

# Floor Concerns

**Non-slip Surface:** Choose tiles with a rough texture or specifically designed outdoor non-slip tiles. Wet conditions can make surfaces slippery, increasing the risk of falls.

**Cushioned Areas:** Consider areas with outdoor play mats or cushioned tiles, especially if children play there frequently.

**Splinters and Nails:** Sand down those splinters and remove those nails that can be reached.

---

<u>**Rooftop Terrace**</u>
Infant/Non-mobile: (Birth - 6 months)
Infant crawl/roll: (5 months - 1 year)
→ **Toddler/Pre-school: (1 year - 4 years)**
→ **School-age: (5 years - 6+ years)**

# Limit Roof Access

**High Locks:** Install locks or latches high up on the access doors, out of children's reach.

**Alarm Systems:** Consider installing alarms that notify you when the door to the terrace is opened.

# Sturdy and Stable Furniture

**Heavy-Duty Furniture:** Choose heavy furniture to prevent tipping over but not too hard or rigid, which could cause injury.

**Low-Centered Gravity:** Furniture with a low center of gravity will be less likely to tip over if a child attempts to climb on it.

**Non-Tipping Chairs:** Choose chairs that have a broad base to prevent tipping, avoiding high stools or chairs that can easily tip over.

**Safety Features:** Furniture with rounded edges and non-toxic finishes are preferable. Avoid glass tables or fragile items.

---



# Plant Safety

**Safe Plants:** Research plants to ensure they aren't toxic. Common plants like oleander can be poisonous if ingested.

**Stable Planters:** Heavy or anchored planters prevent children from tipping them over.

---



# Terrace Electricity Concerns

**Elevated Outlets:** Have outlets installed at a higher level that is out of the reach of children.

**Childproof Covers:** Use safety covers on all outlets to prevent curious fingers from poking inside.

---

# STANDING WATER CONCERNS

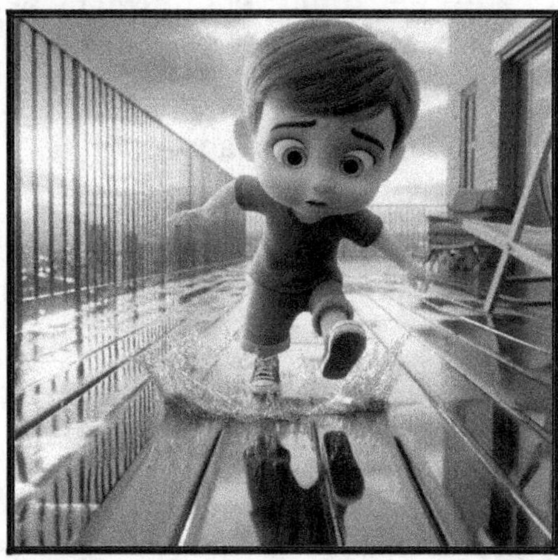

Childproofing a rooftop terrace to address water concerns is a comprehensive process that necessitates close attention to numerous details to prevent accidents and maintain a safe environment.

**Non-Slip Flooring:** Install non-slip flooring to prevent accidents from slips and falls, especially in wet conditions. This could be tiled with a rough texture or wooden decking with adequate grip.

**Drainage Systems:** Ensure that a proper drainage system is in place to prevent water accumulation and puddle formation, which could lead to slips and falls.

**Water-Alert Sensors:** Consider installing water-alert sensors that notify you if there's water accumulation in certain areas, allowing for timely intervention.

**Routine Inspections:** Carry out regular inspections, especially during the rainy season, to check for water stagnation and clear it promptly to prevent accidents.

**Water Features and Pools:** Drowning Remains a Silent Threat. Drowning is the leading cause of injury-related death for children aged 1 to 4 years, with over 3,500 fatalities worldwide each year. (Source: World Health Organization (WHO) – Drowning)

**Fenced Water Features:** If the terrace has water features or a small pool, make sure it is fenced off properly to prevent unsupervised access by children.

**Anti-Slip Mats:** Place anti-slip mats near water features or pools to provide additional traction and prevent slips.

**Covered Water Features:** To prevent drowning hazards, ensure that water features can be covered securely when not in use.

**Safety Equipment:** Keep life-saving equipment like life rings or ropes near water features, even if they are shallow.

## Rainwater Harvesting and Plants

**Secure Rain Barrels:** If rainwater is harvested on the terrace, ensure that the collection barrels are securely covered to prevent children from falling in.

**Safe Plant Watering Systems:** Set up safe plant watering systems that do not create puddles or slippery areas. Consider drip irrigation systems for water efficiency and safety.

**Education and Supervision:** Educate children on the dangers of water bodies and ensure constant supervision when they are near water features or pools.

---

**Rooftop Terrace**
Infant/Non-mobile: (Birth - 6 months)
Infant crawl/roll: (5 months - 1 year)
→ **Toddler/Pre-school: (1 year - 4 years)**
→ **School-age: (5 years - 6+ years)**

# Storage Concerns

**Locked Containers:** All gardening tools, fertilizers, or chemicals should be stored in locked containers or cabinets.

**Organized Play Area:** Designate specific areas for toys and play items. This not only keeps the area tidy but reduces tripping hazards.

---

<u>**Rooftop Terrace**</u>
→ **Infant/Non-mobile: (Birth - 6 months)**
→ **Infant crawl/roll: (5 months - 1 year)**
→ **Toddler/Pre-school: (1 year - 4 years)**
→ **School-age: (5 years - 6+ years)**

# ENVIRONMENTAL CONCERNS

**UV-Protected Areas:** Use UV-protected umbrellas or shades to protect children from harmful sun rays.

**Wind Safety:** Anchor items that might blow away in strong winds, such as lightweight chairs or toys.

<u>**Rooftop Terrace**</u>
→ **Infant/Non-mobile: (Birth - 6 months)**
→ **Infant crawl/roll: (5 months - 1 year)**
→ **Toddler/Pre-school: (1 year - 4 years)**
→ **School-age: (5 years - 6+ years)**

# INSPECT FREQUENTLY

**Monthly Checks:** Dedicate time each month to inspect the entire terrace. Check for loose screws, wobbly railings, or other potential hazards.

**Immediate Repairs:** Address any wear and tear immediately. A small issue can quickly become a significant hazard if left unattended.

<u>**Rooftop Terrace**</u>
Infant/Non-mobile: (Birth - 6 months)
Infant crawl/roll: (5 months - 1 year)
→ **Toddler/Pre-school: (1 year - 4 years)**
→ **School-age: (5 years - 6+ years)**

# EDUCATE AND SUPERVISE

**Safety Rules:** Establish and consistently enforce rules, such as no running on the terrace or no climbing on furniture.

**Constant Supervision:** Even with all safety measures, always supervise children. It's the best way to ensure their safety.

# |Ch. 23| Garage

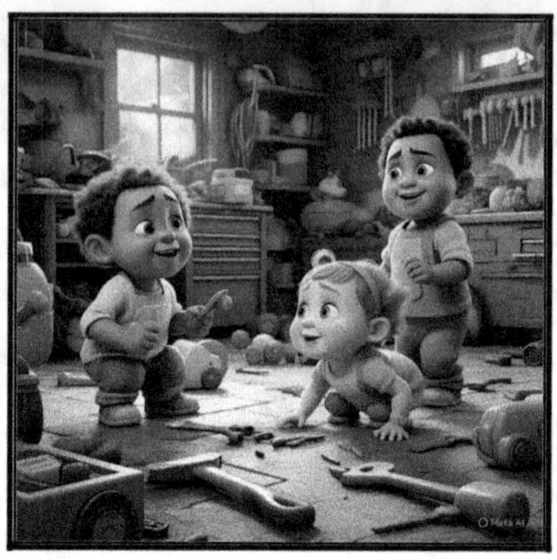

**Introduction:** In the journey of making every nook and cranny of your home a safe haven for your little ones, the garage should not be overlooked. Often considered a storage spot for tools, automobiles, and miscellaneous items, a garage harbors potential dangers that are sometimes underestimated. As we venture into this chapter, we will guide you through the essential steps of childproofing your garage, a place where safety measures are as crucial as in any other part of your home. From securing hazardous materials to ensuring the safe storage of tools and machinery, we aim to help you create a space that is not only functional but also child friendly. Let's embark on this vital aspect of home safety together, fostering a secure environment where your children can grow and explore without bounds.

---

**<u>Garage</u>**
Infant/Non-mobile: (Birth – 6 months)
Infant crawl/roll: (5 months – 1 year)
→ **Toddler/Pre-school: (1 year – 4 years)**
→ **School-age: (5 years – 6+ years)**

# GARAGE TOOL STORAGE

10,000+ children injured yearly by improperly stored tools (CPSC). Lockable cabinets. Store tools properly, sharp edges covered. Keys out of reach. Elevated placement. Organize/label. Teach safe handling. Keep garage locked. Regular inspections.

---

# Booster Seat

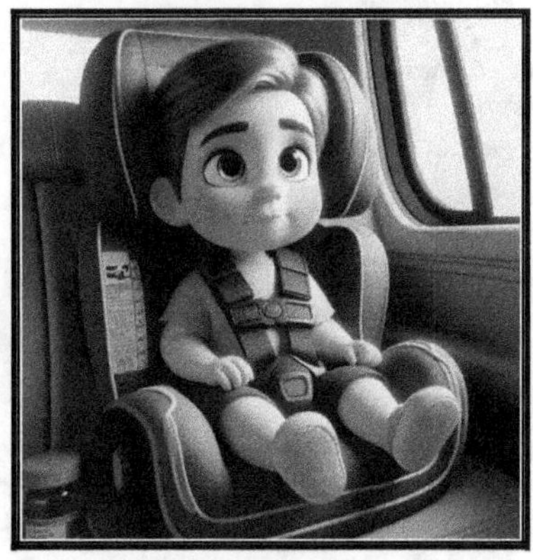

Child safety is of the utmost importance when it comes to booster seats, and choosing and using them correctly is crucial.

**Check for expiration dates:** Like car seats, booster seats have expiration dates. Be sure to check the manufacturer's label or manual for the expiration date and replace the booster seat if it has passed. Expired seats may not provide the necessary protection in case of an accident.

**Proper positioning of the seatbelt:** Ensure that the seat belt fits your child correctly when using a booster seat. The shoulder belt should lie across the chest and shoulder, not the neck or arm, and the lap belt should fit low and snug across the hips, not the stomach.

**Backless vs. High-back Boosters:** There are two main types of booster seats backless boosters and high-back boosters. Backless boosters are suitable for vehicles with headrests and provide a lift to ensure proper seat belt positioning. High-back boosters offer additional head and neck support and are ideal for vehicles without headrests or for children who need extra support.

**Use in the Rear Seat:** Booster seats should always be used in the vehicle's back seat. The rear seat is the safest place for children to ride, and using a booster seat in the front seat may expose them to unnecessary risks from airbags.

---

**Garage**

Infant/Non-mobile: (Birth - 6 months)
Infant crawl/roll: (5 months - 1 year)
→ **Toddler/Pre-school: (1 year - 4 years)**
→ **School-age: (5 years - 6+ years)**

# TOOLBOX

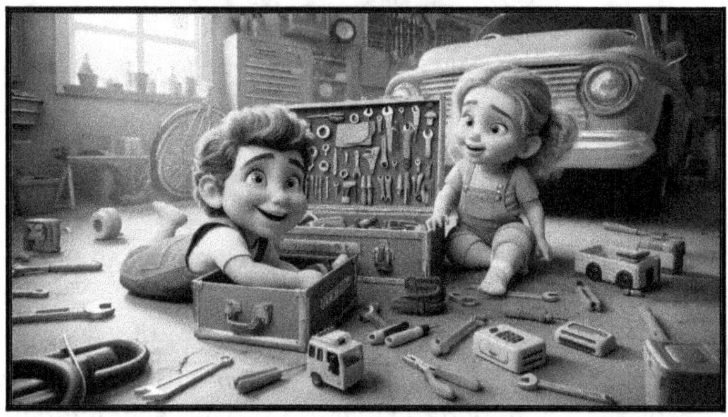

**Lock It Down:** Get a sturdy, lockable toolbox. If it can't be locked, you might as well leave the garage door open, allowing all the tools to come to life like a toy story gone wrong.

**Keep it Out of Reach:** Keep it on a high shelf or locked in a cabinet. Unless your child is Spider-Man, they're unlikely to climb that high.

**Tool Covers:** Sharp tools? Put covers on anything pointy, stabby, or capable of unscrewing your sanity.

**Magnetic Tool Holders:** Tools that stick to the wall with magnets are fantastic for adults but might look like magic to kids. Ensure they are high up or inside a closed area.

**No Power-Play:** If there are power tools, unplug them! Even better, store them in a separate, locked cabinet. A kid with a drill is a disaster movie waiting to happen.

---

# Kid-Free Zone

To create a childproof area in the garage that a child can't access, follow these steps:

**Install Safety Gates:** Place sturdy safety gates or barriers at the entrance of the designated area to prevent children from entering.

**Elevated Shelving:** Utilize high and secure shelving to store items that could be hazardous or easily reached by children.

**Lockable Cabinets:** Store tools, chemicals, or any potentially dangerous items out of children's reach in lockable cabinets or drawers.

**Childproof Latches:** Install childproof latches on any cabinets, drawers, or storage containers within the area.

**Secure Doors and Windows:** Ensure that any doors or windows leading to the childproof area have secure locks to prevent unauthorized access.

**Store Ladders Safely:** If ladders are in the garage, store them vertically or hang them on wall hooks high above children's reach.

**Organize Cords and Wires:** Tuck away and secure any cords or wires, especially those connected to power tools or equipment, to avoid tripping hazards and potential accidents.

**Hazardous Materials:** Store dangerous materials, such as chemicals or flammable substances, in a locked cabinet or a separate area inaccessible to children.

**Label Danger Zones:** Use clear signage or labels to indicate areas that are off-limits to children.

**Keep Floor Clean and Tidy:** Remove any small objects or debris from the floor that children could potentially pick up and put in their mouths.

**Properly Store Garden Tools:** securely Store Garden tools such as rakes, shovels, and shears in designated racks or wall hangers.

**Provide Safe Play Areas:** Create a separate play area for children in the garage with age-appropriate toys and activities away from potential hazards.

---



# Garage Freezer Concerns

Childproofing the freezer in the garage is essential to prevent accidents and ensure the safety of children.

**Lock or Secure the Freezer:** Secure the freezer door with a childproof lock or latch to prevent young children from opening it without adult supervision.

**Elevate the Freezer:** If possible, elevate the freezer to a height that is out of reach of young children. This can be achieved by placing it on a sturdy stand or platform.

**Store Hazardous Items Safely:** If the freezer contains items that could be hazardous to children, such as alcoholic beverages or medications, store them in a separate locked compartment or higher shelf within the freezer.

**Organize Contents:** Keep the freezer organized and tidy so children are less likely to be tempted to explore its contents.

**Teach Safe Habits:** Educate older children about the potential dangers of the freezer and the importance of not playing with the appliance.

**Store Cleaning Products Separately:** If you store cleaning products or chemicals in the garage, ensure they are kept in a locked cabinet or a high shelf away from the freezer.

**Supervise Children:** Always supervise children when they are in the garage or near the freezer to prevent accidents.

**Use Warning Signs:** Consider placing a warning sign on the freezer to remind children that it is off-limits without adult permission.

**Secure Power Cord:** Ensure that the freezer's power cord is securely tucked away and not dangling where children can reach it.

**Regular Maintenance:** Regularly inspect the freezer for any signs of wear or damage and address them promptly.

**Proper Disposal:** If you decide to replace the freezer, dispose of the old one properly, making sure it is inaccessible to children.

---

<u>**Garage**</u>
Infant/Non-mobile: (Birth - 6 months)
Infant crawl/roll: (5 months - 1 year)
→ **Toddler/Pre-school: (1 year - 4 years)**
→ **School-age: (5 years - 6+ years)**

# INSTALL AUTOMATICALLY REVERSING GARAGE DOOR

## (Or make sure yours comes with one)

**Install sensors no higher than 6 inches.** Test frequently. Professional annual inspections. Supervise children. Keep remotes out of reach. Never tie anything to emergency release rope or door handle. 2018–2022: 10.4% of garage door injuries in children 10 and under (Consumer Affairs).

---

<u>**Garage**</u>
Infant/Non-mobile: (Birth - 6 months)
Infant crawl/roll: (5 months - 1 year)
→ **Toddler/Pre-school: (1 year - 4 years)**
→ **School-age: (5 years - 6+ years)**

# NEVER TIE ANYTHING TO THE GARAGE DOOR HANDLE

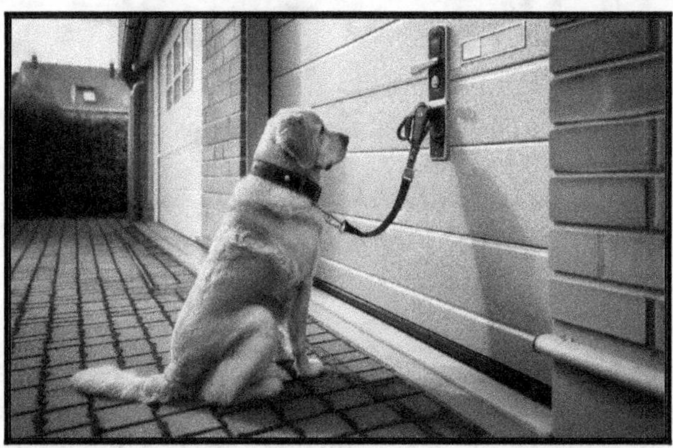

Tying anything to the garage doorknob or handle on the outside of the door is not recommended and can lead to safety hazards and damage to the door. Tying objects on the garage doorknob can **interfere with the door's proper operation** and may prevent it from closing or opening correctly. It can also unnecessarily stress the door mechanism and hardware, leading to potential malfunctions or damage.

Furthermore, tying anything to the garage door from the outside can be seen as an **invitation to potential intruders,** as it may indicate that the garage is not secured correctly.

To ensure the safety and security of your garage and belongings, avoid tying anything to the garage doorknob or handle on the outside. Instead, use appropriate locks and security measures to protect your garage and its contents. If you have specific needs or concerns regarding your garage security, consider consulting a professional locksmith or garage door technician who can provide expert advice, and solutions tailored to your situation.

---

**<u>Garage</u>**
Infant/Non-mobile: (Birth - 6 months)
Infant crawl/roll: (5 months - 1 year)
→ **Toddler/Pre-school: (1 year - 4 years)**
→ **School-age: (5 years - 6+ years)**

# WATER BUCKET CONCERNS

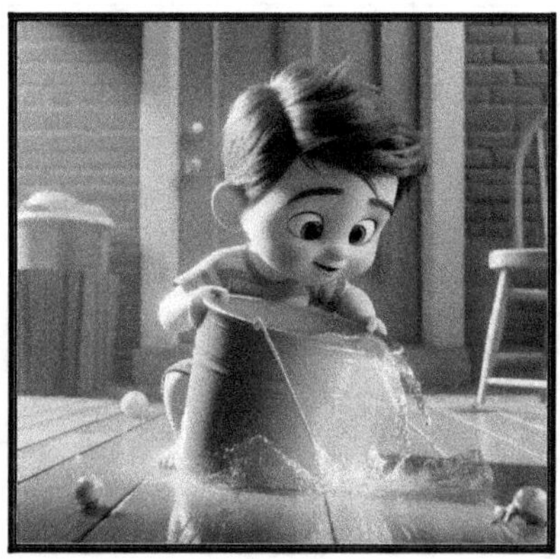

Keeping buckets out of reach of young children is an important safety measure. Buckets can pose various risks to children, especially if they contain liquid or other materials.

> **Drowning Hazard:** Buckets filled with water, cleaning solutions, or any other liquid can be a drowning hazard for young children. Even a tiny amount of water in a bucket can be dangerous if a child accidentally falls into it headfirst.

> **Suffocation Risk:** An empty bucket can become a suffocation risk if a child places it over their head and gets stuck inside. This is especially true for small children who may not have the strength to remove the bucket themselves.

**Ingestion of Harmful Substances:** If a bucket contains chemicals, paints, or any toxic substances, a child may accidentally ingest them if they get access to the bucket.

**Store Buckets Upside Down:** Store buckets upside down to prevent them from collecting water or other liquids, reducing the risk of drowning.

**Keep Buckets in Locked Cabinets:** Store buckets in locked cabinets or on high shelves where young children cannot reach them.

**Empty Buckets Promptly:** Empty any buckets used for cleaning or other purposes immediately after use and store them out of reach.

**Toppling Over:** Children may use buckets as stepping stools or try to climb on them, which can cause the bucket to tip over and cause injuries.

**Supervise Children:** Always supervise young children and keep them away from areas where they store buckets or potentially hazardous items.

**Educate Older Children:** If you have older children, educate them about the potential risks of buckets and the importance of keeping them out of reach of younger siblings.

---

<u>**Garage**</u>
Infant/Non-mobile: (Birth - 6 months)
Infant crawl/roll: (5 months - 1 year)
→ **Toddler/Pre-school: (1 year - 4 years)**
→ **School-age: (5 years - 6+ years)**

# DESIGNATED TOY AREA

Having a designated box in the garage or a shed for children's toys is a fantastic idea to keep the play area organized and create a safe and easily accessible space for children to enjoy their toys.

**Choose the Right Location:** Select a suitable garage or yard location for the toy box or shed. Ensure it is easily accessible to children but also protected from the elements, especially if it's an outdoor shed.

**Toy Box or Shed:** Decide whether a designated toy box or a dedicated shed is more appropriate depending on the number of toys and available space. Both options work well, but a shed provides additional protection from the weather and more storage capacity.

**Child-Friendly Design:** Whether it's a toy box or a shed, make sure the design is child-friendly and safe. Avoid sharp edges, choose childproof locks if needed, and ensure proper ventilation in the shed.

**Organize and Label:** Organize toys in the box or shed by categories or age-appropriateness. Use labels or pictures to help children identify where each type of toy belongs.

**Involve Children:** Involve your children in the setup process. Let them choose the organization and decorations for their toy box or shed, making it a fun and engaging project.

**Rotate Toys:** If space is limited, consider rotating toys periodically. Keep some toys in storage while others are available for play. This helps to keep the play area fresh and encourages creativity.

**Regular Clean-up:** Encourage children to clean up and put their toys back in the designated area after playtime. Make it a routine, and they will develop good habits.

**Safety Precautions:** Ensure that the toy box or shed is secure and childproofed. Lock the shed if it contains items that may be hazardous to children.

**Regular Maintenance:** Regularly inspect and maintain the toy box or shed to ensure it remains safe and in good condition.

---

**Garage**
Infant/Non-mobile: (Birth - 6 months)
Infant crawl/roll: (5 months - 1 year)
→ **Toddler/Pre-school: (1 year - 4 years)**
→ **School-age: (5 years - 6+ years)**

# Golf Clubs

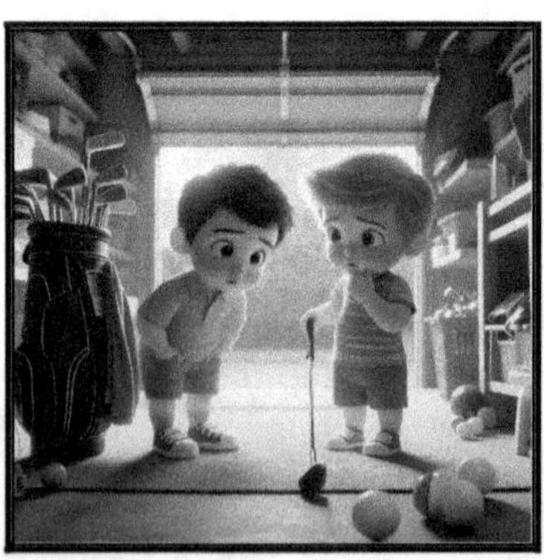

Childproofing golf clubs is important to keep children safe and prevent accidents. Golf clubs can have sharp edges and heavy heads, making them potentially dangerous if not properly stored. Each year, approximately **4,000 children** are injured by improperly stored sporting goods, such as bats, hockey sticks, and balls. (Source: National Safety Council (NSC) - Injury Facts)

**Secure Storage:** Store golf clubs in a locked or secured area, such as a golf bag with a zipper or a locked closet. When not in use, keep them out of the reach of children.

**Use Golf Club Covers:** Invest in golf club headcovers to protect the clubs' sharp edges and prevent scratching or damage.

**Remove Grips:** Remove the grips from the clubs when not in use. This will make them less appealing to children and deter them from trying to play with them.

**Educate Children:** Teach children about the potential dangers of golf clubs and explain that they are not toys. Let them know that golf clubs are for adults to use responsibly.

**Supervise Play:** If you allow children to be near golf clubs or play with plastic toy golf clubs, always supervise their activities to ensure their safety.

**Lock the Golf Bag:** If you keep your golf clubs in a bag, consider using a padlock or a bag with a lockable compartment to prevent unauthorized access.

**Store Out of Sight:** To minimize children's curiosity, keep golf clubs out of sight and out of reach.

**Use Childproof Locks:** If you store your golf clubs in a cabinet or closet, consider using childproof locks to prevent children from opening them.

**Golf Club Organizer:** If you have a golf club organizer or stand, ensure it is stable and securely attached to prevent tipping over.

**Set a Good Example:** Always model responsible behavior with golf clubs when children are around. Demonstrating safe handling will teach them to treat the clubs with respect.

You can ensure that golf clubs are safely stored and handled, reducing the risk of accidents and injuries to children. Remember, child safety should always be a priority, and taking proactive measures can prevent potential hazards.

---

**Garage**
Infant/Non-mobile: (Birth - 6 months)
Infant crawl/roll: (5 months - 1 year)
→ **Toddler/Pre-school: (1 year - 4 years)**
→ **School-age: (5 years - 6+ years)**

# Garage Floor

Clean and seal. Rubber mats or foam tiles. Cover cracks. Non-slip surfaces. Store chemicals locked. Clear clutter. Cover sharp edges. Secure heavy items. Non-slip flooring. Proper lighting (overhead, motion-activated, LED).

---

**Garage**
Infant/Non-mobile: (Birth - 6 months)
Infant crawl/roll: (5 months - 1 year)
→ **Toddler/Pre-school: (1 year - 4 years)**
→ **School-age: (5 years - 6+ years)**

# Vehicle Lighter/Outlet Concerns

Childproofing a car lighter/outlet is essential to prevent children from accidentally engaging or playing with it, as car lighters can get hot and cause burns or other injuries.

**Use a Safety Plug:** Consider using a safety plug or cover specifically designed for car lighters. These plugs will prevent children from inserting objects into the lighter socket and engaging the heating element.

**Educate Children:** Teach children about the car's interior components and explain to them that the car lighter is not a toy and should never be touched or played with.

**Keep Lighter Away:** Store lighters and any other potentially hazardous items out of children's reach, such as in the glove compartment or other secure compartments.

**Child Locks:** If your car model has child safety locks, activate them to prevent children from accessing the front console or lighter area without adult supervision.

**Supervise:** Always supervise children in the car to ensure they don't engage with the lighter or any other controls.

**Use the Lighter with Caution:** If you must use the car lighter to charge devices or for other purposes, do so with caution and keep it out of children's reach when not in use.

**Regular Maintenance:** Ensure that the lighter socket is in good working condition. If it becomes loose or malfunctioning, have it repaired or replaced promptly.

**Teach Emergency Procedures:** If you have older children, teach them about the car's emergency procedures, including the use of the car lighter for emergency purposes only.

**Keep a Spare:** If possible, keep a spare car lighter plug or cover in case the original one gets lost or damaged.

---

<u>**Garage**</u>
Infant/Non-mobile: (Birth - 6 months)
Infant crawl/roll: (5 months - 1 year)
→ **Toddler/Pre-school: (1 year - 4 years)**
→ **School-age: (5 years - 6+ years)**

# LOCK VEHICLE DOORS

**Prevent Unwanted Access:** Locking the garage doors ensures that children cannot enter the vehicle without adult supervision, preventing potential accidents and injuries.

**Avoid Trapped Children:** Children may be curious and inadvertently climb into an unlocked car while playing in the garage, putting them at risk of being trapped inside.

**Prevent Accidental Engaging:** Locking car doors helps prevent children from accidentally engaging controls or equipment inside the car, such as activating the windows or playing with the gearshift.

**Carbon Monoxide Safety:** If the car is running, locking the doors helps prevent children from entering the car and being exposed to carbon monoxide, a dangerous and potentially fatal gas.

**Avoid Car Rolling:** Locking the car doors prevents children from accidentally releasing the parking brake or shifting gears, which could cause the car to roll in the garage.

**Garage Safety:** Locking the car doors adds an extra layer of security to the garage, minimizing the risk of unauthorized individuals gaining access to the car.

**Supervision:** While in the garage, always supervise children and make sure they are away from the car. Locking the car doors is an additional safety measure, but proper supervision is crucial.

**Prevent Theft:** Locking the car doors also helps protect the vehicle from theft, ensuring it remains secure in the garage.

Childproofing is not limited to the home interior, and the garage is an important area to consider. Always prioritize safety and establish good habits, such as locking car doors when in the garage, to keep children safe from potential dangers.

---

<u>**Garage**</u>
→ **Infant/Non-mobile: (Birth - 6 months)**
→ **Infant crawl/roll: (5 months - 1 year)**
→ **Toddler/Pre-school: (1 year - 4 years)**
→ **School-age: (5 years - 6+ years)**

# Car Seat Safety

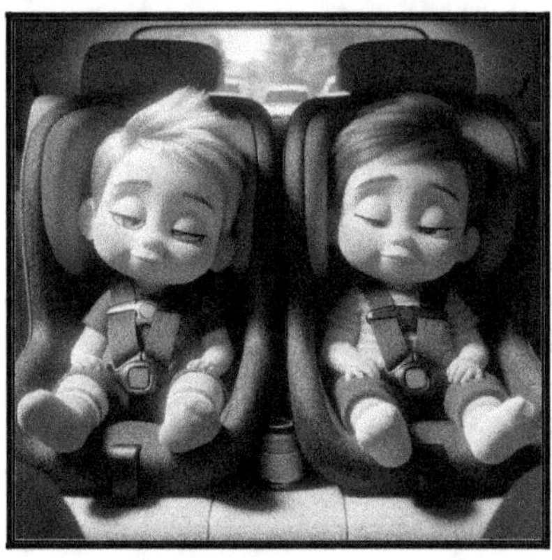

Car seats play a crucial role in keeping children safe while traveling in vehicles.

**Choose the Right Seat:** Select a car seat or booster seat appropriate for your child's age, weight, and height. Follow the manufacturer's guidelines and local regulations to ensure proper fit and safety.

**Rear-Facing Seats for Infants:** Infants should ride in a rear-facing car seat until they are at least two or until they reach the maximum height and weight limit recommended by the car seat manufacturer.

**Forward-Facing Seats for Toddlers:** Use a forward-facing car seat with a harness once your child outgrows the rear-facing seat. Continue using this seat until your child is ready for a booster seat.

**Booster Seats for Older Children:** Transition your child to a booster seat when they outgrow the forward-facing car seat. A booster seat positions the seatbelt correctly over their lap and shoulder.

**Proper Installation:** Ensure that the car seat or booster seat is correctly installed in your vehicle. Follow the installation instructions provided by the car seat manufacturer and your vehicle's owner's manual.

**Tighten Straps Securely:** When using a car seat with a harness, make sure the straps are snug and properly adjusted. The harness should fit snugly against your child's body.

**Position of the Harness:** When using a forward-facing car seat, the harness straps should be at or just above your child's shoulders.

**Secure the Booster Seat:** If you use a booster seat, ensure it is securely installed in the vehicle and that the seatbelt passes correctly through its guides.

**Use the Right Seatbelt:** Ensure that your child uses the vehicle's seatbelt correctly when in a booster seat. The seatbelt should properly fit across their lap and shoulder without crossing the neck or face.

**Check for Recalls:** Regularly check for recalls on your car seat or booster seat to ensure they meet current safety standards.

**Keep Children in the Back:** Always place children in the vehicle's back seat. This is the safest place for them to ride until they reach the appropriate age and size to use a seatbelt without a booster seat.

**Set a Good Example:** Always wear your seatbelt when driving with children to set a positive example for safe behavior.

You can significantly reduce the risk of injuries and ensure that your child is properly protected during car rides. Remember that car seats save lives; using them correctly and consistently is essential.

---

**Garage**
→ **Infant/Non-mobile: (Birth - 6 months)**
→ **Infant crawl/roll: (5 months - 1 year)**
→ **Toddler/Pre-school: (1 year - 4 years)**
→ **School-age: (5 years - 6+ years)**

# WHAT TO PUT IN A TRAVEL SAFETY KIT

A car safety kit is essential to have in your vehicle, especially when traveling with children.

**First Aid Kit:** A well-stocked first aid kit should include bandages, adhesive tape, antiseptic wipes, gauze pads, tweezers, scissors, pain relievers, and any necessary medications specific to your family's needs.

**Emergency Contact Information:** Keep a list of emergency contact numbers, including local emergency services, your pediatrician, and family members or friends who can be reached in case of an emergency.

**Bottled Water and Non-Perishable Snacks:** Include bottled water and non-perishable snacks, like granola bars or dried fruit, to keep everyone hydrated and nourished during unexpected delays or emergencies.

**Blankets or Extra Clothing:** Have blankets or extra clothing, including jackets or sweaters, in case of cold weather or if you need to stay warm during an emergency.

**Flashlight and Extra Batteries:** A flashlight will be useful at night in case of car trouble or to search for items in the car. Make sure you have extra batteries for the flashlight.

**Reflective Triangles or Flares: These can** alert other drivers if your car breaks down on the side of the road, making your vehicle more visible and promoting safety.

**Jumper Cables:** Carry jumper cables in case your car battery dies, and you need a jump-start from another vehicle.

**Tire Jack and Spare Tire:** Ensure your car has a tire jack and a properly inflated spare tire in case of a flat tire.

**Multi-Tool or Swiss Army Knife:** A multi-tool with a knife, screwdriver, and other functions can be handy in various situations.

**Roadside Assistance Information:** Keep information about your roadside assistance coverage and contact numbers accessible.

**Paper Towels and Trash Bags:** Have paper towels and trash bags to clean up spills and keep the car tidy.

**Car Phone Charger:** Keep a car phone charger to ensure your phone is always charged. This allows you to make emergency calls or access navigation.

**Child-Friendly Items:** If you have children, consider adding items like baby wipes, diapers, and children's entertainment (books, toys) to keep them comfortable during a car journey.

Make sure to periodically check and update the items in your car safety kit, especially the first aid supplies and emergency contact information. Being prepared with a well-stocked car safety kit can provide peace of mind and assistance during unexpected situations while traveling with children.

# Garage Wall Concerns

**Cover Sharp Edges:** Inspect the garage walls for any sharp edges or protruding nails. Use edge protectors or corner guards to cover these areas and prevent injuries if children accidentally bump into them.

**Lock Hazardous Items:** Store hazardous items, such as tools, chemicals, and sharp objects, in locked cabinets or on high shelves that are out of children's reach.

**Secure Heavy Items:** Ensure that heavy items, such as bicycles, ladders, or gardening equipment, are securely stored and properly anchored to prevent them from toppling over.

**Install Safety Mirrors:** If the garage has blind spots, consider installing safety mirrors to improve visibility and prevent accidents.

**Use Non-Slip Flooring:** If the garage floor is slippery, consider using non-slip flooring or placing anti-slip mats in areas where children are likely to walk or play.

**Childproof Garage Door:** Install safety sensors and use childproof locks on the garage door to prevent accidental closing while children are near it.

**Create a Designated Play Area:** If you have space in the garage for play, designate a safe play area away from hazardous items and ensure it is well-supervised.

**Check for Mold or Mildew:** To maintain a healthy environment, regularly inspect the walls for signs of mold or mildew and address any issues promptly.

**Secure Electrical Outlets:** If there are electrical outlets in the garage, use childproof outlet covers to prevent children from inserting objects into them.

**Proper Lighting:** Ensure that the garage is well-lit to avoid trips and falls, especially during nighttime use.

**Install a Fire Extinguisher:** Keep one in the garage and teach older children how to use it in case of emergencies.

**Supervise Children:** Always supervise children when they are in the garage to ensure their safety and guide them away from potential hazards.

You can help create a safer garage environment for children by regularly assessing the garage for potential risks and taking appropriate actions to minimize them. Remember, child safety should be a top priority in every area of the home, including the garage.

---

**Garage**
Infant/Non-mobile: (Birth - 6 months)
Infant crawl/roll: (5 months - 1 year)
→ **Toddler/Pre-school: (1 year - 4 years)**
→ **School-age: (5 years - 6+ years)**

# LADDERS

Childproofing ladders are essential to prevent accidents and injuries, as ladders can be dangerous for children if not properly secured or supervised.

**Store Ladders Safely:** When not in use, store ladders in a locked shed, garage, or other secure area where children cannot access them.

**Use Childproof Locks:** If you have a retractable or foldable ladder, consider using childproof locks to prevent children from extending or opening the ladder.

**Secure Non-Retractable Ladders:** For non-retractable ladders, such as extension ladders, secure them in an upright position and use a ladder lock or strap to keep them closed.

**Keep Ladders Out of Reach:** Store ladders in a location that is out of children's reach, such as high shelves or hanging from the ceiling.

**Supervise Children:** Always supervise children when ladders are in use or accessible, ensuring they do not climb on or play with the ladder.

**Teach Ladder Safety:** If you have older children, teach them ladder safety rules and proper ladder usage, emphasizing that ladders are not toys.

**Anchor Ladders Securely:** When using a ladder, ensure it is placed on a stable and level surface and anchored securely to prevent tipping.

**Use Anti-Slip Feet:** Install anti-slip feet on the ladder to provide better stability and reduce the risk of sliding.

**Check for Damage:** Regularly inspect the ladder for any signs of damage, wear, or loose parts. Repair or replace any damaged components promptly.

**Properly Lock Hinges and Spreader Bars:** Before using the ladder, ensure that all hinges and spreader bars are securely locked in place.

**Demonstrate Safe Ladder Use:** Set a good example by using ladders safely and responsibly in front of children.

You can significantly reduce the risk of ladder-related accidents and create a safer environment for children by always prioritizing safety and ensuring that ladders are properly stored, secured, and used under appropriate supervision.

---

<u>**Garage**</u>
Infant/Non-mobile: (Birth - 6 months)
Infant crawl/roll: (5 months - 1 year)
→ **Toddler/Pre-school: (1 year - 4 years)**
→ **School-age: (5 years - 6+ years)**

# CHEMICAL CONCERNS

Childproofing the garage and ensuring the safety of children involves carefully managing and securing all chemicals and hazardous substances.

**Storage of Chemicals:** Store all chemicals, including cleaning solutions, pesticides, fertilizers, paints, and automotive fluids, in locked cabinets or on high shelves that are out of children's reach.

**Secure Lids and Caps:** Ensure that all containers with hazardous substances have secure lids and caps and double-check that they are tightly closed after use.

**Labeling:** Clearly label all chemical containers with their contents and potential hazards. When possible, use childproof and waterproof labels.

**Organize and Separate:** Store chemicals separately from other items in the garage and organize them so that they are easily accessible only to adults.

**Childproof Locks:** Install childproof locks on cabinets containing hazardous substances, making it difficult for young children to open them.

**Dispose of Unused Chemicals:** Properly dispose of any old or expired chemicals following local guidelines and hazardous waste disposal regulations.

**Educate Older Children:** If you have older children, educate them about the potential dangers of chemicals and the importance of not handling them without adult supervision.

**Regular Inspection:** Regularly inspect the garage to ensure that no chemicals or hazardous materials are left unattended or within your children's reach.

**Locking the Garage Door:** Keep the garage door locked when not in use and ensure that children cannot access the garage without adult permission.

**Safety Data Sheets (SDS):** Keep safety data sheets for all chemicals in the garage. These sheets provide essential information on handling, storage, and emergency procedures.

**Childproof Outlets:** If there are electrical outlets in the garage, use childproof outlet covers to prevent children from inserting objects into them.

**Remove Toxic Plants:** If you have plants in the garage, ensure they are non-toxic and safe for children. Remove any poisonous plants from the area.

**Lock Up Tools:** When not in use, keep tools, especially sharp or heavy ones, in locked toolboxes or cabinets.

**Maintain Fire Safety:** Install a fire extinguisher in the garage and teach older children how to use it in case of emergencies.

**Supervision:** Always supervise children when they are in the garage and guide them away from potential hazards.

Childproofing the garage requires vigilance and attention to detail, but it is essential for creating a safe environment for children.

---

**Garage**
Infant/Non-mobile: (Birth - 6 months)
Infant crawl/roll: (5 months - 1 year)
→ **Toddler/Pre-school: (1 year - 4 years)**
→ **School-age: (5 years - 6+ years)**

# GARAGE LIGHTING CONCERNS

Ensuring good garage lighting is crucial for childproofing and overall safety.

**Install Adequate Lighting:** Make sure the garage has sufficient lighting to provide clear visibility throughout the space. Consider installing overhead, wall-mounted, or LED strip lights to brighten the area.

**Motion-Activated Lights:** Consider installing motion-activated lights near the garage entrance and key areas. These lights automatically turn on when someone enters the garage, providing enhanced safety and energy efficiency.

**LED Bulbs:** Use energy-efficient LED bulbs in the garage. They provide bright illumination while consuming less energy and lasting longer.

**Light Switch Accessibility:** Ensure that light switches are easily accessible and conveniently placed, allowing for quick lighting adjustments when entering or exiting the garage.

**Night Lighting:** If the garage is frequently used at night, install night lighting with a lower intensity to provide visibility without disturbing others nearby.

**Task Lighting:** Add task lighting in specific areas, such as workbenches or tool storage areas, to provide focused and adequate illumination for specific activities.

**Clean Light Fixtures:** Regularly clean the light fixtures to remove dust and debris, as dirty fixtures can reduce the effectiveness of the lighting.

**Reflective Surfaces:** Consider using reflective surfaces like white walls or mirrors to bounce light around the garage and improve overall brightness.

**Bright Paint:** If feasible, consider painting the garage walls and ceiling with light-colored, reflective paint to enhance the overall brightness.

**Skylights or Windows:** Add skylights or windows to allow natural light into the garage during the daytime.

**Regular Maintenance:** Regularly inspect and maintain the lighting system, promptly replacing any faulty bulbs or fixtures.

**Emergency Lighting:** Install battery-operated emergency lights or keep flashlights handy in case of power outages.

You create a safer and more child-friendly environment. Proper lighting helps reduce the risk of accidents and allows for better supervision and organization of the space.

---

# Lookout as You Pull In or Out of a Garage

Being aware of your children's whereabouts when pulling in and out of the garage is crucial for their safety.

**Check Surroundings Before Moving:** Always check around and behind your vehicle before moving it. Walk around the car to ensure there are no children or pets nearby.

**Use Rearview Cameras and Sensors:** Many modern vehicles are equipped with rear-view cameras and parking sensors. Utilize these technologies to better view the area behind your car.

**Supervise Children:** Always supervise children when they are in or near the garage. Make sure they are a safe distance away from moving vehicles.

**Teach Children About Garage Safety:** Educate your children about the potential dangers of playing near cars and the importance of staying away from moving vehicles.

**Designate Safe Areas:** Establish specific safe areas in the driveway or garage where children can play, away from moving cars.

**Keep the Garage Door Closed:** Keep the garage door closed when not in use to prevent children from running into the garage unexpectedly.

**Use Visual Aids:** If necessary, use visual aids such as colorful flags or markers in the driveway to remind children to stay away from moving vehicles.

**Teach Children Traffic Safety:** Teach older children about traffic safety, including staying clear of vehicles, looking both ways before crossing driveways, and using designated sidewalks.

**Limit Distractions:** Avoid distractions while driving in the driveway or garage, such as using a cell phone or adjusting the radio.

**Use Reflective Gear:** If children play outside during low-light conditions, have them wear reflective clothing or accessories to be easily visible to drivers.

**Backup Safely:** If you need to exit the garage, do so slowly and cautiously, checking all mirrors and using rear view cameras.

# |Ch. 24| The Yard

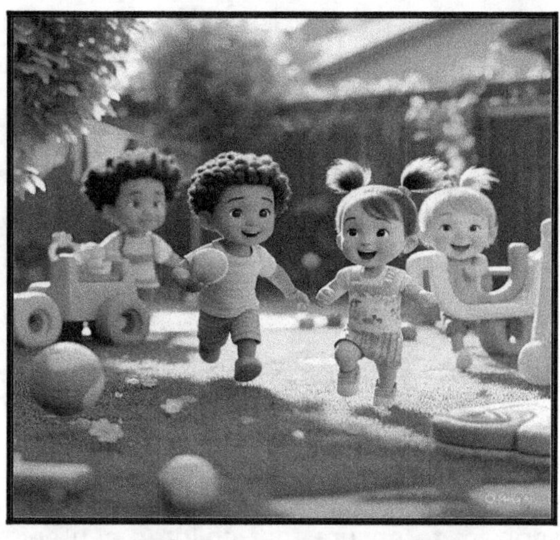

**Introduction**: Playground-related injuries account for **over 300,000 emergency visits annually** in the U.S., with fractures and concussions being the most common types of injuries. (Source: U.S. Consumer Product Safety Commission (CPSC) - Playground Safety) The family yard metamorphoses into a vast realm of endless adventures, from pirate-infested seas to jungles brimming with wildlife. As parents, our role is to foster this rich playground of imagination while ensuring it remains a sanctuary of safety. This chapter guides you through the essential steps to transform your yard into a haven where little explorers can embark on their adventures without any peril. From securing potentially hazardous areas to selecting child-friendly plants and materials, we'll help you craft a yard where children can grow, play, and explore, enveloped in the comforting embrace of safety. Let's embark on this journey to create a yard that harmonizes the spirit of adventure with the peace of mind that comes from knowing your child is safe. Also, I chose to put this statistic in this section, but it applies to the whole house. Each year, **over 100,000 children in the U.S. suffer eye injuries** caused by household objects such as toys, tools, and cleaning supplies. *(Source: Centers for Disease Control and Prevention (CDC) - Eye Injury Statistics)*

---

# Bee Safety

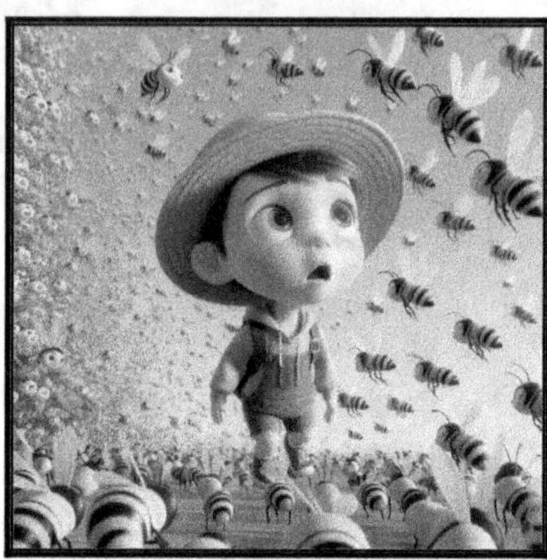

Bee safety is important to ensure that children can enjoy the outdoors and learn about nature while minimizing the risk of bee stings. Bees play a crucial role in pollination and are generally not aggressive unless provoked.

**Educate Children:** Teach children about bees, their importance in nature, and how to observe them from a safe distance. Explain that bees are not interested in stinging unless they feel threatened.

**Avoid Swatting or Agitating Bees:** Instruct children not to swat at bees or try to catch them. Sudden movements may provoke a defensive response from the bees.

**Wear Light-Colored Clothing:** Bees are attracted to dark colors, so encourage children to wear light-colored clothing when spending time outdoors.

**Avoid Fragrances:** Scented products like perfumes, scented lotions, and heavily scented soaps may attract bees. Encourage children to avoid using such products when going outside.

**Choose Appropriate Play Areas:** Avoid setting up play areas near beehives or flowering plants where bees are actively foraging.

**Inspect Play Areas:** Before allowing children to play outside, regularly inspect play areas, tree houses, and outdoor toys for signs of bee activity.

**Cover Food and Drinks:** During picnics or outdoor activities, cover food and drinks to deter bees from being attracted to them.

**Stay Calm:** Teach children to remain calm if a bee comes near them. Panicking or running can increase the likelihood of a bee sting.

**Use Bee Repellents with Caution:** Avoid using bee repellents or insecticides on children unless recommended by a healthcare professional.

**Keep Gardens and Lawns Maintained:** Regularly maintain gardens and lawns to reduce bee nesting sites and minimize bee activity close to play areas.

**Create Bee-Friendly Gardens:** Plant bee-friendly flowers away from play areas to attract bees away from high-traffic zones.

**Supervise Play:** Always supervise young children when they are playing outdoors, especially in areas with flowering plants.

**Avoid Attracting Bees during Feeding:** If bottle-feeding infants outdoors, keep the bottles covered to avoid attracting bees.

**Be Prepared/Know Allergies:** If your child has known bee sting allergies, keep a bee sting kit or other relevant medications on hand.

You can promote bee safety, allowing children to explore and appreciate nature while minimizing the risk of bee stings. Educating children about bees and their behavior is key to fostering respect for these important pollinators and ensuring peaceful coexistence.

---

**Yard**
Infant/Non-mobile: (Birth - 6 months)
Infant crawl/roll: (5 months - 1 year)
→ **Toddler/Pre-school: (1 year - 4 years)**
→ **School-age: (5 years - 6+ years)**

# Tree and Plant Concerns

Each year, **more than 500 children** are injured near chemical plants and industrial areas due to accidental exposure to hazardous substances. (Source: Centers for Disease Control and Prevention (CDC) - Environmental Health) Ensuring the safety of children in a yard filled with nature's greenery involves being aware of the potentially dangerous plants and trees that could cause harm to the little ones.

# Dangerous Plants and Trees:

## Oleander (Oleander Nerium)

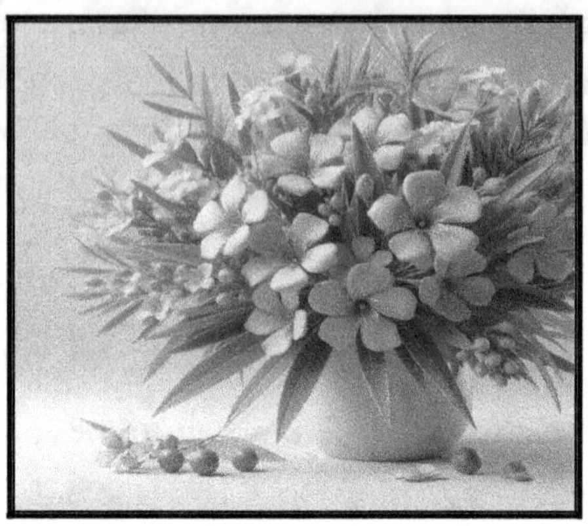

**Description:** A beautiful shrub with glossy leaves and vibrant flowers, usually pink, red, or white.

**Danger:** Every part of this plant is toxic and can cause severe poisoning, resulting in symptoms such as nausea, vomiting, abdominal pain, heart irregularities, and even death.

---

## Castor Bean Plant (Ricinus Communis)

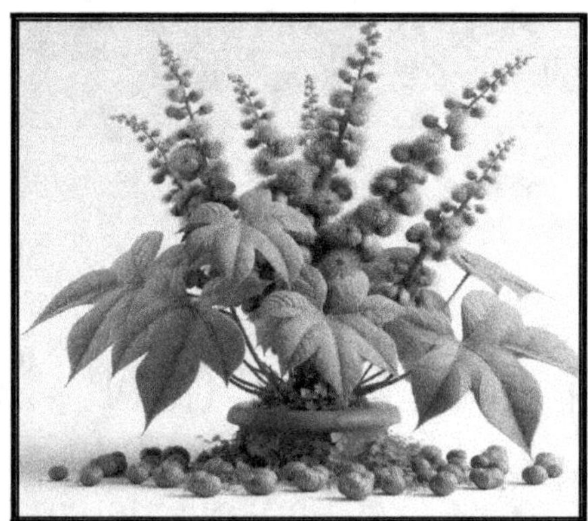

**Description:** A plant with large, glossy leaves and clustered flowers, producing beans that contain seeds.

**Danger:** The seeds are highly toxic if ingested, causing severe abdominal pain, vomiting, diarrhea, and potentially fatal organ damage.

---

# Foxglove (Digitalis Purpurea)

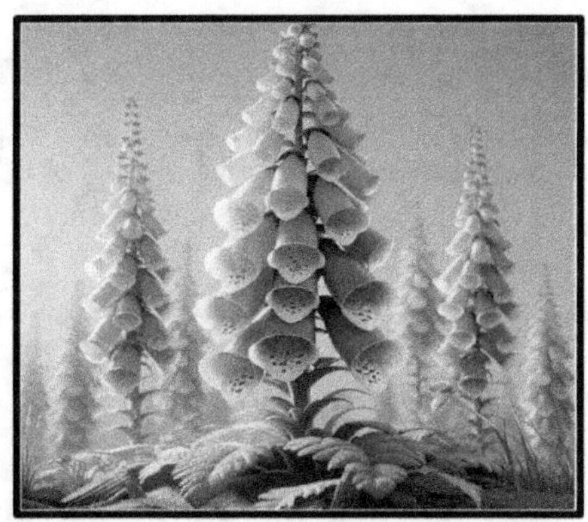

**Description:** A tall plant with a spike of bell-shaped flowers, usually in purple or white.

**Danger:** All parts of the plant are poisonous, leading to symptoms like diarrhea, headache, and convulsions. It affects the heart and can be fatal in high doses.

# Poison Ivy (Toxicodendron Radicans)

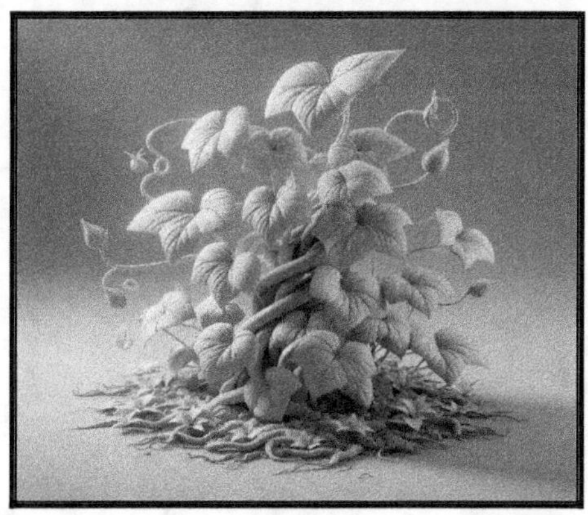

**Description:** A plant with leaves grouped in threes exhibiting a glossy surface. It can grow as a vine or shrub.

**Danger:** Contact can cause skin irritation, intense itching, and blisters due to an oily resin called urushiol present in the leaves. Wash off your skin immediately after contact and wash clothes that were in contact as well.

# Angel's Trumpet (Brugmansia

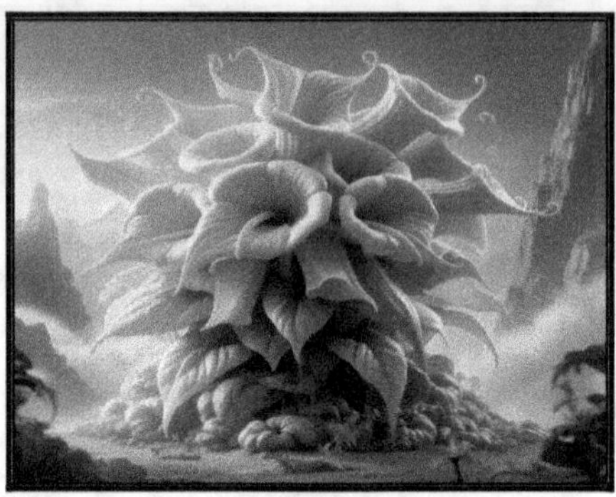

**Description:** A shrub or small tree with large, pendulous flowers that resemble trumpets, typically yellow, pink, or white.

**Danger:** All parts are toxic, causing symptoms like confusion, hallucinations, and potentially fatal respiratory depression if ingested.

# Rosary Pea (Abrus Precatorius)

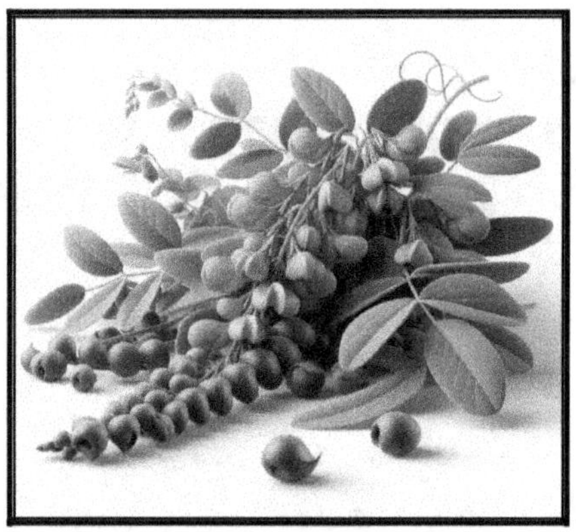

**Description:** A vine with slender stems, light green leaves, and seeds encased in bright red pods.

**Danger:** The seeds are highly toxic if ingested, causing severe nausea, vomiting, and abdominal pain, and can lead to death due to organ failure.

## Daphne (Daphne spp.)

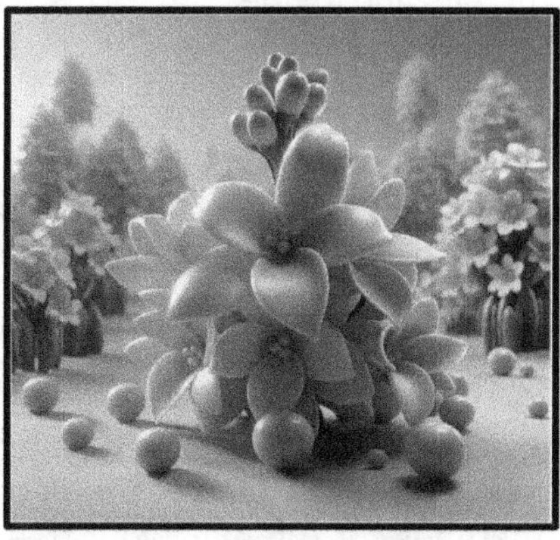

**Description:** A small shrub with clusters of fragrant, tubular flowers, usually pink or white.

**Danger:** The berries are poisonous, causing symptoms like diarrhea, headache, and even coma in severe cases.

**Child Safety Measures:** Remove or fence off these dangerous plants from areas where children play. Educate children about the dangers of touching or ingesting unknown plants. Supervise children closely while they are playing in the yard.

---

**Yard**
Infant/Non-mobile: (Birth - 6 months)
Infant crawl/roll: (5 months - 1 year)
Toddler/Pre-school: (1 year - 4 years)
→ **School-age: (5 years - 6+ years)**

# LIMIT TREE CLIMBING

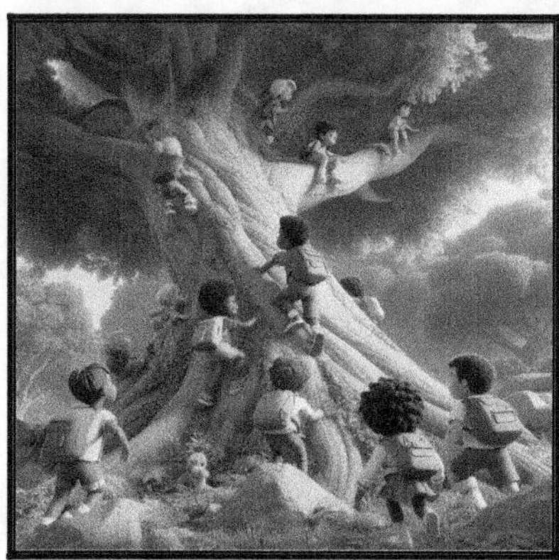

Childproofing your yard by trimming trees to prevent unwanted climbing is critical. Children are naturally curious and may be tempted to climb trees, which can lead to falls and injuries.

## Identifying Risk Factors

**Low Branches:** Identify and trim branches that are low enough for children to reach and attempt to climb.

**Weak Limbs:** Remove weak or rotting limbs, as they can easily break under a child's weight.

**Nearby Structures:** Note any structures near trees, like fences or playsets, that children might use to access higher branches.

## Trimming Techniques

**Professional Consultation:** Consult with a professional arborist to identify the best methods for trimming your trees without damaging them.

**Regular Maintenance:** Regularly trim the trees to prevent the growth of low, accessible branches.

**Proper Tools:** Use the correct trimming tools, such as pruners for small branches and chainsaws for larger limbs, to ensure clean cuts and prevent disease.

## Safe Tree Varieties

**Choosing Safe Trees:** Consider planting trees that don't readily encourage climbing, such as those with smooth bark or densely packed branches.

**Thorny Plants:** If possible, avoid having trees with thorns or spiky leaves that can cause injuries.

## Educational Measures

**Teaching Safety:** Teach children about the dangers of climbing trees and explain why certain trees are off-limits.

**Supervision:** Always supervise young children when they are playing outside to prevent unwanted climbing attempts.

## Creating Safe Play Areas

**Separate Play Areas:** Create designated play areas away from tempting trees to discourage climbing.

**Ground-Level Play:** Encourage ground-level play by providing play equipment like swings and slides, which are safer alternatives to tree climbing.

To ensure children's safety, you must first identify the risk factors, such as low branches and weak limbs that may invite climbing. You must also notice any nearby structures that children might use to gain access to higher branches. Once identified, employ the right techniques for trimming trees.

It is advisable to consult with a professional arborist for guidance on trimming without damaging the trees. Regular maintenance is key to preventing the growth of accessible branches.

Furthermore, you should consider planting tree varieties that do not encourage climbing and avoid trees with thorns or spiky leaves to prevent injuries. At the same time, it's crucial to educate children about the dangers associated with tree climbing and constantly supervise them to prevent unwanted climbing attempts. Creating separate play areas and encouraging ground-level play with safe play equipment can also discourage children from climbing trees.

---

❦ According to Nationwide Children, each year, approximately 2,800 children (up to age 19) are treated in U.S. emergency departments for tree house related injuries, with most injuries involving falls, fractures, and head trauma. **Children under 5 years old are particularly likely to suffer head injuries from these falls.**

---

**Yard**

Infant/Non-mobile: (Birth - 6 months)
Infant crawl/roll: (5 months - 1 year)
**→ Toddler/Pre-school: (1 year - 4 years)**
**→ School-age: (5 years - 6+ years)**

# Slip and Slide

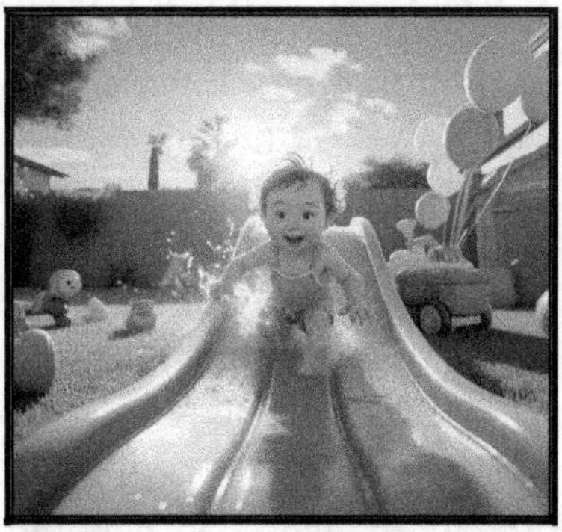

**Supervision:** Always ensure that children are supervised by an adult when using the slip-and-slide. Active supervision can prevent accidents.

**Surface Check:** Before setting up the slip-and-slide, check the ground for sharp objects, rocks, or uneven surfaces that could cause injury. Choose a soft, grassy area free of potential hazards.

**Water Control:** Ensure the water source used to keep the slide slippery is at a safe pressure. Too much water pressure can cause more dangerous slips and falls.

**Age Appropriateness:** Ensure the slip and slide is suitable for the child's age. Some slides have size or age limits, so it's important to follow those guidelines.

**End Padding:** Place a padded surface, like soft mats or inflatable barriers, at the end of the slip and slide to prevent children from sliding into hard surfaces or obstacles like fences or trees.

**No Rough Play:** Establish rules for safe use, such as no running before jumping onto the slide and limiting the number of children using it at once to avoid collisions.

**Sun Protection:** Ensure children wear sunscreen and wear hats or clothing that provides sun protection. A slip-and-slide can keep kids in the sun for long periods.

**Hydration:** Ensure children drink enough water, as outdoor play in the sun can lead to dehydration.

---

**<u>Yard</u>**
Infant/Non-mobile: (Birth - 6 months)
Infant crawl/roll: (5 months - 1 year)
→ **Toddler/Pre-school: (1 year - 4 years)**
→ **School-age: (5 years - 6+ years)**

# Hedges and Bushes Concerns

Keeping hedges and bushes trimmed is crucial for ensuring children's safety in and around the yard. Overgrown vegetation can pose various hazards, from hiding potential dangers to providing easy access to climbing or tripping risks.

**Visibility:** Trim hedges and bushes to maintain clear sightlines throughout the yard. This ensures that hazards, such as toys left out, uneven ground, or sharp objects, are easily visible, reducing the risk of accidents.

**Accessibility:** Overgrown hedges can become inviting hiding spots for children, which may lead to them getting stuck or injured. Regular trimming eliminates such hiding spots and discourages children from venturing into confined areas.

**Thorny or Poisonous Plants:** If you have hedges or bushes with thorns or poisonous berries, it's essential to trim them regularly and keep them at a safe distance from play areas to prevent accidental contact.

**Prevent Overgrowth:** Regular trimming prevents hedges and bushes from becoming overgrown, which could encroach on walkways, play areas, or structures, posing tripping or entanglement hazards.

**Maintain Pathways:** Trim hedges along pathways and walkways to keep them clear and prevent obstruction or potential injuries.

**Prevent Nesting Areas:** Untrimmed hedges may become nesting spots for insects or animals, increasing the risk of stings or bites. Regular maintenance helps reduce this risk.

**Avoid Climbing Risks:** Overgrown bushes with sturdy branches may tempt children to climb. Keeping them trimmed discourages climbing and reduces the risk of falls.

**Avoid Spider Webs:** Trim bushes away from doorways and play areas to reduce the likelihood of encountering spider webs that may cause discomfort or surprise.

**Use the Right Tools:** Use appropriate gardening tools, such as hedge trimmers or pruning shears, to ensure clean and precise cuts while trimming.

**Safety Gear:** When trimming hedges and bushes, wear appropriate safety gear, such as gloves and eye protection.

**Regular Trimming Schedule:** Establish a regular trimming schedule for the hedges and bushes in your yard, usually once or twice a year, depending on the plant's growth rate.

**Proper Disposal:** Dispose of trimmed branches and debris safely to prevent tripping hazards or the risk of children playing with the waste.

**Educate Children:** Explain to children the importance of avoiding hedges and bushes and the potential risks involved.

**Supervision:** Always supervise children when they are playing outdoors, especially in areas with hedges and bushes.

Keeping hedges and bushes trimmed creates a safer outdoor environment for children to play and explore. Regular maintenance of vegetation contributes to a well-maintained yard that minimizes potential hazards and ensures children's safety while enjoying outdoor activities.

# MOSS CONCERNS

Moss is generally not harmful to children and can add a natural and charming element to outdoor spaces. However, some child safety concerns are associated with moss, especially in specific situations.

**Slippery Surfaces:** Moss can make surfaces, such as rocks, stones, or pathways, slippery when it's wet or damp. This may lead to slips and falls, especially for young children who may not have fully developed their balance and coordination. To address this concern, regularly inspect areas with moss and remove it from high-traffic pathways or play areas to reduce the risk of slipping.

**Allergies:** Some children may be allergic to moss or may develop skin irritation after contact with it. If you notice any signs of allergic reactions or skin irritation in your child after contact with moss, avoid direct exposure and seek medical advice if necessary.

**Choking Hazard:** Moss, particularly small and loose pieces, may pose a choking hazard if young children put it in their mouths. Always supervise young children when they are playing in areas with moss to prevent them from doing so.

**Ingestion Concerns:** Ingesting large quantities of moss could cause stomach upset or other gastrointestinal issues. Educate children about the importance of not eating or putting moss in their mouths and regularly remind them to avoid doing so.

**Bacteria and Contaminants:** Moss can sometimes grow in damp and shady areas, possibly accumulating bacteria or contaminants. Regularly inspect areas with moss, especially if it's growing in stagnant water, and promptly address any potential contamination concerns.

**Habitat for Insects:** Moss can provide a habitat for insects, some of which may bite or sting. Inspect areas with moss for insect activity and take measures to control or remove insects, especially those that may pose a threat to children.

**Falling Moss:** Moss may detach and fall in certain situations, particularly on trees or other structures. To prevent injury, keep children away from areas where moss is likely to fall.

**Respiratory Concerns:** Although rare, inhaled spores from certain types of moss may cause respiratory issues in some individuals. If your child has a respiratory condition, consult with a healthcare professional about potential risks and whether precautions are necessary.

While moss can be a beautiful part of the outdoor environment, addressing these child safety concerns and taking appropriate measures to ensure a safe and enjoyable play experience for children in areas where moss is present is essential. Regular maintenance, supervision, and education about potential hazards are key to promoting child safety around moss. This applies equally to algae, which is more likely to be found around ponds and permanent waterways, like drainage ditches or sprinkler systems. Some bleach water and a good blast from the hose should remedy the problem.

---

**Yard**

Infant/Non-mobile: (Birth - 6 months)

→ **Infant crawl/roll: (5 months - 1 year)**

→ **Toddler/Pre-school: (1 year - 4 years)**

→ **School-age: (5 years - 6+ years)**

# Chemically Treated Lawn Concerns

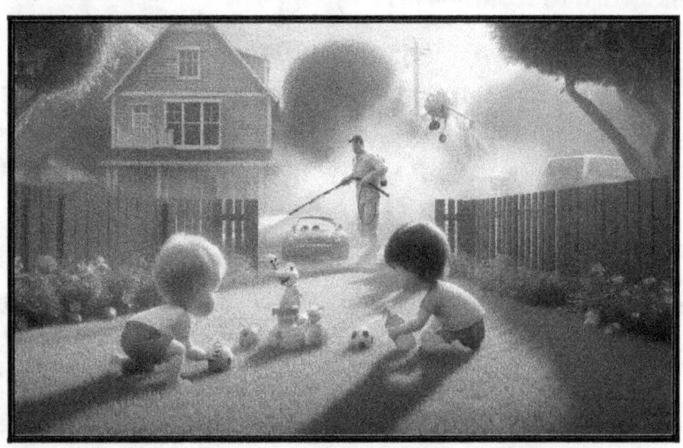

Chemically treated lawns can present several child safety concerns due to the potential exposure to harmful chemicals. Lawn care products, such as herbicides, pesticides, and fertilizers, often contain toxic substances that can be hazardous to children's health.

**Toxic Exposure:** Children may come into direct contact with chemically treated lawns while playing or crawling on the grass, leading to skin irritation, eye irritation, or more severe health issues if they accidentally ingest or inhale the chemicals. Avoid using chemical lawn care products in areas where children play frequently. Opt for organic or natural lawn care alternatives that are safer for children and pets.

**Accidental Ingestion:** Young children may inadvertently put their hands in their mouths after playing on chemically treated lawns, leading to the ingestion of harmful chemicals.

**Keep children away from chemically treated lawns** for at least 24-48 hours after application to allow the chemicals to dry or dissipate. Encourage children to wash their hands thoroughly after playing outdoors, especially on chemically treated lawns.

**Contaminated Play Equipment:** Chemicals used on the lawn may transfer to play equipment, toys, or other outdoor items, increasing the risk of exposure to children. Clean and rinse play equipment regularly to remove any chemical residues. Store toys and play equipment away from chemically treated areas when not in use.

**Runoff and Water Contamination:** Rainwater or irrigation can wash chemicals from the lawn into nearby water sources, such as ponds, streams, or storm drains, contaminating the water. Follow application instructions carefully and avoid overusing lawn care products. Water lawns conservatively to minimize runoff and prevent chemicals from leaching into the soil.

**Respiratory Irritation:** Children with respiratory conditions like asthma may be more sensitive to airborne chemical particles from chemically treated lawns. To minimize the risk of chemical particles becoming airborne, avoid applying lawn care products on windy days. Consider using natural lawn care methods that reduce the potential for respiratory irritation.

**Educate and Post Warnings:** If you use chemical lawn care products, post visible warnings to keep children and pets away from treated areas until it's safe. Educate children about the potential hazards of chemically treated lawns and the importance of not touching or playing on treated grass.

**Switch to Safer Alternatives:** Consider switching to non-toxic and eco-friendly lawn care products that are safer for children, pets, and the environment.

You can minimize child safety concerns associated with chemically treated lawns and create a healthier and safer outdoor environment for children to enjoy. Always prioritize the safety of children when choosing lawn care products and methods.

**Yard**
Infant/Non-mobile: (Birth - 6 months)
Infant crawl/roll: (5 months - 1 year)
→ **Toddler/Pre-school: (1 year - 4 years)**
→ **School-age: (5 years - 6+ years)**

# Garden Safety

**5,000+ children injured yearly by garden tools** (CPSC). Choose non-toxic plants. Childproof fencing. Lock sharp tools. Chemical-free gardening. Safety fence around water. Secure containers. Non-slip flooring. Sun protection.

---

**Yard**
Infant/Non-mobile: (Birth - 6 months)
Infant crawl/roll: (5 months - 1 year)
→ **Toddler/Pre-school: (1 year - 4 years)**
→ **School-age: (5 years - 6+ years)**

# Deck/Patio Safety

Railings 36+ inches high, gaps under 4 inches. Secure furniture. No-climb zones. Self-closing gates. Slip-resistant surface. Proper lighting. Supervise.

---

**Yard**
→ **Infant/Non-mobile: (Birth - 6 months)**
→ **Infant crawl/roll: (5 months - 1 year)**
→ **Toddler/Pre-school: (1 year - 4 years)**
→ **School-age: (5 years - 6+ years)**

# Allow your Home Address to be Seen (Lighting)

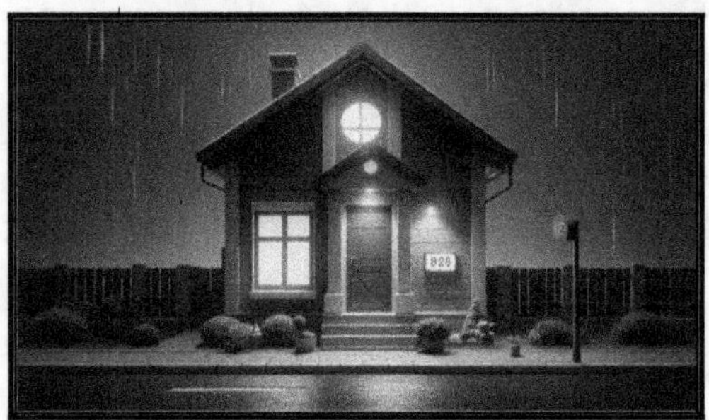

Ensure the Home Address is Visible to Emergency Responders. Having a marked home address is crucial for emergency responders to locate your home quickly during an emergency.

**Use large, reflective numbers** that are a contrasting color from your home. Dark numbers on a light background are ideal.

**Position address numbers near the street** on your home, mailbox, or driveway entrance should be easily seen from the road.

**Make sure address numbers are not obstructed** by trees, shrubs, decorations, or anything else. Trim back any foliage blocking visibility.

**Install adequate lighting** to illuminate your address at night. Use spotlights or solar-powered numbers.

**Add reflective address stickers on your mailbox** to identify it from both directions. Post your address number at the end of your driveway if your home is not visible from the road. Childproofing extends beyond the interior of your home; it also involves ensuring that help can reach you swiftly in case of emergencies. Making sure your home address is easily visible both during the day and at night is a critical part of this.

### Visibility During the Day

**Contrasting Colors:** Use large numbers in a color that contrasts sharply with the background. This will make the numbers stand out clearly. For example, if your home is painted in a light color, use dark numbers and vice versa.

**Proper Placement:** Place the numbers where they are easily visible from the road. This could be near the street, your home's facade, the mailbox, or the driveway entrance.

**Unobstructed View:** Ensure that the view of the numbers is not obstructed by trees, shrubs, or decorations. Regular trimming of foliage and prudent placement of decorations can help maintain clear visibility.

**Weather-Resistant Materials:** Use materials that can withstand various weather conditions without fading or wearing out.

### Visibility at Night

**Illumination:** Install adequate lighting to illuminate the numbers during the night. This could be in the form of spotlights or light fixtures directed at the numbers. Solar-powered numbers that glow in the dark can also be a great option.

**Reflective Materials:** Use reflective materials for the numbers so they can be seen easily under the beam of headlights.

**Additional Markings:** In addition to the main display, add reflective stickers to the mailbox or other noticeable areas that can be seen from both directions of the street.

**Driveway Posting:** If the house is not visible from the road, consider placing a sign with the house number at the end of the driveway.

**Routine Checks:** Perform routine checks to ensure that the numbers are always clean and visible.

**Updates after Renovation:** Ensure that the numbers' visibility has not been compromised after any renovation or landscaping activity.

**Multi-directional Visibility:** Ensure the numbers can be seen from multiple directions, enhancing the chances of quick identification.

In an emergency, every second counts. A visible home address can ensure that help arrives without unnecessary delays, potentially safeguarding the lives and well-being of your children.

---

**Yard**

Infant/Non-mobile: (Birth - 6 months)
Infant crawl/roll: (5 months - 1 year)
→ **Toddler/Pre-school: (1 year - 4 years)**
→ **School-age: (5 years - 6+ years)**

# WATER WELL CONCERNS

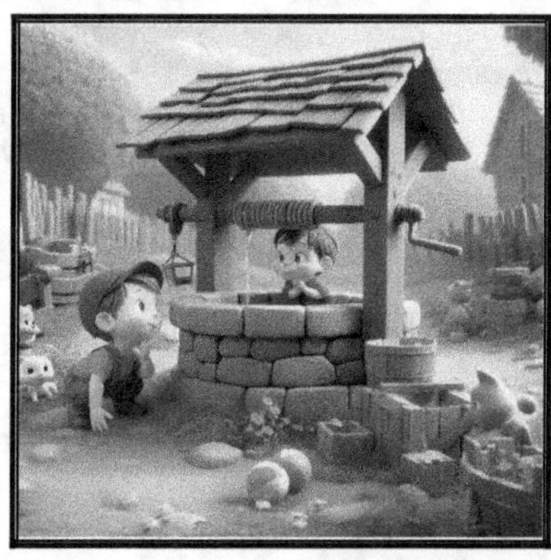

**Install a weatherproof cover** over the window well. Look for heavy-duty metal or fiberglass covers that can be locked or screwed in place. This prevents kids from falling in or climbing into the well.

**Consider installing vertical bars** or grates over the window well opening. Space the bars no more than 4 inches apart to prevent children from slipping through, and the bars need to be securely installed.

**Use a sturdy grate** or mesh screen over the window well. The openings should be too small for a child's head to fit through, and the screens should be tightly fastened.

**Plant thorny bushes** like roses or pyracantha around the inside perimeter of the window well. The thorns will deter kids from climbing down into the space.

**Place large rocks**, gravel, or wood chips in the bottom of the well to make the area uninviting for play and provide safer footing.

**Check that the window well cover is locked** and secure at all times. Conduct regular inspections and maintenance.

**Keep toys, chairs, etc., away from window wells** so kids are not tempted to stand on them to look inside.

**Attach a safety ladder inside** the window well so anyone who falls in can climb out.

**Talk to children and explain the dangers** of window wells so they understand to stay away.

Taking proper precautions with covers, barriers, and signage can help prevent tragic window well accidents involving curious kids. Be vigilant!

---

🦉 The most visceral danger in your book should be the "orphan" or abandoned well. **There are an estimated millions of abandoned wells in the U.S. alone**. Because of changes in property lines and farm consolidations, many of these are "lost". Hidden under brush, rotted plywood, or thin layers of turf. An old hand-dug well can be 3 to 5 feet wide and dozens of feet deep. To a child, a patch of soft ground or a "wooden lid" looks like a platform. If it collapses, the child disappears into a narrow, dark shaft with limited oxygen and cold water at the bottom. While rare, these incidents are almost always fatal or result in multi-day, high-stakes rescues. In many states, landowners are not legally required to "plug" (seal with concrete) these wells until they are discovered. *-National Ground Water Association (NGWA) / Iowa State University Extension.*

---

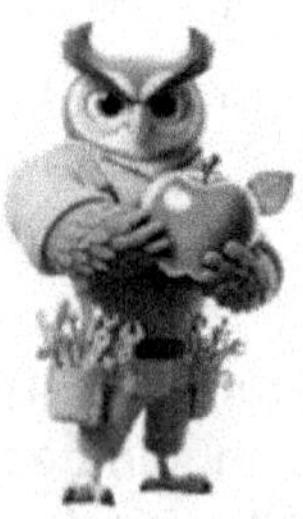

# FENCE CONCERNS

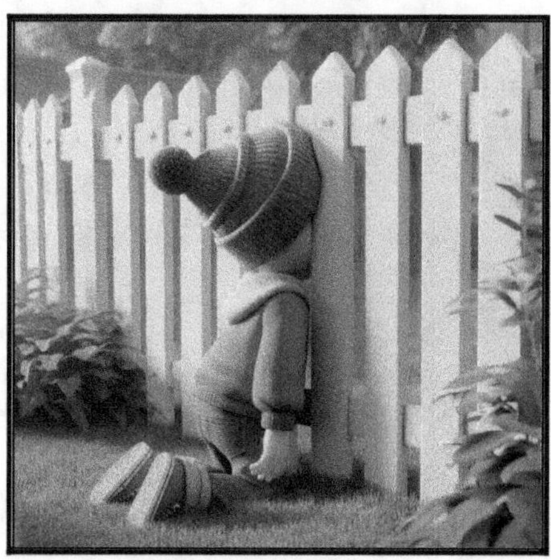

Childproofing your yard fence requires meticulous planning and execution to ensure the safety of your children.

## Material and Structure

**Smooth Surface:** Choose fencing materials with smooth surfaces to prevent splinters and other injuries. Avoid fences with sharp edges or points.

**Sturdy Construction:** The fence should be constructed with solid materials to withstand pressure or force, preventing it from collapsing or being easily climbed.

**Non-Toxic Materials:** Ensure that the materials used are non-toxic and do not have the potential to harm children if they happen to chew or lick the fence.

## Design and Layout

**Visibility:** While privacy is important, consider having sections of the fence where you can easily see through to monitor your children as they play.

**Height:** The fence should be tall enough to prevent children from climbing over it. Generally, a height of 4 feet or more is recommended.

**Gaps and Openings:** Make sure that there are no gaps or openings where children can squeeze through. Any slats should be spaced closely to prevent kids from getting their heads or limbs stuck.

### Gate and Locking Mechanism

**Self-Closing and Self-Latching Gates:** Install self-closing and self-latching gates to prevent children from accidentally leaving the yard unsupervised.

**Locks and Alarms:** Consider installing locks and alarms on the gates that notify you if they are opened.

### Surrounding Area

**Climbable Objects:** Ensure that no climbing objects are near the fence that children can use to scale it.

**Vegetation:** Be cautious about the type of vegetation near the fence. Avoid thorny or poisonous plants that could harm children.

### Maintenance

**Regular Inspections:** Conduct regular inspections to check for any damage or wear and tear that might create a safety hazard.

**Quick Repairs:** Address any issues promptly to maintain the safety of the fence.

### Education and Supervision

**Educate Your Children:** Teach your children about the importance of staying inside the fence and not attempting to climb it.

**Supervision:** Always supervise your children while they are playing in the yard, especially if they are very young.

Childproofing your yard fence is an ongoing process that requires regular checks and maintenance to ensure it remains safe and secure.

---

🍎 *According to the CPSC* From 1990–2010, about **37,673 children under age 7 were treated in U.S. emergency departments yearly due to injuries from gates and barriers,** averaging roughly 1,800 cases per year.

Children ages 2–6 were more likely injured by gate contact (e.g., pinches, cuts), whereas toddlers under 2 more often suffered falls due to gate collapses

---

# PICNIC TABLE SAFETY

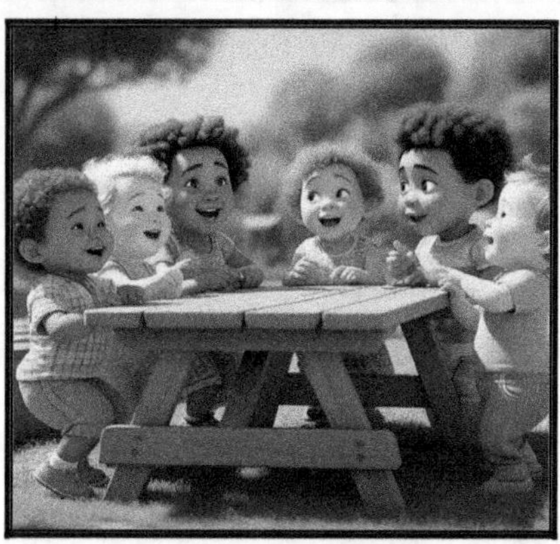

Secure the table to the ground. This will prevent it from tipping over if a child climbs on it.

**Ground Anchors:** These are metal spikes that you drive into the ground and then attach the table to them.

**Tiedowns:** These are straps that you can wrap around the table legs and secure to a tree or other solid object.

**Remove loose Items:** Remove loose items when they are not being used like tablecloths, placemats, and chairs. Make sure small items are not left on the table which could be a choking hazard for young children.

**Block Access to Sharp Edges:** If the table has any sharp edges, you can cover them with tape or rubber edging.

**Install Corner Guards:** These are plastic or rubber bumpers that you can attach to the corners of the table to prevent children from getting hurt if they bump into them.

**Keep the Table Clean and Free of Debris:** This will help to prevent children from tripping or slipping.

**Always Supervise Children:** Even if you have taken all of these precautions, it is still important to supervise children closely when they are near the table.

**If you have a dog,** make sure that the table is not accessible to them. Dogs can knock over tables and injure children.

**If you have a pool or other water feature** nearby, make sure that the table is not located too close to it. Children could climb on the table and fall into the water.

---

<u>Yard</u>
Infant/Non-mobile: (Birth - 6 months)
Infant crawl/roll: (5 months - 1 year)
→ **Toddler/Pre-school: (1 year - 4 years)**
→ **School-age: (5 years - 6+ years)**

# Yard Tool Safety

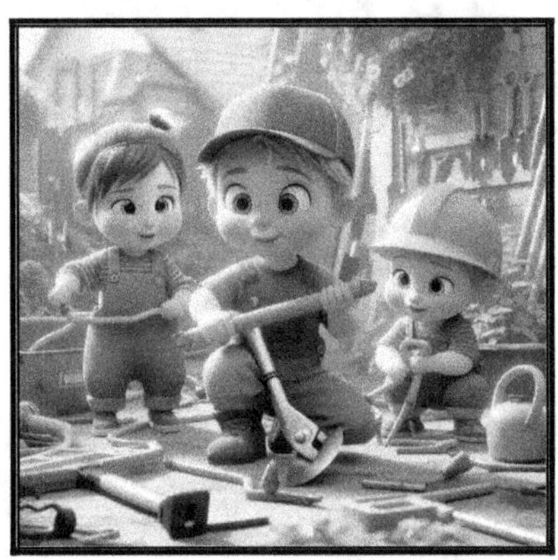

Yard tools can be very dangerous, and childproofing is essential in preventing accidents and ensuring the safety of your children.

## <u>Dangers</u>

**Sharp Edges:** Tools like saws, pruners, and shears have sharp edges that can cause cuts and severe injuries.

**Heavy Objects:** Heavy tools such as hammers and axes can cause bruises or more severe injuries if dropped or mishandled.

**Chemical Exposures:** Tools like sprayers may contain residues of harmful chemicals that can be dangerous if ingested or come in contact with skin.

**Tripping Hazards:** Tools left lying around can create tripping hazards, leading to falls and injuries.

**Electrical Tools:** Electric yard tools can cause electrocution if not handled correctly or if they are faulty.

## Precautions

**Designated Storage Area:** Create a designated storage area for all yard tools, ideally locked to prevent children from accessing them.

**Tool Covers:** Use tool covers to shield sharp edges and prevent accidents when tools are not in use.

**Secure Heavy Tools:** Store heavy tools so that they cannot be pulled down or tipped over.

**Supervision:** Never use potentially dangerous yard tools when children are around without another adult supervising them.

**Safety Gear:** When children are old enough to use yard tools, ensure they are wearing appropriate safety gear, including gloves, eye protection, and helmets as necessary.

**Education:** From an early age, teach children about the dangers associated with yard tools and instruct them never to touch these tools without adult supervision.

**Demo Safety Measures:** As children grow, demonstrate the correct way to handle tools safely, instilling good habits early on.

## Maintenance

**Regular Maintenance:** Ensure all tools are well maintained to prevent accidents due to malfunction or breakage.

**Electric Tool Safety:** When it comes to electrical tools, teach children the importance of keeping them away from water and the proper way to handle them to avoid electrocution.

## First Aid

**First Aid Kit:** Keep a first-aid kit readily accessible in the yard to immediately address minor injuries.

**Emergency Plan:** Have an emergency plan in place, and ensure children know what to do if they see someone getting hurt with a yard tool.

---

🍎 *According to Stanford Medicine Children's Health,* **over 5,900 young children (ages 0–5) are injured every year in the U.S. by yard tools.** About 4,800 from lawn mowers alone, and another 1,100+ from trimmers, rakes, shovels, and other equipment. Among toddlers (under 5), nearly 42% of mower injuries are burns, and lawn mowers cause around 600 amputations annually. It's a chilling reminder. Even simple yard chores carry serious risks for little ones.

---

# LAWNMOWER SAFETY

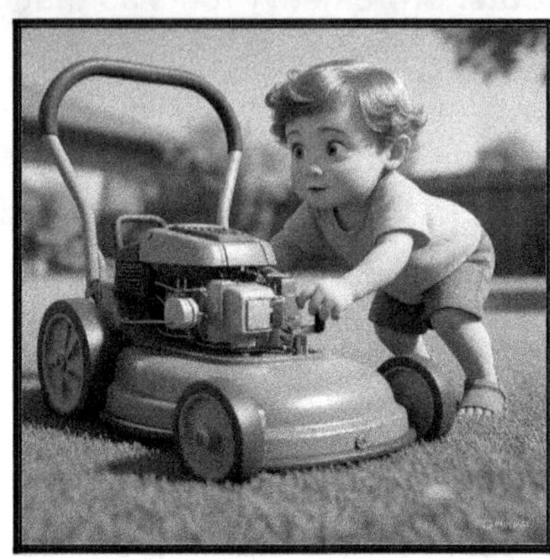

Children should never be in the yard or on a riding mower while it is being operated. According to the U.S. Consumer Product Safety Commission (CPSC). **More than 800 young children are run over or backed over by riding mowers each year**. This can happen when children fall off the mower while being given rides or when they approach the operating mower and are not seen until it is too late.

**Riding mowers can be very dangerous,** even for adults. They can weigh hundreds of pounds and have blades that can rotate at high speeds.

**Children are especially vulnerable** to riding mower injuries. They are small and may not be seen by the operator, and they may not be able to get out of the way of the mower in time.

**Even if you are not using the mower,** children should not be allowed in the yard while it is running. Even if it is not moving, the mower can still be a hazard.

<u>**It is Important to Take Steps to Keep Children Safe Around Riding Mowers**</u>

- **Never give children rides on a riding mower.**
- **Never allow children to operate a riding mower.**
- **Keep children away from the mower when it is running.**
- **Be aware of your surroundings** when you are mowing. Ensure no children or pets are in the area before you start mowing.

- **If you see a child** or pet in the area, stop the mower immediately. Do not start mowing again until the child or pet is safely away.

Many children suffer severe burns to their hands and arms when they touch the hot muffler of running or recently running engines. Keep children away from power equipment.

This also applies to hedge trimmers, where the noisy motor blocks out the sound of an approaching child.

---

<u>**Yard**</u>
Infant/Non-mobile: (Birth - 6 months)
Infant crawl/roll: (5 months - 1 year)
→ **Toddler/Pre-school: (1 year - 4 years)**
→ **School-age: (5 years - 6+ years)**

# YARD TOY SAFETY

Childproofing yard toys is important for creating a safe outdoor environment where children can play freely without the risk of injury. By understanding potential hazards and implementing preventive measures, you can ensure that your yard is a secure space for children to enjoy.

## Choking Hazards

**Small Parts:** Yard toys with small, detachable components, like building blocks or action figures, can pose a significant choking risk, especially for younger children who are prone to putting objects in their mouths.

**Balloons:** Broken balloon pieces can be particularly dangerous as they can easily get lodged in a child's throat, leading to choking.

## Strangulation Hazards

**Strings & Ropes:** Toys that include long strings, ropes, or cords, such as jump ropes or pull toys, can be a strangulation risk if they become wrapped around a child's neck.

**Bike Helmets:** While helmets are crucial for safety when riding, children should not wear them during other play activities as the straps can get caught on playground equipment or branches, posing a strangulation hazard.

## Tip and Fall Hazards

**Uneven Surfaces:** Toys that create an uneven playing surface, like toy trucks or wagons left on the ground, can cause children to trip and fall.

**Wet Toys:** Toys that become slippery when wet, such as plastic slides or inflatable pools, increase the risk of falls and injuries.

## Chemical Hazards

**Toxic Paints & Materials:** Some older or cheaply made toys may contain harmful chemicals or toxic paints, which can be hazardous if ingested or absorbed through the skin.

**Batteries:** Battery-operated toys can pose a risk if the batteries leak harmful chemicals or if small batteries like button cells are swallowed.

**Projectile Hazards:** Toys that shoot projectiles, such as darts, arrows, or balls, can cause serious injuries, particularly to the eyes.

**Heat-Related Hazards:** Toys with metal components can absorb heat from the sun and become hot enough to cause burns, especially in warm climates.

## Prevention Strategies

**Proper Storage:** Use weather-resistant storage bins to keep toys organized and prevent them from becoming tripping hazards. Proper storage also protects toys from weather damage. Store toys with metal parts in shaded areas to keep them cool and prevent burn injuries.

**Supervision:** Always supervise children, especially when they are playing with toys that have small parts, long strings, or can shoot projectiles. This ensures immediate intervention if a dangerous situation arises.

**Safe Toy Selection:** Choose toys suitable for your child's age and developmental level. This helps reduce the risk of choking, strangulation, and other injuries. Select toys made from non-toxic, BPA-free materials, and ensure any paints or finishes are lead-free and safe for children.

**Regular Inspections:** Regularly check toys for wear and tear, such as cracks, sharp edges, or loose parts. Discard or repair any damaged toys immediately. Routinely inspect battery-operated toys to ensure batteries are intact and not leaking. Replace worn-out batteries promptly.

**Education:** Educate children on the importance of safe play. Teach them not to put toys in their mouths, to be mindful of others when playing with projectiles, and to play cautiously to avoid trips and falls. Make sure children know how to seek help in an emergency, such as finding an adult if they or another child are hurt.

**Surface Safety:** Install soft surfaces like grass, mulch, or rubber mats in play areas to cushion falls and reduce the severity of injuries. Regularly clear the play area of debris, toys, and other obstacles that could cause trips and falls.

**First Aid:** Keep a well-stocked first aid kit easily accessible in the yard. Include bandages, antiseptic wipes, and other essentials to quickly address any minor injuries.

---

🍎 *U.S. Consumer Product Safety Commission (CPSC).* In backyards across America, an estimated **208,000 young children** (ages 0–6) are treated in emergency rooms every year for injuries caused by yard toys. Everything from trampolines and ride-on scooters to playsets and bounce houses. That's over **22 kids every hour, injured while doing something as innocent as playing outside.**

---

<u>Yard</u>
Infant/Non-mobile: (Birth - 6 months)
Infant crawl/roll: (5 months - 1 year)
→ **Toddler/Pre-school: (1 year - 4 years)**
→ **School-age: (5 years - 6+ years)**

# SANDBOX SAFETY

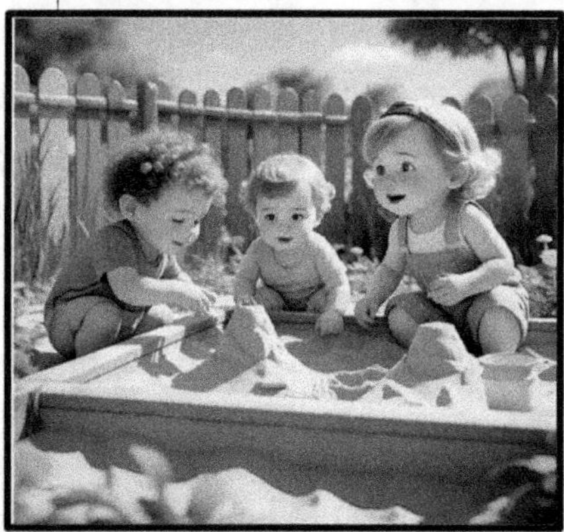

A sandbox can provide endless fun and sensory play for children, but it also comes with some child safety concerns that need to be addressed.

**Sandbox Location:** Choose a suitable location away from direct sunlight to prevent overheating during hot weather. Also, avoid placing it under trees or near overhanging branches that could drop debris into the sandbox.

**Cover When Not in Use:** When not in use, cover the sandbox with a secure and well-fitting lid or tarp to prevent animals from using it as a litter box and keep it free from debris and rainwater.

**Inspect for Hazards:** Before allowing children to play, regularly inspect the sandbox for broken glass, sharp objects, or other potential hazards.

**Clean Sand:** Use clean and washed play sand without any contaminants, chemicals, or harmful substances.

**Sun Protection:** Provide shade or use a sun umbrella to protect children from the sun's harmful UV rays while playing in the sandbox.

**Proper Clothing:** Encourage children to wear appropriate clothing, such as hats and closed-toe shoes, to protect them from the sun and sand.

**No Eating or Drinking:** Teach children not to eat or drink while playing in the sandbox to prevent the ingestion of sand and potential health issues.

**Supervision:** Always supervise young children while they play in the sandbox to prevent them from engaging in unsafe behaviors or sharing sand toys that may pose choking hazards.

**Insect Control:** Take measures to control insects in the sandbox to avoid stings or bites.

**Allergies:** Be aware of any allergies to sand or outdoor elements that your children may have and take appropriate precautions.

**Clean Hands:** Encourage children to wash their hands thoroughly after playing in the sandbox, especially before eating.

**Keep Cats Away:** To prevent cats from using the sandbox as a litter box, consider using natural deterrents or placing physical barriers around it.

**Size and Depth:** Ensure the sandbox is appropriate in size and depth, allowing enough room for children to play comfortably without overcrowding.

**Regular Maintenance:** Regularly rake and maintain the sand to keep it clean and free from debris.

**Sand Toy Safety:** Provide age-appropriate and safe sand toys that are free from sharp edges or small parts that could pose choking hazards.

---

# HIDE 'N SEEK

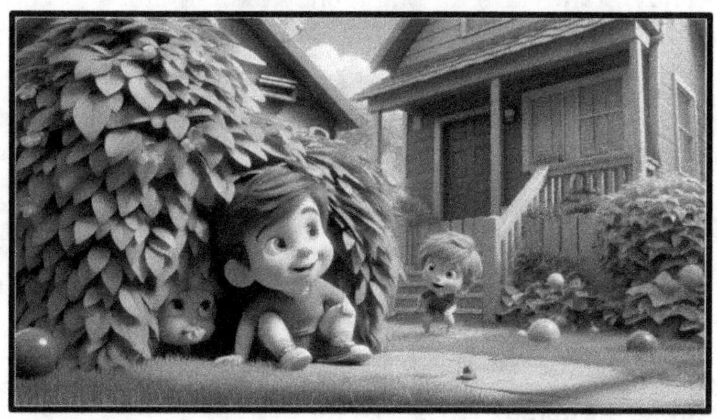

Hide and Seek is a classic and enjoyable game that children love to play. However, to ensure a fun and risk-free experience, it's essential to consider child safety while playing this game.

**Choose Safe Hiding Places:** Encourage children to hide in safe and visible areas. Avoid places with potential hazards, such as near traffic, bodies of water, or sharp objects.

**Set Boundaries:** Establish clear boundaries for the game to ensure that children do not wander too far from the play area.

**Supervision:** Always have adult supervision during the game, especially for younger children. The supervisor can ensure that all participants are safe and following the rules.

**Avoid Enclosed Spaces:** To prevent accidental lock-ins or entrapment, discourage children from hiding in enclosed spaces, such as locked rooms, large containers, or small cabinets.

**Communication:** Teach children to communicate clearly and calmly if they are in distress or need help during the game.

**Avoid Darkness:** Avoid playing hide-and-seek in dark or poorly lit areas to reduce the risk of falls and injuries.

**Check Before Seeking:** Before counting and seeking, ensure that all children are in safe hiding spots, not dangerous areas.

**Play with Familiar Playmates:** Play Hide and Seek with children who are familiar with the game's rules and safety guidelines.

**Age-Appropriate Boundaries:** Set different boundaries for older and younger children to ensure a safe level of challenge for each age group.

**Emergency Plan:** Have an emergency plan in place in case a child gets hurt or lost during the game. Make sure all participants know what to do in case of an emergency.

**Inclusive Play:** Consider the abilities and limitations of all players to ensure that the game is inclusive and accessible for everyone.

**Respect Private Areas:** Teach children to respect private areas or spaces that are off-limits for hiding.

**Be Mindful of Furniture:** Avoid hiding behind or inside furniture that may tip over or cause injury.

**No Climbing:** Discourage children from climbing on structures or trees during the game.

**Fair Play:** Encourage fair play and sportsmanship among participants.

Ensuring adult supervision, setting clear boundaries, and teaching children about safe hiding places are essential elements for promoting child safety during this popular game.

---

<u>Yard</u>
Infant/Non-mobile: (Birth - 6 months)
Infant crawl/roll: (5 months - 1 year)
→ **Toddler/Pre-school: (1 year - 4 years)**
→ **School-age: (5 years - 6+ years)**

# WELL-DRAINED YARD PLAY AREA

A well-drained play area is crucial for child safety, especially during outdoor activities.

**Preventing Puddles and Water Accumulation:** A well-drained play area ensures that rainwater and other liquids do not accumulate, preventing the formation of puddles that could pose slipping hazards for children.

**Reducing Trip and Fall Hazards:** Proper drainage helps keep the play area dry and free from mud, reducing the risk of trips and falls.

**Preventing Mosquito Breeding:** Standing water can become a breeding ground for mosquitoes carrying diseases. A well-drained play area minimizes the risk of mosquito infestations.

**Maintaining Play Equipment Integrity:** Water accumulation around play equipment can lead to rust and deterioration, compromising its safety and longevity.

**Site Selection:** Choose a location that naturally allows water to flow away from the play area. Avoid areas with poor drainage, low spots, or places prone to flooding.

**Grading and Sloping:** Grade the play area to slope slightly away from the play structures. This allows water to drain away naturally.

**Install Drainage Systems:** For areas with more significant drainage challenges, consider installing drainage systems such as French drains, swales, or catch basins to direct water away from the play area.

**Use Permeable Materials:** For the playing surface, opt for permeable materials such as rubber tiles, mulch, or gravel. These materials allow water to pass through, reducing runoff and promoting better drainage.

**Regular Maintenance:** Keep the play area clear of debris, leaves, and other materials that can clog drainage systems or impede water flow.

**Inspect and Repair:** Regularly inspect the play area for any drainage issues and promptly address any problems, such as clogged drains or erosion.

Ensuring proper drainage in the play area creates a safer and more enjoyable environment for children to play and explore without concerns about water accumulation or slipping hazards.

---

**Notes:**

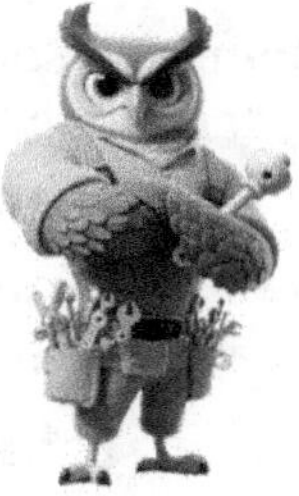

# SWING SET SAFETY

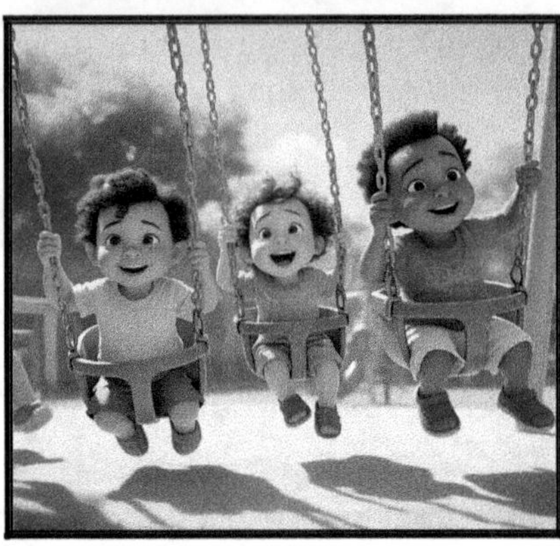

Play area safety is paramount to protect children while they engage in outdoor play. Let's address the specific safety concerns related to tubes on swing sets and sand underneath swings.

## <u>Tubes on Swing Sets</u>

**Entrapment Hazards:** Ensure that the tubes on swing sets have appropriate openings or are designed to prevent the entrapment of children's heads, limbs, or clothing.

**Secure Installation:** Check that the tubes are securely fastened to the swing set frame to prevent them from loosening or detaching during play.

## <u>Sand Underneath Swings</u>

**Depth and Cushioning:** Ensure that the sand under the swings is of an adequate depth to provide sufficient cushioning in case of falls. A depth of at least 12 inches is recommended to help absorb impact.

**Maintain Sand Level:** Regularly inspect and maintain the sand surface to ensure it remains at the appropriate depth. Rake and level the sand as needed to prevent uneven surfaces.

**Free of Debris:** Keep the sand area free from any debris, sharp objects, or rocks that could cause injuries during play.

**Impact Zones:** Establish a clear zone around the swings where children should not be standing or playing to avoid collisions with other swinging children.

**Supervision:** Always provide adult supervision during playtime to quickly respond to any emergencies or potential hazards.

**Age-Appropriate Play:** Ensure that the play area and equipment are suitable for the children's age and developmental level.

**Regular Inspections:** Regularly inspect the play area, including swing sets and other equipment, for signs of wear, damage, or potential hazards. Address any issues promptly.

**Soft Surfaces:** Consider using soft surfaces like rubber tiles, wood chips, or rubber mulch under play equipment to provide cushioning in case of falls.

**Sun Protection:** Provide shade or use sun umbrellas to protect children from excessive sun exposure during outdoor play.

**Proper Use:** Educate children on how to use play equipment safely and enforce rules to promote safe play behaviors.

**Clear Space:** Ensure there is ample clear space around play equipment to avoid collisions with other children or nearby objects.

---

**Yard**

Infant/Non-mobile: (Birth - 6 months)
Infant crawl/roll: (5 months - 1 year)
→ **Toddler/Pre-school: (1 year - 4 years)**
→ **School-age: (5 years - 6+ years)**

# BUILDING A BETTER PLAY AREA

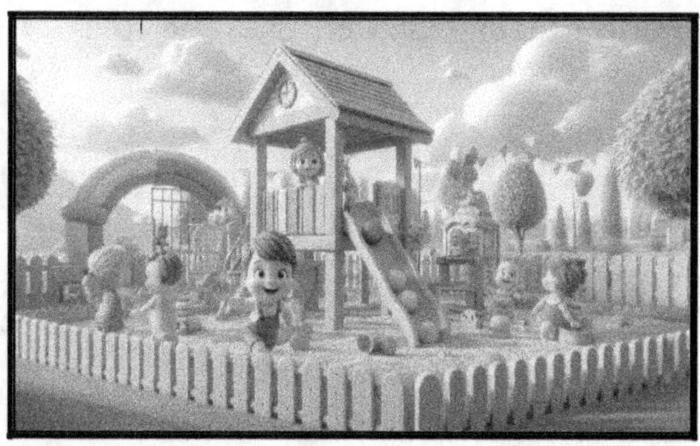

**Choose a Safe Location:** Select a flat and level area away from traffic, water features, and potential hazards. Ensure there are no overhanging branches or obstacles that could pose a risk.

**Proper Ground Surface:** Under play equipment, use a soft and impact-absorbing ground surface like rubber tiles, wood chips, or rubber mulch to cushion falls and reduce the risk of injuries.

**Age-Appropriate Equipment:** Install age-appropriate play equipment that suits the children's developmental level and abilities.

**Sturdy and Well-Maintained Equipment:** Ensure that all play equipment is sturdy, properly anchored, and free from sharp edges or protruding parts. Regularly inspect and maintain the equipment to keep it safe.

**No Trip Hazards:** Keep the play area free from tripping hazards such as rocks, tree roots, or debris.

**Fence the Play Area:** Consider fencing the play area to prevent unauthorized access and to keep children safely contained.

**Safe Entry and Exit Points:** Install easy-to-use entry and exit points for children, such as ramps or steps with handrails, to ensure secure access to the play area.

**Shade and Sun Protection:** Provide shade structures or use sun umbrellas to protect children from sunburn and overheating during hot weather.

**Water Safety:** If there is a water play feature, ensure proper supervision and age-appropriate safety measures to prevent drowning.

**Supervision:** Always have adult supervision during playtime to monitor children's activities and quickly respond to any emergencies.

**Age-Appropriate Rules:** Teach children the rules of safe play and enforce them consistently.

**Safe Swings:** If including swings, make sure they have appropriate seat restraints, and provide enough space between swings to prevent collisions.

**Avoid Toxic Materials:** Use non-toxic and child-safe materials for construction and avoid any chemicals that could be harmful to children.

**Accessibility:** To promote inclusive play, consider making the playground accessible to children of all abilities, including those with physical disabilities.

**Emergency Plan:** Establish an emergency plan and ensure that all caregivers and supervisors are aware of it

To create a safe play area, choose a suitable location and use proper ground surfaces. Install age-appropriate equipment, maintain equipment regularly, and eliminate trip hazards. The area should be fenced with safe entry and exit points. It should offer shade and sun protection. Ensure water safety, avoid toxic materials, and use safe swings and equipment. Always supervise children, enforce age-appropriate rules, and consider accessibility. Make sure you have an emergency plan in place.

---

**Yard**

Infant/Non-mobile: (Birth - 6 months)
Infant crawl/roll: (5 months - 1 year)
→ **Toddler/Pre-school: (1 year - 4 years)**
→ **School-age: (5 years - 6+ years)**

# Bicycle/Scooter/Skateboard Safety

**Bicycle injuries:** 100,000+ ER visits yearly (CDC). Always wear helmets. Proper bike size. Traffic rules. Safe areas. Supervise. Reflectors/lights.

**E-bikes:** battery hazards, heavier, faster, complex—store securely, lowest speed setting.

**Scooters/skates/boards:** 10,000 injured yearly (NEISS-CDC). Protective gear. Smooth surfaces. Avoid high speeds. Supervise.

---

**Yard**

Infant/Non-mobile: (Birth - 6 months)
Infant crawl/roll: (5 months - 1 year)
→ **Toddler/Pre-school: (1 year - 4 years)**
→ **School-age: (5 years - 6+ years)**

# Trampoline Safety

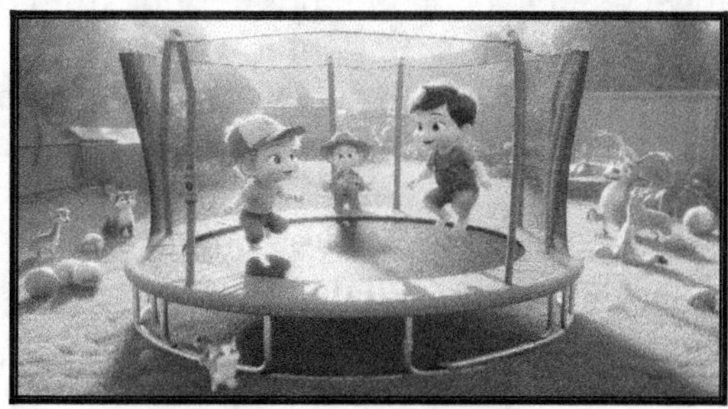

**100,000 children treated yearly (CDC).** Always supervise. Age restrictions. One jumper at time. No flips. Safety enclosures. Proper setup. Soft landing surface. Regular inspections. No jumping from height. Time limits.

# GARDEN HOSE CONCERNS

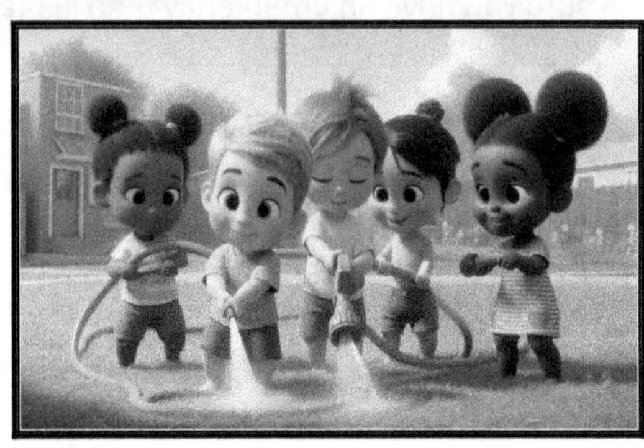

Childproofing a garden hose is important for preventing accidents and ensuring that children are kept safe while in outdoor spaces. Key precautions include storing the hose properly, using a hose reel or wall-mounted holder to keep it neatly coiled and off the ground, which minimizes tripping hazards. Elevating the hose using hooks or hangers also helps to keep it out of children's way. Regularly inspecting the hose for sharp edges, kinks, and wear and tear is crucial, as damaged areas can cause injuries or disruptions in water flow. Additionally, removing nozzles and spray attachments when not in use prevents children from accidentally turning on the water, which could lead to soaking or injury. Reducing water pressure around children adds another layer of safety by preventing high-pressure accidents.

Further steps involve teaching children not to drink from the garden hose due to potential contaminants or water temperature issues. Using childproof hose bib attachments ensures that children cannot turn the water on unsupervised. It is also important to store watering tools such as sprinklers or spray nozzles out of reach when not in use and opt for child-friendly designs. Always supervise children during use and keep them at a safe distance when watering plants. Additionally, regularly inspecting and maintaining the hose, as well as educating children on safe usage, reinforces the importance of safety around garden hoses. **Annually, approximately 1,000 children are injured by lawn sprinklers and irrigation systems**, including trips and falls. (Source: U.S. Consumer Product Safety Commission (CPSC) - Outdoor Equipment Safety)

❦ This is the most immediate physical danger. A hose left in the summer sun is effectively a **solar water heater**. Water inside a garden hose exposed to direct sunlight can reach temperatures of **140°F to 150°F. At $140°F, it takes only 5 seconds** for an adult to sustain a third-degree burn. Because a child's skin is significantly thinner, a "full-thickness" (third-degree) burn can occur almost instantly. **The Scenario:** A parent turns on the hose to fill a kiddie pool or spray a child; the initial "slug" of stagnant, superheated water hits the child before the cool water from the underground pipes arrives. *Safe Kids Worldwide / Burn Foundation statistics on "Solar-Heated Water Scalding."*

<u>**Yard**</u>
Infant/Non-mobile: (Birth - 6 months)
Infant crawl/roll: (5 months - 1 year)
→ **Toddler/Pre-school: (1 year - 4 years)**
→ **School-age: (5 years - 6+ years)**

# Bird Bath Concerns

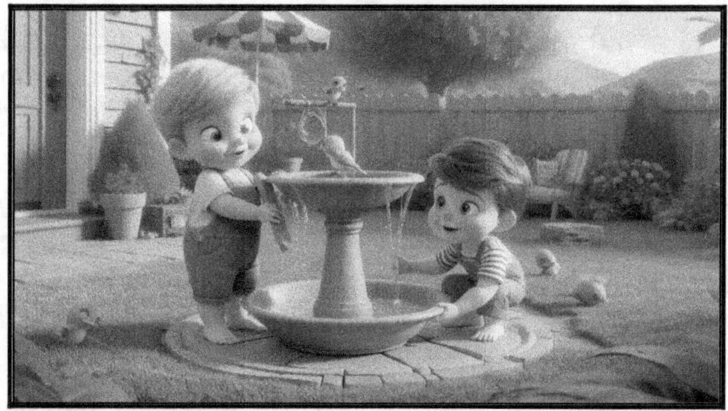

**Elevate the Bird Bath:** Consider elevating the bird bath on a sturdy pedestal or platform to keep it out of reach of young children. This will help prevent accidental falls or splashing.

**Smooth Edges:** Ensure that the edges of the bird bath are smooth and rounded to minimize the risk of cuts or injuries.

**Safe Material:** Choose a bird bath made of child-safe materials, such as non-toxic resin, stone, or ceramic, to avoid any potential harm from harmful chemicals.

**Stability and Weight:** The bird bath should be stable and heavy enough to prevent tipping or toppling over if a child tries to climb on it.

**Secure Placement:** To minimize the risk of children colliding with it, place the birdbath away from play areas or high-traffic zones.

**No Deep Water:** Avoid filling the bird bath with deep water, which may pose a drowning risk to young children. Keep the water level shallow, allowing birds to bathe safely without creating a hazard for kids.

**Keep It Clean:** Regularly clean the bird bath to prevent the growth of algae or bacteria that could be harmful if children come into contact with the water.

**No Chemicals:** Do not use chemical additives or treatments in the bird bath water, as children might accidentally touch or ingest them.

**Cover when Not in Use:** When the bird bath is not in use, consider covering it with a childproof cover or net to prevent curious children from exploring it.

**Supervision:** Always supervise children around the bird bath to ensure their safety and to prevent them from touching the water or any decorative elements.

**Educate About Birds:** Teach children about the importance of bird baths and the significance of leaving them undisturbed to attract and nurture birds.

**Inspect for Hazards:** Regularly inspect the bird bath for any signs of wear, damage, or potential hazards. Repair or replace any issues promptly.

**Secure Surrounding Area:** To prevent accidents, keep the area around the bird bath free of tripping hazards, such as toys or garden tools.

**Use Child-Friendly Bird Baths:** If possible, choose bird baths with child-friendly designs, smooth surfaces, and no small parts that might pose choking hazards.

You can make the bird bath area safer for children and create a welcoming environment for both birds and kids to enjoy the outdoors responsibly.

---

# WATER FEATURE CONCERNS

Fencing around water features is a critical child safety measure to prevent accidents and protect young children from potential hazards.

**Drowning Prevention:** The most significant concern is drowning, which is a leading cause of accidental death in young children. Fencing creates a physical barrier between children and the water, reducing the risk of accidental entry and drowning incidents.

**Curiosity and Exploration:** Children are naturally curious and may be drawn to the water feature, unaware of its dangers. Fencing acts as a deterrent, limiting access and discouraging unsupervised exploration.

**Fast Access to Water:** Children can move quickly and reach a water feature before parents or caregivers intervene. Fencing provides an additional layer of protection and buys valuable time to react and prevent accidents.

**Unpredictable Behavior:** Young children can exhibit unpredictable behavior, such as climbing or reaching for objects near the water feature. A fence can prevent them from accidentally falling in or getting too close to the water.

**Preventing Climbing:** Fencing should be designed to avoid climbing. Children might try to climb over the fence, so it's crucial to ensure it is tall enough and doesn't have any footholds or objects nearby that could aid climbing.

**Protection from Accidental Falls:** Water features like ponds or waterfalls may have slippery surfaces or uneven terrain surrounding them, increasing the risk of accidental falls. Fencing keeps children at a safe distance away from such areas.

**Supervision Limitations:** Even with diligent supervision, accidents can happen. A fence provides an additional safety measure, reducing the reliance solely on adult supervision.

**Unsupervised Access:** In settings like public parks or community areas, a fence helps prevent unauthorized or unsupervised access to water features, ensuring they are enjoyed responsibly.

**Compliance with Regulations:** In many jurisdictions, installing fencing around certain types of water features is required by law to meet safety standards.

**Education and Awareness:** Fencing also serves as a visual reminder for children and adults about the potential dangers of the water feature and the importance of staying away when unsupervised.

Fencing helps keep children safe by creating a physical barrier and allows for worry-free enjoyment of water features under appropriate supervision. It is a responsible and effective way to protect young children and ensure they can explore and play safely in their surroundings.

---

**Yard**
→ **Infant/Non-mobile: (Birth - 6 months)**
→ **Infant crawl/roll: (5 months - 1 year)**
→ **Toddler/Pre-school: (1 year - 4 years)**
→ **School-age: (5 years - 6+ years)**

# Septic Tanks and Water Well Security

Child safety concerns related to wells and septic tanks are significant due to their potential dangers to young children.

## Water Wells

**Water Well Caps and Covers:** Ensure wells have secure and child-resistant caps or covers. The cover should be durable, lockable, and capable of withstanding a child's weight to prevent accidental falls into the well.

**Regular Inspections:** Conduct regular inspections of the well cover to check for damage or wear. If any issues are identified, repair or replace the cover immediately.

**Fencing and Barriers:** Install a fence or barrier around the well to restrict access and prevent children from getting too close to the opening. The fence should be at a safe distance from the well to avoid accidents.

**Supervision:** Always supervise young children when they are playing outside to prevent them from wandering near the well.

**Educate Children:** Teach children about the dangers of wells and the importance of staying away from them. Create clear rules about not playing around wells.

**No Play Equipment Near Wells:** Keep play equipment, such as swings or slides, away from the well area to prevent children from accidentally falling into the well.

### Septic Tanks

**Tank Covers and Lids:** Ensure that septic tank covers and lids are secure and child resistant. Consider using lockable covers to prevent unauthorized access.

**Clear Signage:** Display clear and visible warning signs near the septic tank area to indicate the presence of a hazardous site.

**Fencing and Barriers:** Install a fence or barrier around the septic tank area to prevent children from accessing it.

**Regular Inspections:** Regularly inspect the septic tank covers and lids to check for any signs of damage or wear. Repair or replace them promptly if needed.

**Supervision:** Supervise young children when they are playing outside to ensure they do not go near the septic tank area.

**No Digging:** Instruct children not to dig or play in the ground near the septic tank area, as this could damage the tank or cause accidents.

**Safe Landscaping:** Choose landscaping materials, such as thorny bushes or gravel, that deter children from playing near the septic tank area.

**Proper Maintenance:** Ensure the septic tank is properly maintained and emptied regularly to reduce the risk of overflows or leaks.

**Educate Children:** Teach children about the potential dangers of septic tanks and the importance of staying away from them.

Overall, taking these safety measures seriously is crucial to protect children from potential hazards associated with wells and septic tanks. Regular maintenance, proper covers and barriers, and constant supervision are crucial to ensuring child safety around these areas.

---

🏵 Septic tanks and wells can hide lethal dangers right in your backyard. While no U.S. data isolates toddlers, legal records estimate about **50 child fatalities per year from unsecured septic tanks. In one Florida county, a child under 5 lost their life in such a tank.** Add wells and cisterns, and you're looking at an under reported but unmistakable threat to young children. *-House Digest*

---

# Teach Your Child to Swim

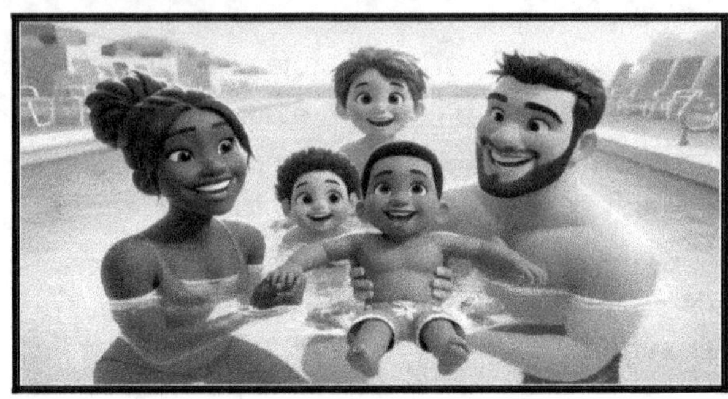

Start your child's water safety journey early by introducing them to swimming at a young age. Some believe that newborns have an innate ability to swim to the surface, and many community centers offer swim lessons tailored for infants, toddlers, and school-aged children. Seize this opportunity to instill a love for swimming and ensure your kids are equipped for a lifetime of summer fun. However, it's essential to remember that even proficient swimmers are not entirely safe when alone in a pool. Shockingly, according to the U.S. Consumer Product Safety Commission (CPSC) swimming pools rank as the second-leading cause of death in children under five years old. It takes less than four minutes for a person to drown, emphasizing the critical importance of constant supervision and vigilance around water.

If your child ever goes missing, always **check the pool first** in case of an accident. Never underestimate the potential risks of water, even if your child appears confident in swimming. Enroll them in formal swimming lessons but remember that adult supervision and proper pool safety measures are equally indispensable in ensuring your child's safety in and around water.

---

**Yard**
Infant/Non-mobile: (Birth - 6 months)
Infant crawl/roll: (5 months - 1 year)
→ **Toddler/Pre-school: (1 year - 4 years)**
→ **School-age: (5 years - 6+ years)**

# PFD's (Life Jacket) Information

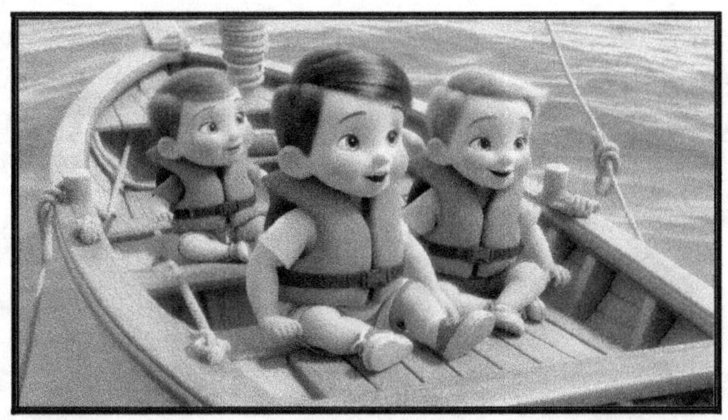

**Life jackets should be U.S. Coast Guard approved, correct type and size for each child's weight. Check straps and buckles periodically.** The reaching pole should be non-conductive (fiberglass or plastic), 12 to 16 feet long with securely attached Shepherd's Crook. Keep phone in waterproof pouch well away from pool, charged and labeled "EMERGENCY PHONE." First aid kit should be waterproof, stored with phone, including bandages, gauze, tape, antiseptic wipes, antibiotic ointment, gloves, CPR mask, emergency blanket, trauma pads, tweezers, scissors, and cold packs. Safety signs made of durable materials placed prominently: depth markers, NO DIVING warnings, pool rules, emergency numbers, CPR instructions. Fencing at least 4 feet high with self-closing, self-latching gates. Inspect regularly, consider installing alarm. Actively watch children in pool. Never leave unsupervised, even briefly. Adults avoid distractions like phones.

---

**Yard**
Infant/Non-mobile: (Birth - 6 months)
→ **Infant crawl/roll: (5 months - 1 year)**
→ **Toddler/Pre-school: (1 year - 4 years)**
→ **School-age: (5 years - 6+ years)**

# Don't Be Overconfident!

**Swimmies and floaties are fantastic aids for beginners, ensuring those little smiling faces have help staying afloat and visible in the water.** However, it's crucial to remember that these floatation devices are not a substitute for vigilant su pervision. While they provide valuable support, they should never replace the watchful eye of an adult. **Arm floaties, rubber duckies, or even life jackets are not enough to ensure a child's safety without proper supervision.** These accessories are designed to assist in swimming but should always be accompanied by responsible adult supervision. Even the most proficient swimmers need someone to watch over them to prevent accidents.

**So, don't rely solely on floatation devices when enjoying water activities with your little ones.** Be the lifeguard they need by always keeping a close eye on them. Together with the right safety gear and vigilant supervision, you can create a safe and enjoyable water experience for your children.

---

<u>Yard</u>
Infant/Non-mobile: (Birth - 6 months)
Infant crawl/roll: (5 months - 1 year)
→ **Toddler/Pre-school: (1 year - 4 years)**
→ **School-age: (5 years - 6+ years)**

# Pool Gates

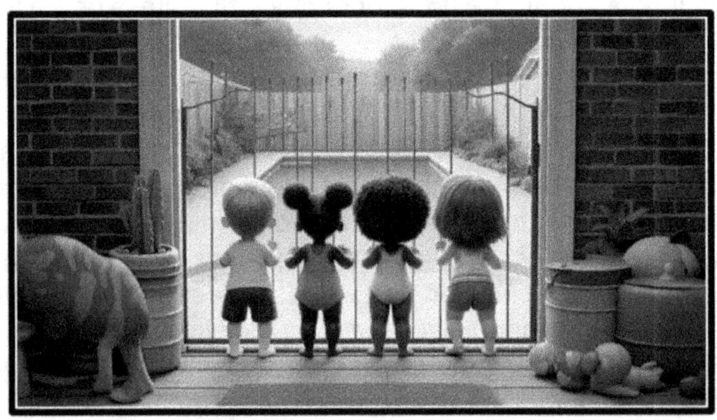

Gating a pool is of utmost importance for child safety and is essential in preventing accidents and potential tragedies.

**Drowning Prevention:** Drowning is a significant risk for young children, especially those under the age of five. Gating a pool acts as a physical barrier that keeps children from accessing the pool area unsupervised, significantly reducing the risk of accidental drowning.

**Preventing Unsupervised Access:** Children are naturally curious and may be drawn to water without understanding the dangers it poses. A pool gate with a secure latch ensures that children cannot access the pool area without adult supervision.

**A Layer of Protection:** A pool gate is an additional layer of protection that complements adult supervision. Even with vigilant monitoring, a moment of distraction can occur, and a closed and locked gate provides an extra barrier to prevent unsupervised entry.

**Safety Compliance:** In many jurisdictions, installing a pool gate is required by law to meet safety standards. Failure to comply with these regulations can result in legal consequences and, more importantly, jeopardize the safety of children.

**Types of Pool Gates:** Pool gates come in various designs, including self-closing and self-latching options. Choose a gate at least four feet high with a latch that children cannot open easily.

**Gating Additional Water Features:** If your pool has additional water features, such as fountains or spas, make sure to gate these areas as well to prevent access when not in use.

**Fence Material:** To deter children from attempting to scale the fence, consider using a fence material that is difficult to climb, such as smooth vinyl or metal.

**Education and Rules:** Educate children about pool safety and establish clear rules regarding pool access. Teach them never to attempt to open the gate without adult permission.

**Supervision Reminders:** Never leave children unattended around the water, even with a pool gate. Constant adult supervision is vital, and the gate should serve as an added safety measure, not a substitute for supervision.

**Regular Maintenance:** Inspect the pool gate regularly to ensure it is in good condition. Check for damage, loose parts, or malfunctioning latches and address issues promptly.

Gating a pool is a critical safety measure to protect children from the risks associated with water. By providing a physical barrier, gating ensures that children can only access the pool area under adult supervision, significantly reducing the chances of accidents and providing parents and caregivers with peace of mind. Always prioritize water safety and remember that a pool gate is just one piece of the comprehensive safety measures needed to create a safe and enjoyable swimming environment for children.

---

<u>Yard</u>
→ **Infant/Non-mobile: (Birth - 6 months)**
→ **Infant crawl/roll: (5 months - 1 year)**
→ **Toddler/Pre-school: (1 year - 4 years)**
→ **School-age: (5 years - 6+ years)**

# CPR (Cardiopulmonary Resuscitation)

Child safety and the importance of CPR (Cardiopulmonary Resuscitation) go hand in hand, as CPR can be a life-saving skill in emergencies.

**Rapid Response in Emergencies:** Accidents and medical emergencies can happen at any time, and children, in particular, are vulnerable to injuries. Knowing CPR enables adults to provide immediate assistance while waiting for professional medical help to arrive.

**Preventing Brain Damage and Death:** In critical situations like drowning, choking, or cardiac arrest, CPR can help maintain blood flow to vital organs, especially the brain, until emergency services arrive. Early initiation of CPR increases the chances of a positive outcome and reduces the risk of permanent brain damage or death.

**Common Childhood Emergencies:** Children are prone to various accidents and medical emergencies, such as choking on small objects, near-drowning incidents, or sudden cardiac events. Being trained in CPR empowers caregivers to respond appropriately.

**Immediate Action Matters:** In cardiac arrest cases, the survival rate drops by approximately 10% for every minute that passes without CPR. Quick and effective CPR can make a significant difference in the outcome.

**Peace of Mind:** Knowing CPR provides parents, caregivers, and teachers with confidence and a sense of empowerment to handle emergencies effectively, creating a safer environment for children.

**Safety at Home and in Public Places:** CPR skills are valuable both at home and in public spaces. Children spend considerable time in various environments, and CPR-trained individuals can respond effectively in any setting.

**Complementing Professional Help:** While waiting for emergency medical services to arrive, CPR acts as a bridge to maintain blood circulation and oxygen supply, improving the child's chances of survival.

**Standard First Aid Training:** CPR training is a standard in first aid courses, which also teach participants how to manage injuries and medical emergencies specific to children.

**Community Awareness:** Widespread knowledge of CPR within a community increases the likelihood that someone nearby can assist in an emergency, making communities safer for children.

**Empowerment for Teenagers:** Teaching CPR to teenagers can empower them to respond effectively in emergencies and even become responsible babysitters or caregivers for younger siblings.

CPR is a critical skill that plays a significant role in child safety. Being trained in CPR enables adults to respond promptly and effectively during emergencies, improving the chances of positive outcomes and reducing the severity of potential injuries. CPR education should be accessible to all caregivers, parents, teachers, and older children to create a safer environment for children and foster a community that is well-prepared to handle emergencies.

---

**Yard**
→ **Infant/Non-mobile: (Birth - 6 months)**
→ **Infant crawl/roll: (5 months - 1 year)**
→ **Toddler/Pre-school: (1 year - 4 years)**
→ **School-age: (5 years - 6+ years)**

# LIFE-SAVING EDUCATION

Taking a child life-saving course is a proactive and responsible step to ensure the safety of children in various situations. These courses typically cover essential skills, techniques, and knowledge necessary to respond effectively to emergencies involving children.

**CPR and First Aid Skills:** Child life-saving courses teach essential CPR, and first aid skills explicitly tailored to respond to emergencies involving infants, toddlers, and older children. Participants learnhow to provide immediate assistance in critical situations, such as choking, drowning, or cardiac arrest.

**Accident Prevention:** Child life-saving courses often include valuable information on accident prevention, highlighting potential hazards at home, at school, and in public spaces. Understanding and addressing these risks can significantly reduce the likelihood of accidents.

**Quick and Confident Response:** Knowing how to respond promptly and confidently in emergencies can make a life-saving difference for a child. Child life-saving courses help build the necessary skills and boost participants' confidence in handling challenging situations.

**Preparedness for Caregivers:** Parents, grandparents, teachers, babysitters, and anyone responsible for children can greatly benefit from child life-saving courses. Being prepared to handle emergencies increases children's safety and provides caregivers with peace of mind.

**Specialized Techniques:** Child life-saving courses often cover specialized techniques, such as caring for children with specific medical conditions, dealing with allergic reactions, or managing pediatric injuries.

**Emergency Scenarios Practice:** These courses often include practical exercises and simulations of emergency scenarios involving children. This hands-on experience helps participants apply their knowledge and skills in a controlled setting.

**Community Safety:** Widespread participation in child life-saving courses enhances overall community safety. The more people trained in life-saving skills mean that there is a higher likelihood of someone nearby being able to respond effectively in an emergency.

**Certification:** Many children's life-saving courses offer certification upon successful completion, which can be valuable for certain professions or when seeking babysitting or caregiving opportunities.

Individuals can actively promote child safety and well-being within their families and communities by taking a child life-saving course. Being prepared to respond effectively in emergencies involving children can save lives and make a positive difference in critical situations.

---

<u>Yard</u>
→ **Infant/Non-mobile: (Birth - 6 months)**
→ **Infant crawl/roll: (5 months - 1 year)**
→ **Toddler/Pre-school: (1 year - 4 years)**
→ **School-age: (5 years - 6+ years)**

# KEEP RESCUE EQUIPMENT AND A PHONE NEAR THE POOL

**Life jackets should be U.S. Coast Guard approved, correct type and size for each child's weight.** Check straps and buckles periodically. The reaching pole should be non-conductive (fiberglass or plastic), 12 to 16 feet long with securely attached Shepherd's Crook. Keep phone in waterproof pouch well away from pool, charged and labeled "EMERGENCY PHONE." First aid kit should be waterproof, stored with phone, including bandages, gauze, tape, antiseptic wipes, antibiotic ointment, gloves, CPR mask, emergency blanket, trauma pads, tweezers, scissors, and cold packs. Safety signs made of durable materials placed prominently: depth markers, NO DIVING warnings, pool rules, emergency numbers, CPR instructions. Fencing at least 4 feet high with self-closing, self-latching gates. Inspect regularly, consider installing alarm. Actively watch children in pool. Never leave unsupervised, even briefly. Adults avoid distractions like phones.

---

<u>**Yard**</u>
Infant/Non-mobile: (Birth - 6 months)
→ **Infant crawl/roll: (5 months - 1 year)**
→ **Toddler/Pre-school: (1 year - 4 years)**
→ **School-age: (5 years - 6+ years)**

# Proper Pool Cover

**A proper pool cover is an essential safety measure to prevent accidents and protect children around pools.** By providing a physical barrier between children and the pool, a pool cover can significantly reduce the risk of accidental drownings.

**Benefits of Using a Pool Cover:** Pool covers prevent unsupervised access, maintain water quality, reduce evaporation, and improve water temperature. Safety covers (vinyl or mesh) prevent children from accessing pool. Solar covers maintain temperature. Choose safety coverage for young children. Ensure proper installation and maintenance. Loose or damaged covers compromise safety.

---

❦ **This is the most critical distinction for your readers:** Solar covers (bubble wrap) and winter tarps are NOT safety devices. **The Shocking Truth:** If a child falls onto a floating solar cover, it does not support them; it wraps around them. The weight of the child creates a "cocoon" effect. As they struggle, the suction of the water against the plastic makes it nearly impossible for them to break the surface or even move their limbs. **The "Invisible" Factor:** Unlike a splash in an open pool, a child slipping under a cover makes almost no sound. Furthermore, because the cover remains on top of the water, a parent looking out the window may see a "still pool" and not realize their child is underneath the plastic. *CPSC (Consumer Product Safety Commission) - Safety Alert: "The Dangers of Floating Pool Covers."*

---

<u>**Yard**</u>
Infant/Non-mobile: (Birth - 6 months)
Infant crawl/roll: (5 months - 1 year)
→ **Toddler/Pre-school: (1 year - 4 years)**
→ **School-age: (5 years - 6+ years)**

# Remove the Ladder from Above Ground Pool

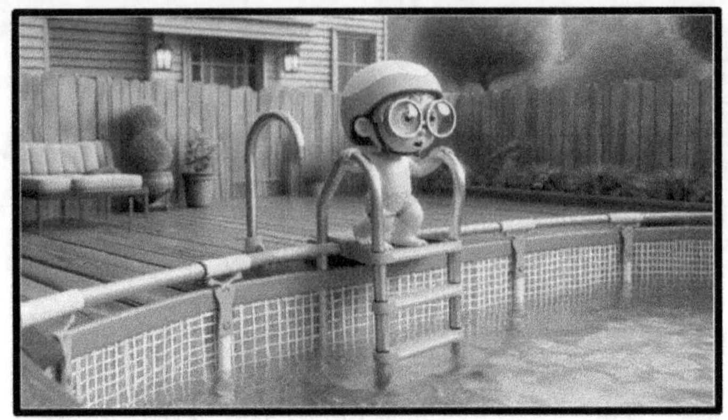

Remove ladder immediately after use. Store securely where children cannot access. Check no residual steps remain. Retractable ladders fully retracted and locked. Use safety cover or fence as supplementary security. Constant supervision during pool use. Educate older children never to access pool without adult supervision. Regular checks ensure protocol followed consistently.

---

**Yard**
Infant/Non-mobile: (Birth - 6 months)
Infant crawl/roll: (5 months - 1 year)
→ **Toddler/Pre-school: (1 year - 4 years)**
→ **School-age: (5 years - 6+ years)**

# SEPARATE PLAY AND POOL AREAS

Reduces drowning risk. Creates physical barrier between play activities and pool. Allows focused supervision. Minimizes distractions. Establish clear boundaries using fences, hedges, or barriers. Install fence with self-closing, self-latching gates. Use pool safety covers and alarms. Designate age-appropriate play areas. Educate children about rules. Use visual cues and signs. Regular maintenance of fences and barriers. Adult supervision and communication protocols.

---

**Yard**
Infant/Non-mobile: (Birth - 6 months)
Infant crawl/roll: (5 months - 1 year)
→ **Toddler/Pre-school: (1 year - 4 years)**
→ **School-age: (5 years - 6+ years)**

# BATTERIES OVER POOL OUTLETS

If any of the pool equipment is not working properly, keep everyone out of the water. This includes underwater lights, pumps, and filters. If any of these device's malfunction, they could create a stray electrical current that could be fatal.

**Use only battery-operated appliances in and around the swimming pool.** This includes radios, fans, and water toys. If you must use an electrical appliance, make sure it is plugged into a GFCI outlet. GFCI outlets have built-in safety features that will cut off the power if there is a problem.

**Designate a Water Watcher** to supervise children in the swimming pool. The Water Watcher should be an adult who is not distracted by anything else and can always pay attention to the children.

**Teach children about the dangers of electricity and swimming pools.** They should know not to touch electrical equipment near the pool and never swim alone.

Have your pool professionally inspected and maintained every year. This will help ensure that all of the electrical equipment is in good working order. Keep the pool area clear of clutter. This will help prevent people from tripping over objects and falling into the water. Post warning signs around the pool. These signs should alert people to the dangers of electricity and swimming pools.

---

**Yard**
Infant/Non-mobile: (Birth - 6 months)
Infant crawl/roll: (5 months - 1 year)
→ **Toddler/Pre-school: (1 year - 4 years)**
→ **School-age: (5 years - 6+ years)**

# TOYS NEAR THE POOL CONCERNS

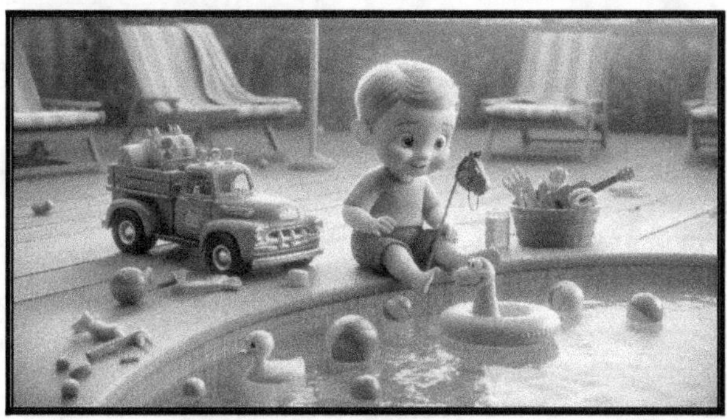

Never leave children unattended with riding toys near pool. Ensure right size toy. Use only in shallow water. Teach how to exit if they fall. Be aware of weather. Check for damage before use. Store away from pool when not in use. Teach not to run near pool.

# SECURE POOL CHEMICALS

Use lockable cabinet for hazardous materials. Store high and dry, out of children's reach. Keep different chemicals separate, clearly labeled. Original containers with labels intact. Well-ventilated area. Dry, cool, shaded storage. Childproof latches. Read labels and instructions. Wear protective equipment when handling. Secure waste disposal per local regulations. Educate older children about dangers. First aid kit and emergency contacts readily available.

---



# POOL RULES

**Never leave unattended. Continuous supervision essential. Safe, level location away from hazards.** Childproof fence or barrier around area. Appropriate water depth for child's age and height. Empty immediately after use. Cover drainage to prevent entrapment. Non-slip mat around pool. No running rule. Safe, age-appropriate toys without small parts. Sun protection with shade structures. Regular water changes for hygiene. Childproof latches if cover present. Educate on safety rules. First aid kit nearby.

---



# WINTER SAFETY

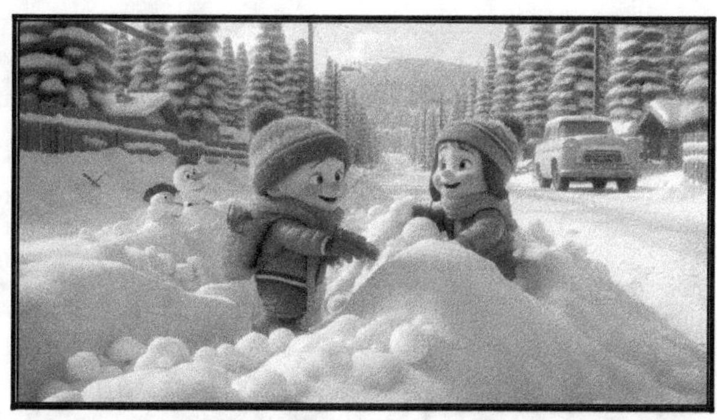

**<u>Never Allow Children to Play on a Snowbank by the Road!</u>**

**Traffic hazards:** snowbanks obstruct driver visibility. Unpredictable child behavior near roads. Slippery surfaces. Limited driver reaction time. Distractions for drivers. Snow removal equipment operating nearby. Unknown road conditions under snow. Encourage designated play areas away from roads: yards, parks, playgrounds. Always supervise outdoor play. Educate about road dangers. Communicate about hazards. Install barriers if feasible.

---

**<u>Yard</u>**
Infant/Non-mobile: (Birth - 6 months)
Infant crawl/roll: (5 months - 1 year)
→ **Toddler/Pre-school: (1 year - 4 years)**
→ **School-age: (5 years - 6+ years)**

# FROSTBITE AND FROST NIP

**Layer clothing:** moisture-wicking base (Made from materials that pull moisture away from the body and allow to evaporate), insulating middle (fleece or wool), waterproof and windproof outer. Protect extremities with gloves, mittens, socks, hat, neck gaiter or scarf. **Stay dry:** adjust layers to avoid sweating, change wet clothes promptly. **Keep moving:** stay active, wiggle toes and fingers regularly. Stay hydrated and eat nutritious foods. Limit time outdoors in extreme cold. Seek shelter if too cold or experiencing numbness. **Know frost nip signs:** cold, pale skin, tingling. **Act promptly:** warm with body heat. For frostbite, seek medical attention immediately. Use sunscreen on exposed skin. Lip balm with SPF. Insulated, waterproof footwear. Warm sleeping gear for camping.

---

<u>**Yard**</u>
Infant/Non-mobile: (Birth - 6 months)
Infant crawl/roll: (5 months - 1 year)
→ **Toddler/Pre-school: (1 year - 4 years)**
→ **School-age: (5 years - 6+ years)**

# Sledding Safety

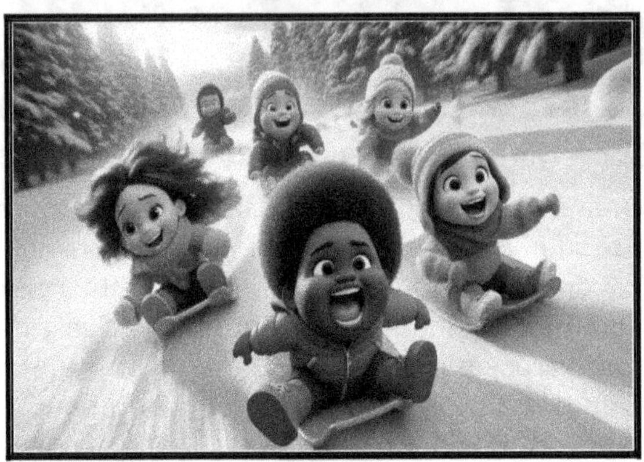

Ensure gentle slope without obstacles: trees, rocks, fences. Far from roads or water. Not too crowded. Toddlers wear helmets. Warm, layered, water-resistant clothing. Secure gloves, boots, hats. Toddler-appropriate sled with wide, stable base and steering if possible. Avoid difficult-to-control or overly fast sleds. Always supervise closely, standing at bottom to help guide or stop. Frequent breaks if tired or cold.

---

<u>**Yard**</u>
Infant/Non-mobile: (Birth - 6 months)
Infant crawl/roll: (5 months - 1 year)
**Toddler/Pre-school: (1 year - 4 years)**
**School-age: (5 years - 6+ years)**

# Ice Skating Safety

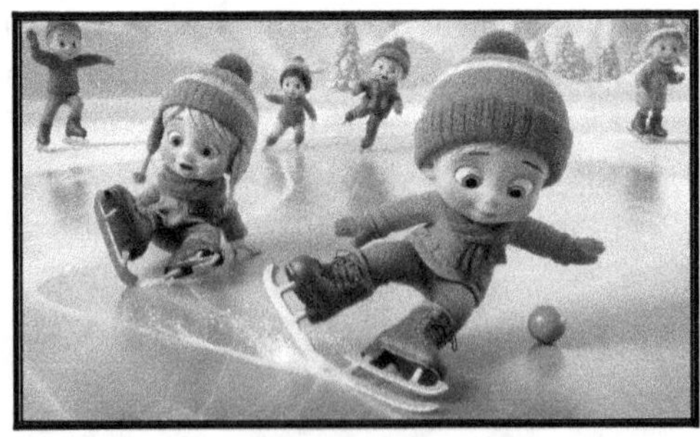

Choose rink with festive decorations, quality ice, safe surroundings.

Festive yet warm clothing. Protective gear: helmets, knee pads, elbow pads. Warm accessories. Supervised skating. Skating lessons to music. Designate "Safety Elf" to ensure rules followed. Warm cocoa treats afterward. Holiday gift bags for safe skating. First aid station. Emergency contact list.

---

🐝 **The Shocking Truth:** The biggest threat to a child who falls isn't the fall itself—it's the other skaters.

**The Danger:** A common instinct for a fallen child is to keep their hands flat on the ice to push themselves up. In a crowded rink, an approaching skater may not see the child's small hand. A steel skate blade carries the full weight of an adult (often 150–200 lbs concentrated on an edge just 3 mm wide. **The Result:** This pressure can result in clean-cut finger amputations or deep tendon lacerations that cause permanent loss of movement. *American Academy of Pediatrics (AAP) / Mass General Brigham Emergency Medicine.*

---

**Yard**

Infant/Non-mobile: (Birth - 6 months)
Infant crawl/roll: (5 months - 1 year)
→ **Toddler/Pre-school: (1 year - 4 years)**
→ **School-age: (5 years - 6+ years)**

# SNOWMOBILE CONCERNS

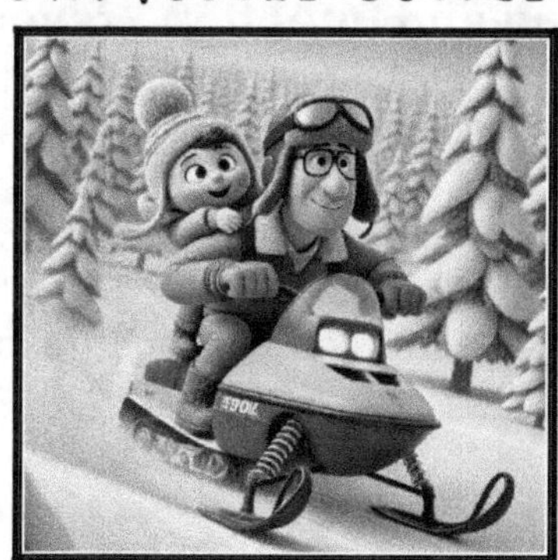

DOT-approved helmets fitting snugly. **Eye protection:** clear shields or goggles. Water-resistant layers, brightly colored for visibility. Good quality gloves and boots. Age-appropriate snowmobiles. **Routine checks:** brakes, lights, safety features. Speed limiter if possible. Enroll in safety courses. Always supervise, never ride alone. Educate on safe routes avoiding thin ice, open water, obstacles. **Emergency kit:** band-aids, warm blankets, whistle. Communication device. Teach safe stop and start. No stunts. Maintain safe distance from others. Respect wildlife.

---

<u>**Yard**</u>
→ **Infant/Non-mobile: (Birth - 6 months)**
→ **Infant crawl/roll: (5 months - 1 year)**
→ **Toddler/Pre-school: (1 year - 4 years)**
→ **School-age: (5 years - 6+ years)**

# SUNSCREEN PROTECTION
## (It's especially Serious!)

SPF 30 to 50, broad spectrum. Mineral-based for children. Avoid oxybenzone. Fragrance-free. Apply generously 20 to 30 minutes before sun. Reapply every 2 hours or after swimming/sweating. Sunglasses with UV protection. Wide-brimmed hats, cover-ups. Seek shade during peak hours (10 AM to 4 PM). Avoid sunscreen on babies under 6 months; use protective clothing and shade. Test for allergies. Lip balm with SPF. Educate on importance. Teach self-application as they grow.

---

<u>**Yard**</u>
Infant/Non-mobile: **(Birth - 6 months)**
→ **Infant crawl/roll: (5 months - 1 year)**
→ **Toddler/Pre-school: (1 year - 4 years)**
→ **School-age: (5 years - 6+ years)**

# PET WASTE CONCERNS
## (Hygiene and Infection Prevention)

Encourage frequent hand washing after playing where pets have been. Supervise young children. Clean up promptly using gloves. Safe disposal in secure bin. Separate play areas for children and pets. Clear garden of waste. Place litter boxes inaccessibly. Clean daily. Educate about dangers. Report concerns. Regular parasite control for pets. Regular vet visits. Monitor air quality; dried feces can cause respiratory issues.

---

<u>**Yard**</u>
Infant/Non-mobile: (Birth - 6 months)
Infant crawl/roll: (5 months - 1 year)
→ **Toddler/Pre-school: (1 year - 4 years)**
→ **School-age: (5 years - 6+ years)**

# HELP PREVENT LYME DISEASE

Use educational materials about Lyme disease and tick dangers. Teach to recognize ticks. Long sleeves and pants in wooded or grassy areas. Light-colored clothing to spot ticks. Child-safe repellents applied by adults.

Regular lawn mowing, remove tall grass and brush. Establish tick-safe play area with wood chips separating from woods. Routine tick checks after outdoor play: head, neck, skin folds. Use bath time for checks. Keep tick-removal kit, know safe removal. If tick embedded, seek medical advice. Regularly check pets. Veterinary advice on tick control. Advocate school programs. Community engagement.

---

**Yard**
Infant/Non-mobile: (Birth - 6 months)
Infant crawl/roll: (5 months - 1 year)
→ **Toddler/Pre-school: (1 year - 4 years)**
→ **School-age: (5 years - 6+ years)**

# FILLING HOLES IN THE YARD

The backyard often serves as a primary play area for children to explore, play, and connect with nature. However, it can also house certain dangers, especially if it is not well-maintained. One such danger is the presence of holes in the yard, which can pose several risks to children. Here, we explore why it's vital to fill up these holes with an eye for detail.

## Potential Risks

**Tripping Hazards:** Holes can create uneven ground, increasing the risk of tripping and falling. Children often run around without paying full attention to the ground, making them more prone to accidents caused by holes.

**Pest Infestation:** Holes can act as breeding grounds for pests like rodents and insects. These pests can potentially carry diseases and infections which can be harmful to children.

**Water Accumulation:** Holes can accumulate water and create puddles, encouraging mosquito breeding. Puddles can turn into messy, muddy pits and can be a slipping hazard.

## Preventive Measures

**Regular Yard Maintenance:** Conduct routine inspections of the yard to identify and fill up any holes. Once identified, take immediate action to fill the holes to prevent any accidents.

**Proper Filling Materials:** Use appropriate material to fill the holes, ensuring that it is compacted well to prevent recurrence. Make sure the ground is leveled properly to prevent tripping hazards.

**Education and Supervision:** Educate children about the dangers of playing near or in holes. Ensure that children are supervised by an adult while playing in the yard.

**Engaging a Professional:** If the yard has multiple holes or more significant depressions, engaging a professional landscaping service might be beneficial to ensure the yard is safe and well-maintained.

Ensuring a yard is free of holes is a critical step in childproofing your outdoor space. It prevents potential physical injuries and keeps pests and related diseases at bay. A level, well-maintained yard provides a safe and enjoyable environment where children can play without risks. By taking the steps outlined above, you can create a fun and safe yard for children.

---

<u>**Yard**</u>
Infant/Non-mobile: (Birth - 6 months)
Infant crawl/roll: (5 months - 1 year)
→ **Toddler/Pre-school: (1 year - 4 years)**
→ **School-age: (5 years - 6+ years)**

# Fire Pit/Bonfire Safety

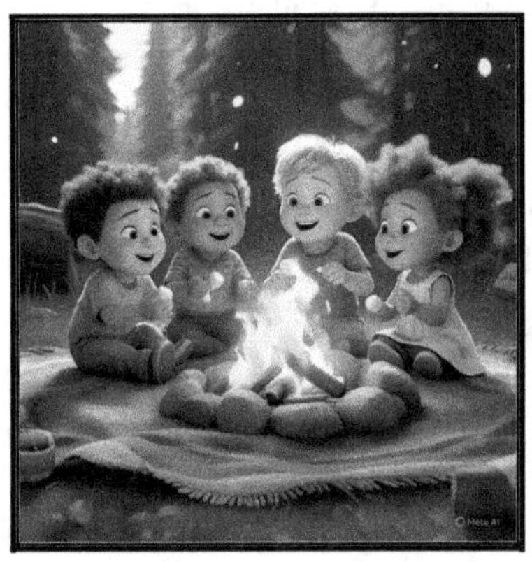

Approximately 700 children injured yearly by portable fire pits (NFPA). Burns and scalds: children get too close, touch flames or embers. Clothing can catch fire. Smoke and fume inhalation causes respiratory issues. Burning certain materials releases toxic fumes. Fire can spread to nearby flammables. Install physical barrier: fence or gate. Clear zone around fire with no flammable materials. Constant supervision. Educate on dangers, establish safe behavior rules. Fire extinguishers readily available, know how to use. Emergency numbers accessible. Use safe fire starters, avoid gasoline or dangerous accelerates.

---

<u>Yard</u>
→ Infant/Non-mobile: (Birth - 6 months)
→ Infant crawl/roll: (5 months - 1 year)
→ Toddler/Pre-school: (1 year - 4 years)
→ School-age: (5 years - 6+ years)

# APPLY INSECT REPELLENT DURING PROPER SEASONS

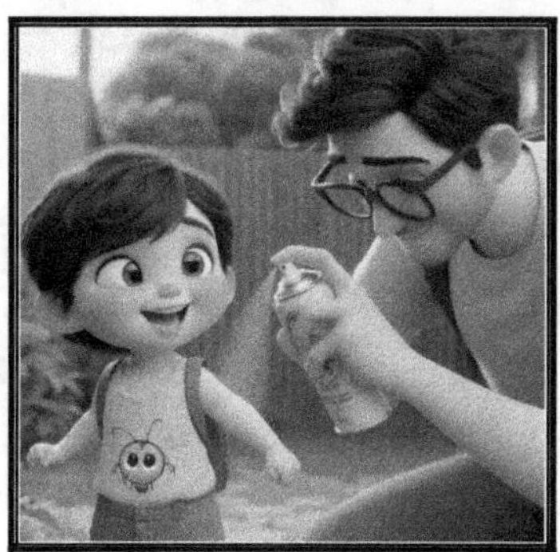

In the delightful journey of childhood, where every stone unturned is a new adventure, it's crucial to safeguard children from the potential hazards of bug bites. Bug bites are not just itchy and uncomfortable—they can also pose significant health risks. Some insects carry serious diseases, and for children with sensitive skin or allergies, a simple bite can lead to severe reactions. That's why using bug repellent is not just a matter of comfort, but a vital step in ensuring children's health and safety. Let's explore why bug repellent is important and how to use it wisely. Understanding the Risks

**Bug bites can lead to both immediate discomfort and long-term health issues.** Children are naturally curious and tend to spend time exploring gardens, parks, and outdoor trails—all of which increase their exposure to insects.

**Disease Transmission** is a primary concern.

**Mosquitoes** are more than just a nuisance; they can transmit malaria, dengue, West Nile virus, and Zika virus.

**Ticks**, often found in grassy or wooded areas, are known carriers of Lyme disease and Rocky Mountain spotted fever.

**Flies**, though often overlooked, can spread diseases such as leishmaniasis, especially in certain regions. Allergic Reactions are another important risk. Some children may experience intense allergic responses, which can range from mild swelling to more severe complications like hives or even anaphylaxis.

**Scratching bug bites can lead to secondary infections,** especially if the skin is broken and bacteria enter the wound. These infections can require antibiotics or other treatments, further stressing a child's immune system.

**Choosing the Right Bug Repellent.** When selecting a bug repellent, it's important to choose products that are both safe and effective for children. Not all repellents are created equal, and some ingredients may not be suitable for younger age groups.

**Age Appropriateness** should always be the first consideration. For infants under two months, avoid repellents altogether. Instead, use protective clothing, mosquito nets, and stroller covers to keep insects away. For older children, choose repellents that are specifically labeled as safe for pediatric use, and always check the recommended age range on the label. **Ingredients** also play a key role in safety and effectiveness.

**DEET** is one of the most effective repellents but should be used in **concentrations of 10–30% for children**. Higher concentrations do not offer better protection, just longer duration.

**Picaridin** is a **gentle, non-greasy alternative to DEET**, and is considered safe for children when used as directed. Oil of Lemon Eucalyptus, although natural, should not be used on children under 3 years old due to its potency.

**Correct application is just as important as choosing the right product. Ensure even coverage on all exposed skin**, avoiding broken or irritated skin.

**For facial application**, spray the repellent into your hands first, then gently rub it onto the child's face, steering clear of the eyes and mouth. **Avoid overapplication** More product does not mean better protection. Follow the instructions on the label carefully. **Apply repellent to clothing** (especially socks and cuffs) for additional protection, but avoid treating undergarments. After outdoor play, wash treated skin with soap and water to reduce the risk of irritation or residue buildup.

Understanding the significance of bug repellent in protecting children from insect-borne illnesses is a key part of responsible parenting. Taking the time to select the right repellent and apply it correctly ensures children can enjoy the outdoors with minimal risk. In the grand adventure of growing up, preventing a bug bite is far easier and healthier than treating one. So let's nurture children's curiosity and spirit of exploration by prioritizing their safety and well-being with thoughtful use of bug repellent.

<u>**Yard**</u>
Infant/Non-mobile: (Birth - 6 months)
Infant crawl/roll: (5 months - 1 year)
→ **Toddler/Pre-school: (1 year - 4 years)**
→ **School-age: (5 years - 6+ years)**

# Install "Watch for Children" Signs in the Front Yard

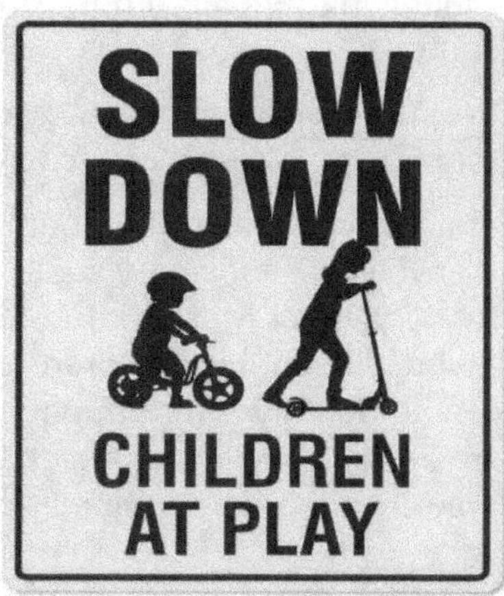


Setting up kid warning signs is an indispensable safety measure when it comes to childproofing a yard, particularly in homes close to roads. These signs alert drivers to slow down and be extra vigilant, as children could be playing nearby.

## <u>Selection of the Correct Signs</u>

**Visual Appeal:** Opt for signs in bright colors such as fluorescent yellow or green to catch drivers' attention easily. Choose signs made with reflective materials to ensure visibility even in low light conditions.

**Message Conveyed:** The wording on the sign should be clear and direct, like "Caution: Children at Play." Signs with pictures of children playing can visually communicate the message swiftly.

**Strategic Placement of Signs:** Set up the signs at a distance, visible to oncoming traffic but not too close to the road where children might venture out.

**Height and Angle:** Ensure the signs are installed at an appropriate height, where they are clearly visible to the driver. The signs should also be angled so that drivers can read them from a distance and have ample time to slow down.

**Maintenance of the Signs:** Regularly check the signs for any wear and tear and replace them as necessary. Keep the signs clean so that they remain visible and their message clear.

**Safety Education:** Teach children the importance of staying within the boundaries of the yard. Educate children on the purpose of the signs and why they should adhere to safety rules.

### Additional Tips

**Fencing:** Consider installing fencing around the yard to provide an additional layer of safety.

**Supervision:** Ensure that children are always supervised while playing in the yard, particularly when close to a road.

Setting up a kids' warning signs near the road is a vital aspect of childproofing a yard. It involves choosing visually appealing and clear signs, placing them strategically for maximum visibility, and maintaining them well. Coupled with educating children on road safety and implementing other complementary safety measures, these signs can significantly enhance the safety of a yard where children play, fostering a secure and worry-free play environment for them.

---

**Yard**
Infant/Non-mobile: (Birth - 6 months)
Infant crawl/roll: (5 months - 1 year)
→ **Toddler/Pre-school: (1 year - 4 years)**
→ **School-age: (5 years - 6+ years)**

# RETRACTABLE DRIVEWAY GUARD

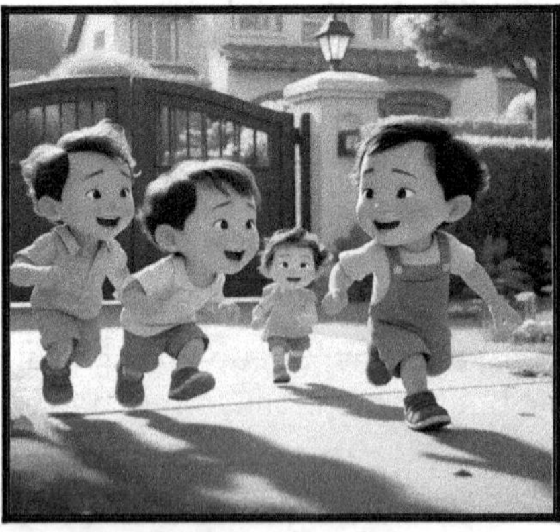

Childproofing demands attention to every potential risk factor in a child's environment. One important aspect that often goes unnoticed is securing the driveway, and this is where retractable driveway guards come into play. Let us delve into the multifaceted benefits and importance of installing a retractable driveway guard in homes with children.

### Understanding a Retractable Driveway Guard

A retractable driveway guard is a barrier, often made of durable netting or similar material, that can be extended across the driveway to prevent children from running into the street and deter vehicles from entering the play area.

## Advantages of Installing a Retractable Driveway Guard

### Child Safety

**Preventing Accidents:** Children often get engrossed in play and may not notice an approaching vehicle. A guard acts as a physical barrier, preventing kids from accidentally running onto the road.

**Defining Play Zones:** Helps demarcate safe play areas and teach children boundaries early on.

### Driver Awareness

**Visual Alert:** This signal acts as a visual cue for drivers to slow down and be alert as they approach your residence.

**Preventing Driveway Turnarounds:** Deters drivers from using your driveway as a turnaround, ensuring the safety of playing children.

### Easy to Use

**Retractability:** Can be easily retracted when not in use, which does not obstruct driveway access for family vehicles.

**Ease of Installation:** These guards are relatively easy to install and do not require any specialized equipment or expertise.

## Selecting the Right Driveway Guard

### Consider the Following

**Width:** Ensure the guard is wide enough to cover the entire width of your driveway.

**Height:** The height should be sufficient to act as a visual and physical barrier for children and vehicles alike.

**Material:** This should be made of durable, weather-resistant materials to ensure longevity.

### Additional Feature

**Reflective Strips:** Opt for guards with reflective strips for better visibility during nighttime.

**Lockable Feature:** A guard with a lockable feature would prevent unauthorized removal or tampering.

## Maintenance and Upkeep

### Regular Inspection

**Inspect Regularly:** Regular inspection to check for any wear and tear is essential to ensure its effectiveness.

**Cleanliness:** Keeping the guard clean ensures visibility and functionality over time.

### Informing Family Members

**Usage:** Educate family members, especially children, on the importance and proper use of the driveway guard.

**Emergency Protocols:** Establish protocols for quick removal in case of emergencies.

A retractable driveway guard is a significant addition to your childproofing measures, offering both a physical barrier and a visual cue to enhance safety in the driveway area. It assists in preventing accidents, delineating play zones, and fostering a safer environment for children. Making a choice based on width, height, and material, coupled with regular maintenance, can help optimize its efficacy for a long time. Moreover, educating family members, especially children, about its usage and importance can go a long way in ensuring a safer play area.

---

**Yard**
Infant/Non-mobile: (Birth - 6 months)
Infant crawl/roll: (5 months - 1 year)
→ **Toddler/Pre-school: (1 year - 4 years)**
→ **School-age: (5 years - 6+ years)**

# BARBECUE/GRILL SAFETY

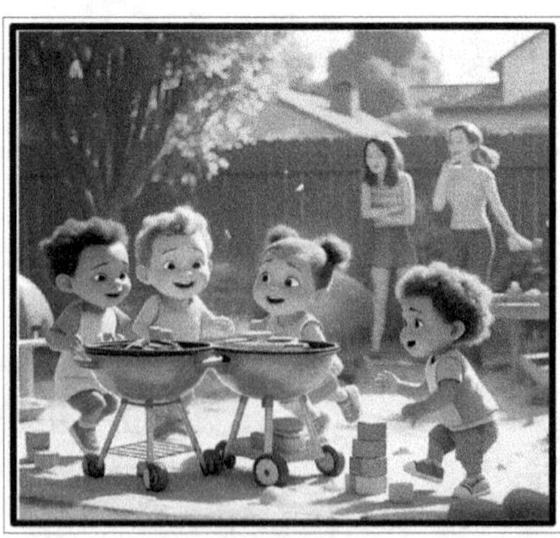

When enjoying outdoor gatherings and delicious grilled meals, it's essential to prioritize child safety around barbecues and grills.

**Location Matters:** Set up the barbecue or grill in a safe and well-ventilated area away from high foot traffic, play zones, and flammable materials like dry leaves or paper. Keep a minimum distance of 10 feet from any structure or overhanging branches.

**Stable Surface:** To prevent tipping, ensure the grill is placed on a level and stable surface. Use a grill pad or heat-resistant mat underneath to protect the ground from heat and grease.

**Supervision is Key:** Always have a responsible adult present when grilling. Children should never be left unattended near a hot grill, even for a moment.

**Keep Kids Away:** Establish a "no-play" zone around the grill. Use physical barriers like a safety fence or cones to mark the area where kids are not allowed.

**Proper Attire:** Encourage everyone, especially children, to wear appropriate clothing while near the grill. Loose sleeves, flowing clothes, and long apron strings can easily catch fire.

**Utensil Safety:** Teach kids to use long-handled utensils to avoid getting too close to the heat. Keep grilling tools out of their reach when not in use.

**Hot Surfaces:** Emphasize the importance of not touching any part of the grill, as it gets extremely hot during and after cooking. Use oven mitts or heat-resistant gloves.

**Fire Safety:** Keep a fire extinguisher or a bucket of sand nearby in case of flare-ups or emergencies. Educate children on how to use them if necessary.

**Gas Cylinder Safety:** Before using a gas grill, check the gas cylinder for leaks. Keep cylinders upright, secure, and away from direct sunlight or heat sources.

**Charcoal Safety:** If using a charcoal grill, ensure the charcoal is completely cool before disposing of ashes. Store unused charcoal in a dry, cool place.

**Lighting Precautions:** Teach children to stay away from the grill when it's being lit. Use long-reach lighters to ignite the grill and avoid lighter fluid if possible.

**Cleanliness Matters:** Regularly clean grease and food build-up from the grill's grates and trays. Empty grease trays fter each use to prevent flare-ups.

**Safe Food Handling:** Educate children about the importance of proper food handling and cooking temperatures to avoid foodborne illnesses.

**After Grilling:** Once grilling is done, turn off the gas and let the coals cool down. Ensure that the grill is properly extinguished before leaving the area.

**Storage Safety:** Store grilling equipment, utensils, and fuel sources out of children's reach in a locked storage area.

**Model Safe Behavior:** Set an example by following all safety practices and rules yourself. Children are more likely to adopt safe habits if they see adults prioritizing safety.

---

<u>**Yard**</u>
→ **Infant/Non-mobile: (Birth - 6 months)**
→ **Infant crawl/roll: (5 months - 1 year)**
→ **Toddler/Pre-school: (1 year - 4 years)**
→ **School-age: (5 years - 6+ years)**

# BEST AGE TO GET A DOG... 8-10

According to ASPCA and Humane Society, waiting until child reaches around 8 to 10 years ensures developed cognitive, emotional, and physical abilities needed to responsibly care for and interact with pet. Younger children may have difficulty understanding responsibilities and handling tasks. Waiting allows better match between child's capabilities and pet's needs.

**Approximately 50,000 children bitten or scratched by pets yearly, requiring medical attention (CDC).**

---

<u>**Yard**</u>
Infant/Non-mobile: (Birth - 6 months)
Infant crawl/roll: (5 months - 1 year)
→ **Toddler/Pre-school: (1 year - 4 years)**
→ **School-age: (5 years - 6+ years)**

# DOGHOUSE SAFETY

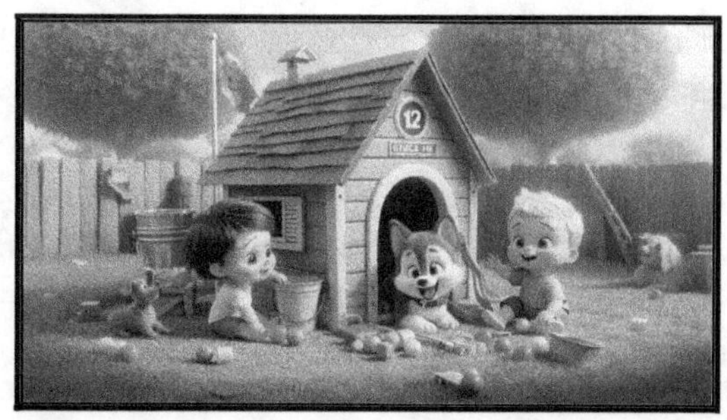

**Choose location away from high-traffic areas and play zones.** Well-ventilated, shaded spot. Sturdy, well-built construction. No sharp edges, protruding nails, or splinters. Appropriate size for pet. Raised flooring keeps pet dry and minimizes pests. Teach child to respect dog's space, not block entrance/exit. Always supervise child's interactions inside doghouse. It's private space for pet. No climbing or sitting on doghouse. Regular cleaning of doghouse and surrounding area. Non-toxic, safe materials. Secured roof to prevent collapses. Educate about dog behavior, signs when dog wants to be alone. Approach gently and respectfully. Foster positive interactions within doghouse area.

---

<u>Yard</u>
Infant/Non-mobile: (Birth - 6 months)
Infant crawl/roll: (5 months - 1 year)
→ **Toddler/Pre-school: (1 year - 4 years)**
→ **School-age: (5 years - 6+ years)**

# BEWARE OF DOG LEASHES BOTH OUTSIDE AND INSIDE

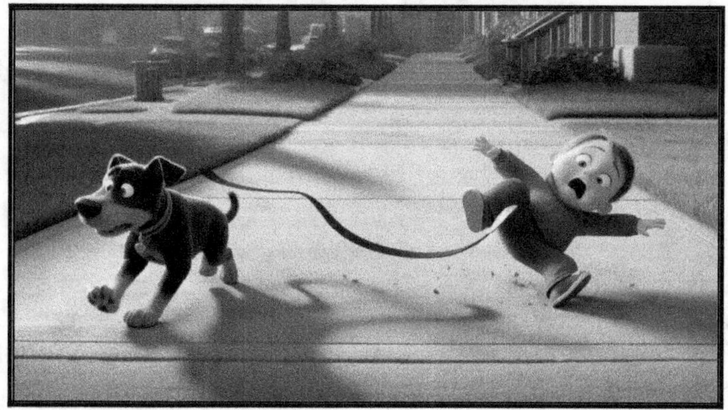

**Inside:** Supervise interactions when dog leashed. Store leashes out of reach. Teach child to respect dog's space when leashed. Keep away from blind cords, curtain ties, other cords (strangulation risk).

**Outside:** Always control leash. Avoid dangling loosely (tripping hazard). Instruct child not to wrap leash around hands, arms, body. Teach proper holding with both hands. No tugging. Adult guides dog's movements.

**Be mindful of surroundings;** leash doesn't entangle with objects. Use leash without loop handle if possible (reduces strangulation risk if child puts head through). Age-appropriate discussions about caution around leashed dogs. Ask permission before interacting with unfamiliar dogs. Properly train dog to walk without excessive pulling.

---

<u>**Yard**</u>
Infant/Non-mobile: (Birth - 6 months)
→ **Infant crawl/roll: (5 months - 1 year)**
→ **Toddler/Pre-school: (1 year - 4 years)**
→ **School-age: (5 years - 6+ years)**

# Teach Children that a Pet Isn't a Toy

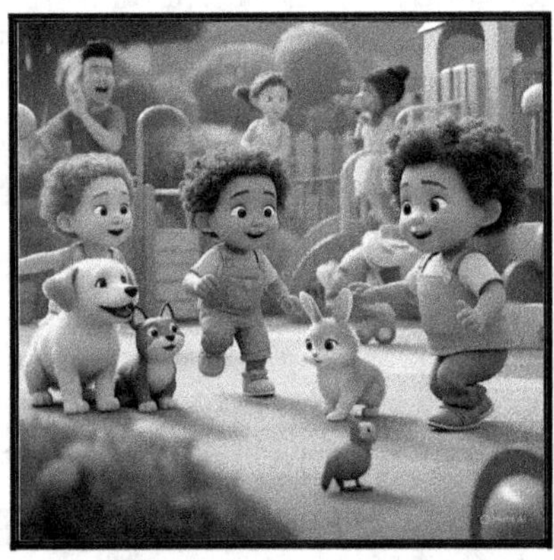

**Age-appropriate conversations about treating pets with kindness and respect.** Explain pets have feelings, sensitive ears, tails, bodies. Demonstrate and encourage gentle touch: soft stroking without sudden movements. Model appropriate behavior. Always supervise interactions, especially young children. Use books, videos, resources depicting respectful pet interactions. Praise gentle behavior. Positive reinforcement. Teach pets have personal space. Recognize signs pet is uncomfortable or stressed (moving away, lowered ears). Cultivate empathy: ask how they'd feel if someone pulled their ears. Encourage gentle play with toys or treats instead of physical pulling. Teach pets should associate them with positive experiences. Redirect inappropriate behavior calmly. Supervise friends' interactions. Consistency key. Continuously reinforce importance of kindness.

---

# KEEP DOG FOOD DISHES OUT OF REACH

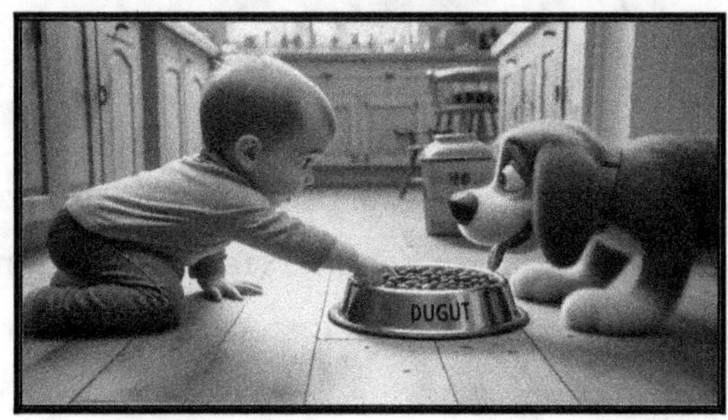


**Choking hazard:** small kibbles.

**Unwanted interaction:** children may disturb dog while eating. Hygiene concerns: transferring germs.

**Preventing food sharing:** children might share inappropriate food. Set designated feeding area not accessible to young children. Elevated feeding stations or wall-mounted holders. Create "pet-only zone." Establish feeding schedule. Supervise feedings.

**Teach respectful behavior:** let dog eat in peace. Positive reinforcement for respecting space. Pet-proof gates or barriers. Store food in secure, child-resistant container. Incorporate mealtime into consistent routine. Teach proper hygiene around pets.

---



# DO NOT BOTHER A DOG WHEN THEY ARE RESTING, SLEEPING, OR EATING

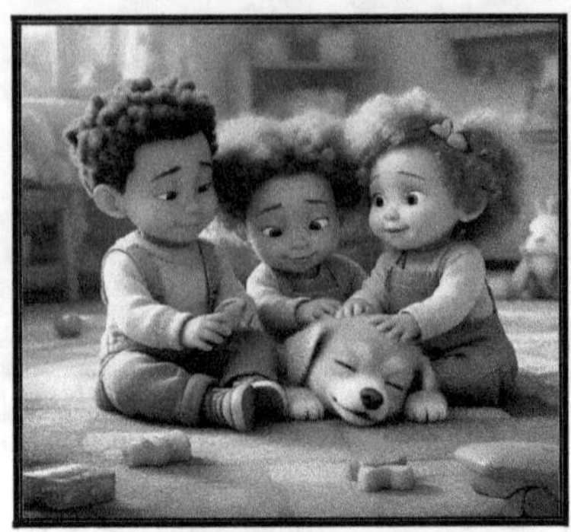

**Health and stress:** interrupting rest causes stress, anxiety.

**Preventing aggression:** dogs can become startled or defensive.

**Bond and trust:** allowing peaceful rest fosters stronger bond.

**Educate about importance:** dogs need rest like people.

**Recognize signs:** closed eyes, relaxed body, quiet demeanor. Create resting zones: designated areas like bed or cushion.

**Teach mealtime etiquette:** dogs need space to eat. Always supervise.

**Set boundaries:** don't approach when resting or sleeping. Use "Do Not Disturb" sign. Positive reinforcement. Schedule playtimes when awake and energetic.

**If dog needs awakening, gentle approach:** call name softly. Explain personal space concept. Model respectful behavior. Consistency.

---

<u>Yard</u>
Infant/Non-mobile: (Birth - 6 months)
→ **Infant crawl/roll: (5 months - 1 year)**
→ **Toddler/Pre-school: (1 year - 4 years)**
→ **School-age: (5 years - 6+ years)**

# Train Your Dog to Tolerate Kids

**Basic obedience training:** sit, stay, come, leave it. Positive associations: treats, toys, praise when calm around children.

**Gradual exposure:** start with calm, older children. Supervised encounters always.

**Teach children to recognize dog's body language:** stress signs like growling, lip licking, stiff posture. Desensitization: expose to child-related sights and sounds, reward calm behavior. Positive reinforcement. Redirect attention to you when children around.

**Teach "go to place" command:** designated spot like mat. Crate training as positive retreat. Socialization in child-friendly environments. Model gentle behavior. Teach "no jumping." Consistency. If aggression or fear toward children, seek professional guidance.

---

<u>**Yard**</u>
→ **Infant/Non-mobile: (Birth - 6 months)**
→ **Infant crawl/roll: (5 months - 1 year)**
→ **Toddler/Pre-school: (1 year - 4 years)**
→ **School-age: (5 years - 6+ years)**

# BEWARE OF MIXED BREED DOGS

**Research and observe physical attributes, size, coat, behavior to understand heritage.** Inquire about known or suspected breeds in lineage. Delve into temperament traits associated with breeds. Remember each dog unique; can display range of characteristics. Knowledge helps foster informed, secure interactions.

---

**Yard**
 **Infant/Non-mobile: (Birth - 6 months)**
→ **Infant crawl/roll: (5 months - 1 year)**
→ **Toddler/Pre-school: (1 year - 4 years)**
→ **School-age: (5 years - 6+ years)**

# BEWARE OF DOGS THAT BITE FREQUENTLY

Recognize warning signs: growling, baring teeth, raised hackles, stiff posture, intense staring. Ask owners about behavior and biting history. Maintain distance if uncertain. Avoid unsupervised interactions with bite-prone dogs. Respect dog's space; don't approach without permission. Teach gentle interaction. Avoid aggravating situations: eating, chewing toy, caring for puppies. Seek professional help if known biting history. Report aggressive dogs to animal control. Educate children about caution. Promote responsible ownership. Combination of awareness, education, respectful interaction. **Roughly 50,000 children under 6 visit ERs yearly after dog bites.** About half of pediatric dog-bite cases. Bite injuries often on head and neck. **Over 70% of serious bites to kids under 5** -DogsBite.org

---

<u>Yard</u>
→ Infant/Non-mobile: (Birth - 6 months)
→ Infant crawl/roll: (5 months - 1 year)
→ Toddler/Pre-school: (1 year - 4 years)
→ School-age: (5 years - 6+ years)

# BETTER DOG BREEDS FOR CHILDREN

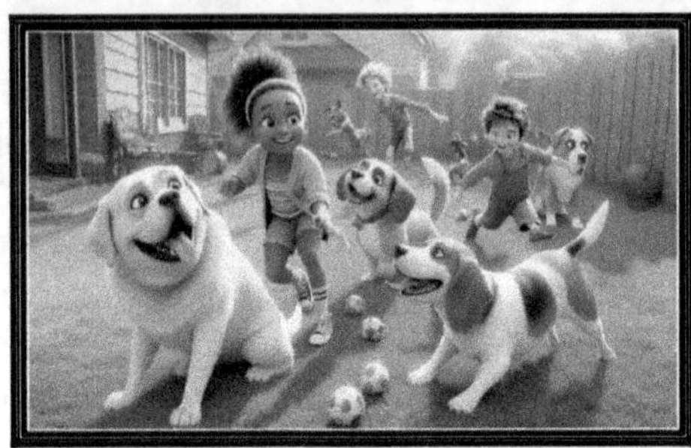

**Golden Retriever:** friendly, tolerant, patient, loyal.

**Labrador Retriever:** playful, outgoing, gentle, patient. Beagle: energetic, friendly, smaller size. Bulldog: calm, gentle, less high-energy.

**Poodle:** intelligent, versatile, hypoallergenic.

**Boxer:** energetic, playful, protective without aggression.

**Collie:** gentle, loyal, strong herding instincts.

**Newfoundland:** affectionate, calm, patient, natural swimmers.

**Cavalier King Charles Spaniel:** affectionate, adaptable. Pug: charming, affectionate, easygoing. Consider temperament, size, energy level, trainability, allergies. Each dog individual; proper socialization, training, supervision essential.

---

<u>Yard</u>
→ Infant/Non-mobile: (Birth - 6 months)
→ Infant crawl/roll: (5 months - 1 year)
→ Toddler/Pre-school: (1 year - 4 years)
→ School-age: (5 years - 6+ years)

# DECLAW YOUR CAT?

**Declawing (onychectomy) involves surgical removal of claws and last bone of each toe.** Painful, lasting effects on behavior and comfort. Consider alternatives: regular nail trimming, scratching posts, soft nail caps. Consult veterinarian or behaviorist. Educate child about appropriate interaction. Establish nail trimming routine. Provide scratching outlets: multiple posts, different materials. Use soft nail caps. Supervise interactions. Positive reinforcement. Regular vet checkups. Create safe spaces for cat. Declawing last resort after exhausting alternatives.

---

<u>Yard</u>
Infant/Non-mobile: (Birth - 6 months)
→ **Infant crawl/roll: (5 months - 1 year)**
→ **Toddler/Pre-school: (1 year - 4 years)**
→ **School-age: (5 years - 6+ years)**

# GERBILS/RATS/RABBITS SAFETY

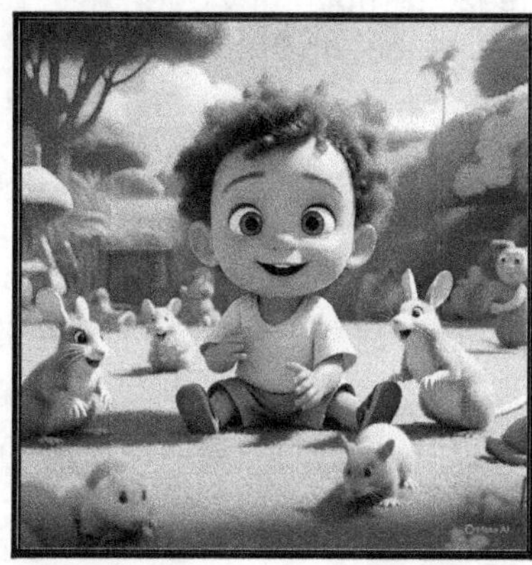

Introducing small pets like gerbils, rats, and rabbits into your household can be a rewarding experience for children. However, it's important to prioritize the safety of both your little ones and the furry members of your family.

**Gerbils/Rats/Rabbits Safety:** Research each animal's temperament, care requirements, health risks. Always supervise interactions. Teach gentle, calm handling. Avoid sudden loud noises. Secure cages with locks. Escape-proof design. Avoid sharp edges. Use safe substrate. Teach hand washing before and after handling. Don't share food with pets. Regular vet checkups. Follow vaccination and preventive care. Designated play area under supervision. Teach respect for boundaries, empathy. Age-appropriate responsibilities with supervision and guidance.

## <u>Proper Handling and Interaction</u>

**Supervise All Interactions:** Always supervise children when they are interacting with these pets to prevent accidental harm to both the child and the animal.

**Gentle Handling:** Teach your children to handle gerbils, rats, and rabbits gently and calmly. Quick movements or rough handling can startle or stress these animals.

**No Sudden Loud Noises:** Avoid sudden loud noises or shouting around the pets, as it can cause stress or fear.

## Cage and Habitat Safety

**Secure Cages and Enclosures:** Ensure that cages and enclosures are securely locked and properly closed to prevent accidental escapes or tampering by curious children.

**Escape-Proof Design:** Choose cages with escape-proof designs, as small pets can squeeze through tiny openings. Rats, in particular, are skilled at escaping, so select an appropriate enclosure.

**Avoid Sharp Edges:** Check the cage for sharp edges, protruding wires, or rough surfaces that could harm pets or children.

**Safe Substrate:** Use appropriate bedding materials that are safe for the animals and free from chemicals. Be cautious if using materials that can cause allergies or respiratory issues in children.

## Feeding and Hygiene

**Hand Washing:** Teach children to wash their hands before and after handling the pets or cleaning their habitats to prevent the spread of germs.

**Food Handling:** Instruct children not to share their food with pets, as some human foods can be harmful to small animals.

## Health and Hygiene

**Regular Vet Check-ups:** Schedule regular veterinary check-ups for your pets to ensure their health and well-being.

**Vaccinations and Preventive Care:** Follow your veterinarian's recommended vaccination and preventive care guidelines.

## Safe Playtime and Interaction

**Designated Play Area:** Create a designated play area where children can interact with the pets under supervision. This helps prevent pets from wandering into areas where they may encounter hazards.

## Teaching Empathy and Responsibility

**Respect for Animals:** Teach children to respect the pets' boundaries and signals. Encourage empathy and understanding of the pets' needs and behaviors.

**Age-Appropriate Responsibilities:** Assign age-appropriate responsibilities to children, such as feeding, cleaning, and interacting with pets. Supervise and guide them in these tasks. You can ensure a harmonious and safe environment for your children and small pets by teaching responsible pet ownership, empathy, and proper handling.

---

<u>**Yard**</u>
Infant/Non-mobile: (Birth - 6 months)
Infant crawl/roll: (5 months - 1 year)
→ **Toddler/Pre-school: (1 year - 4 years)**
→ **School-age: (5 years - 6+ years)**

# FARM ANIMALS

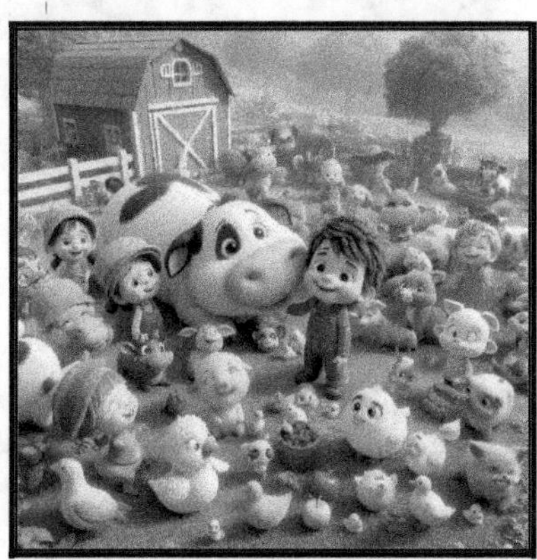

**Educational farm tour about different animals, behaviors, safe interaction.** Always supervise closely. Set clear boundaries and designated areas. Teach animal behavior: recognize stress, aggression, discomfort signs. Encourage participation in age-appropriate chores under guidance. Teach proper feeding practices. Animal-specific safety guidelines. Safety gear for larger animals: helmets, gloves. Secure fencing and enclosures. No rough play or teasing. Train in proper handling techniques. Emphasize hand washing. Develop emergency protocol. Involve in routine health checks. Teach respect for personal space. Safe interaction with young animals. Appropriate play. Supervised feeding. Socialize animals with children from young age.

---

**Notes:**

# |Ch. 25| Wild Animals

<u>Yard</u>
→ Infant/Non-mobile: (Birth - 6 months)
→ Infant crawl/roll: (5 months - 1 year)
→ Toddler/Pre-school: (1 year - 4 years)
→ School-age: (5 years - 6+ years)

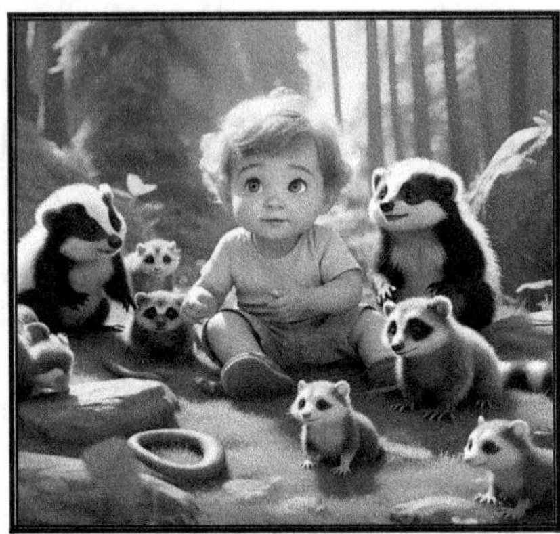

## Keeping Little Ones Safe from Wild Animals

**Common wild animals visiting yards:** raccoons, skunks, snakes, squirrels, coyotes (some areas), opossums, rats, mice. Attracted to food, shelter, water.

**Secure trash cans:** animal-proof or tight lids. Remove food sources: secure pet food, bird seed. Seal entry points: block holes around pipes, vents. Keep yard clean: debris, leaves, weeds attract animals. Install fencing.

**Teach children ages 4 to 6:** stay away from wild animals, don't feed, what to do if they see one (stay calm, back away, find adult). For children under 4: always supervise, watch for hazards, keep close.

**In case of encounter:** stay calm, keep child close, back away slowly, seek shelter if necessary, call 911 or animal control if aggressive. Be aware of common animals in area. Keep child informed as they grow. Prepare for emergencies.

# |Ch. 26| Holidays

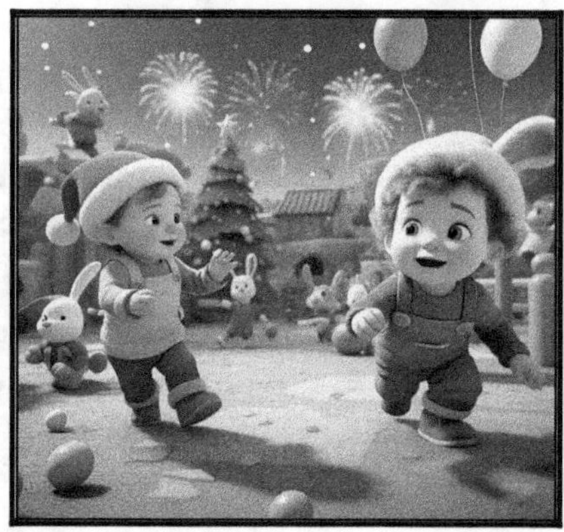

**Introduction**: Holidays are a time of joy, celebration, and family gatherings filled with laughter and love. Homes are adorned with twinkling lights, fragrant candles, and festive decorations, creating a magical atmosphere that delights both adults and children alike. However, amidst the enchantment and excitement, the holiday season also brings unique safety challenges that parents must navigate to ensure their little ones can celebrate safely and joyously.

---

**Christmas**
Infant/Non-mobile: (Birth - 6 months)
Infant crawl/roll: (5 months - 1 year)
**Toddler/Pre-school: (1 year - 4 years)**
**School-age: (5 years - 6+ years)**

## CHRISTMAS DECORATION SAFETY

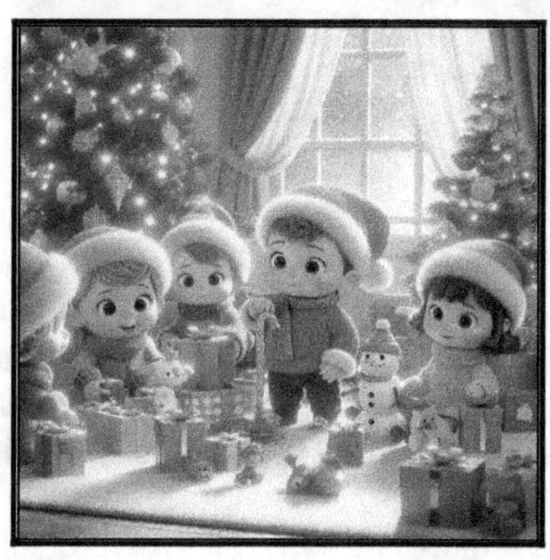

Choose secure tree location away from high-traffic areas. **Anchor properly.** Use shatterproof, child-friendly ornaments. Avoid fragile or sharp. Hang securely. Keep tinsel and garlands out of reach. Inspect lights for frayed wires. Keep lights and cords out of reach. Place candles on sturdy surfaces out of reach; consider flameless alternatives. Opt for non-toxic, child-safe ornaments. Place larger ornaments lower, small ones higher. Secure tree skirt. Non-toxic artificial snow out of reach.

**Be cautious with edible decorations**. Store wrapping materials out of reach. Use outdoor-rated extension cords; not tripping hazards. Caution with holiday plants: poinsettias, holly, mistletoe toxic.

**Place fragile decor high.** Avoid decorations obstructing windows/doors. Use age-appropriate toy decorations. Secure stair railings. Use childproofing accessories like safety gates. Always supervise. Store decorations safely: small parts, batteries, sharp objects out of reach in containers with secure lids.

---

<u>**Christmas**</u>
Infant/Non-mobile: (Birth - 6 months)
Infant crawl/roll: (5 months - 1 year)
→ **Toddler/Pre-school: (1 year - 4 years)**
→ **School-age: (5 years - 6+ years)**

# CHRISTMAS STOCKING SAFETY

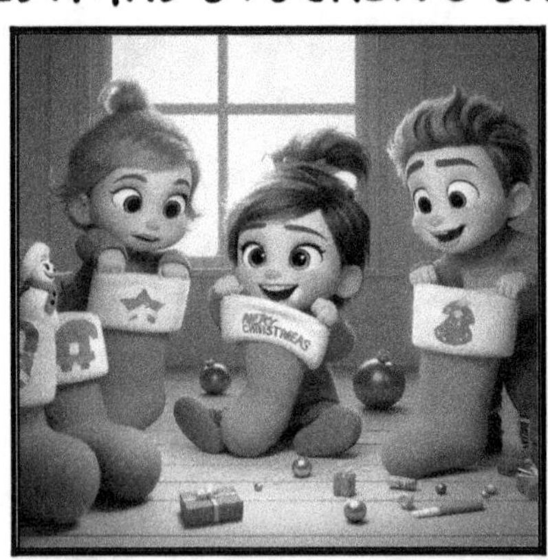


**Hang securely using safely attached hooks. Height out of young children's reach. Be cautious with small decorations, trinkets, toys (choking hazards). Avoid sharp objects.** Ensure battery compartments securely closed. Choose age-appropriate edible treats without choking risk. Avoid hard candies, small snacks. Supervise when exploring stockings. Be mindful of cords, strings, ribbons. Personalized stockings prevent mix-ups. Use child-safe wrapping, avoid excessive tape. Tailor contents to age and stage. Balance weight to prevent falling. Cautious with decorative elements like buttons, beads. Scented items securely enclosed. Don't block emergency exits. Use childproofing techniques. Regular inspections for hazards. Safe removal when taking down.



# ANCHOR THE CHRISTMAS TREE TO THE WALL TO PREVENT FALLING

**Choose stable location away from high-traffic, heavy furniture. Sturdy, wide tree stand.** Purchase tree anchor kit or wall hook. Measure distance from stand top to wall. Install wall bracket with screws. Attach anchor strap to stand top. Extend and connect to wall bracket. Tighten snugly. Conceal strap with garlands or ribbons. Distribute ornaments evenly for balance. Teach children not to pull, tug, or climb tree. Regular checks throughout season. Extra precautions for active children or pets. Applies to artificial trees too.



# CONSIDER GETTING AN ARTIFICIAL TREE

Sturdy **construction with stable base, balanced branches.**

**Fire safety:** flame-resistant materials. No needle shedding (choking hazard). Allergen-free. Customizable height and design. Hassle-free maintenance. Reduced mess.

**Longevity:** reusable, cost-effective, eco-friendly. Easy decoration with hinged branches. Avoiding outdoor hazards.

**Personalization:** built-in lights option. Child-friendly decorating activities. Practicality without compromising festive spirit.

Christmas
→ Infant/Non-mobile: (Birth - 6 months)
→ Infant crawl/roll: (5 months - 1 year)
→ Toddler/Pre-school: (1 year - 4 years)
→ School-age: (5 years - 6+ years)

# LED Decorative Lights

**Place out of reach: high shelves or fixtures.** Secure cords with covers or clips (tripping hazards). Choose sturdy, non-fragile materials. Check for small parts. Consider battery-powered to reduce electrical hazards. Always supervise when lights on. Teach safety: avoid touching lights or cords. Regularly inspect for damage.

---

Christmas
→ Infant/Non-mobile: (Birth - 6 months)
→ Infant crawl/roll: (5 months - 1 year)
→ Toddler/Pre-school: (1 year - 4 years)
→ School-age: (5 years - 6+ years)

# Beware of Lead Candles

**Lead toxic, harmful when ingested or inhaled.** Young children more susceptible. Lead exposure causes developmental, cognitive issues, behavioral problems, learning disabilities. Lead in wicks may not be visible. Can deteriorate while burning. Many countries restrict lead in wicks; imported or older candles may not adhere. Check labels for "lead-free" or "non-toxic."

**Inspect wicks:** avoid metal core or thick wick. Opt for cotton, soy, beeswax candles. Proper ventilation. Limit exposure. Keep out of reach, never unattended. Supervise. Educate children about dangers. Regular cleaning: dust surfaces.

---

Halloween
→ Infant/Non-mobile: (Birth - 6 months)
→ Infant crawl/roll: (5 months - 1 year)
→ Toddler/Pre-school: (1 year - 4 years)
→ School-age: (5 years - 6+ years)

# Use Flame Retardant Costumes and Reflective Components

Each holiday season, over 3,000 children under 15 treated for burns related to flammable costumes. Toddlers comprise majority (pre-1970s:

clothing ignition accounted for half of pediatric burn injuries).

**Flame retardant costumes:** treated with chemicals slowing fire spread. Reduced fire risk in candlelit environments. Avoiding accidents from brushing against flames.

**Reflective components:** enhanced visibility at night. Street crossing safety. Group safety. Look for "flame retardant" or "fire-resistant" labels. Choose costumes with reflective strips or accents.

**DIY:** opt for flame-retardant fabrics (wool, polyester). Sew or attach reflective tape. Incorporate into accessories. Test flame resistance.

**Be visible in dark areas:** carry flashlight or glow sticks.

---

🐝 Each holiday season, more than **3,000 children under age 15** are treated in U.S. emergency rooms for burns related to flammable costumes. And toddlers often comprise the majority of these cases. Before the 1970s, clothing ignition accounted for half of pediatric burn injuries. Thanks to today's flame-resistance rules, such incidents are now less common, but not entirely gone.

---

<u>Halloween</u>
→ **Infant/Non-mobile: (Birth - 6 months)**
→ **Infant crawl/roll: (5 months - 1 year)**
→ **Toddler/Pre-school: (1 year - 4 years)**
→ **School-age: (5 years - 6+ years)**

# CANDLE LIT JACK-O'-LANTERNS

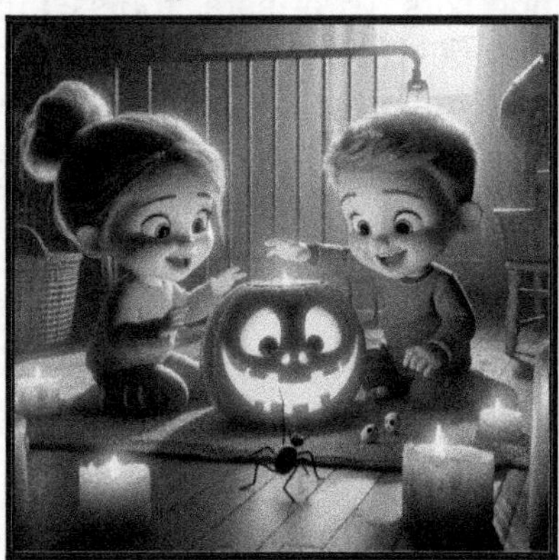

Fire hazard near flammable materials. Children's curiosity: touching flame increases burn risk. Tipping and accidents. Smoke and fumes irritate eyes, respiratory system. Safer alternatives: battery-operated LED lights or flameless candles, glow sticks, string lights, glow paints. If using real candles: secure location away from children's reach, always supervise, place at height to prevent knocking over, well-ventilated area, fire extinguisher or water nearby, never unattended. After Halloween: properly dispose, extinguish candles, place away from flammables. Avoiding candle-lit jack-o'-lanterns, opting for safer alternatives creates festive atmosphere without fire hazards.

---

<u>**Halloween**</u>
Infant/Non-mobile: (Birth - 6 months)
Infant crawl/roll: (5 months - 1 year)
→ **Toddler/Pre-school: (1 year - 4 years)**
→ **School-age: (5 years - 6+ years)**

# WHEN CARVING A PUMPKIN, DO NOT USE A KNIFE

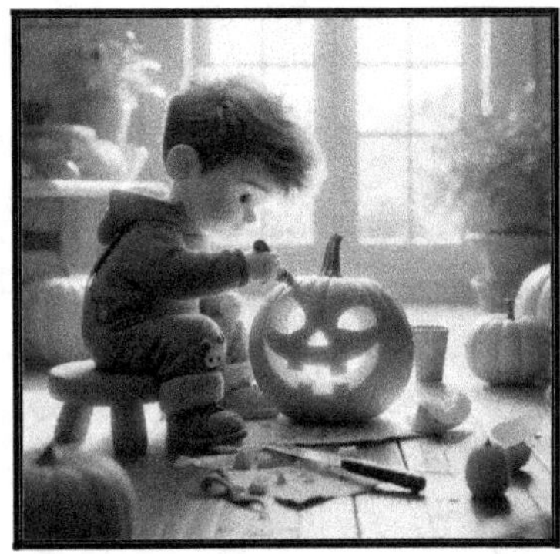

**Sharp object hazard:** Knives cause cuts, punctures. Slip and cut risk. Children's inexperience with fine motor skills. Alternate methods: pumpkin decorating kits with safe tools, pumpkin scoopers or scrapers, stencil and poke method, battery-operated pumpkin drills, stickers and paint. **If using a knife:** adult supervision with proper skills. Safety gear: gloves, goggles. Educate and demonstrate techniques. Pre-carved pumpkins available. Parental assistance always present. Avoiding knives, choosing alternatives creates safe, enjoyable pumpkin activity.

---

<u>**Halloween**</u>
Infant/Non-mobile: (Birth - 6 months)
Infant crawl/roll: (5 months - 1 year)
→ **Toddler/Pre-school: (1 year - 4 years)**
→ **School-age: (5 years - 6+ years)**

# COSTUME PROP CONCERNS

Inspect props for sharp edges, protruding parts, hazards. Avoid metal or hard materials. Choose lightweight, soft, flexible. Smooth, rounded edges. Avoid pointed objects. Flexible, bendable props. Secure attachments. Appropriate size for child's age and size. Avoid functional weapons. Test prop before event. Teach mindful use. Supervision. Remove sharp components. Use **child-friendly alternatives:** foam replicas, soft toys, inflatable props. **Ensure comfort:** doesn't hinder seeing, walking, moving. **Emergency awareness:** teach responsible handling.

---

**Halloween**
Infant/Non-mobile: (Birth - 6 months)
Infant crawl/roll: (5 months - 1 year)
→ **Toddler/Pre-school: (1 year - 4 years)**
→ **School-age: (5 years - 6+ years)**

# AVOID USING DRY ICE

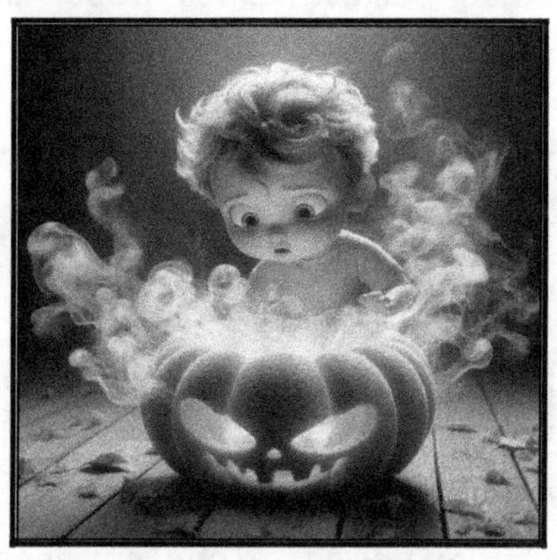

Temperature extremes: extremely cold, causes cold burns or frostbite. Ingestion hazard: not edible, releases CO2, causes discomfort. Choking hazard. Carbon dioxide buildup in enclosed areas: difficulty breathing, dizziness, unconsciousness. Spills and splashes: vigorous bubbling causes burns. Safe alternatives: place in separate container outside punch bowl. Supervision and education. Proper handling: wear gloves, use tongs. Emergency preparedness. While dry ice creates effect, prioritize safety. Use alternative methods for misty effect.

---

Infant/Non-mobile: (Birth - 6 months)
Infant crawl/roll: (5 months - 1 year)
→ **Toddler/Pre-school: (1 year - 4 years)**
→ **School-age: (5 years - 6+ years)**

# BEWARE OF VIOLENT MOVIES

**Emotional impact:** children developing understanding of reality vs. fantasy. Nightmares and sleep disturbances.

**Behavioral changes:** irritability, anxiety, aggression. Desensitization to violence. Developmental stage considerations. Overstimulation. Positive role models important.

**Open communication:** discuss themes, content, reactions. Content ratings and reviews. Preview content when possible. Choose alternatives promoting positive values. Supervision and discussion. Being vigilant, making thoughtful choices creates safe, nurturing media environment supporting emotional development.

---

**Birthdays**
Infant/Non-mobile: (Birth - 6 months)
Infant crawl/roll: (5 months - 1 year)
→ **Toddler/Pre-school: (1 year - 4 years)**
→ **School-age: (5 years - 6+ years)**

# BLOCK ALL EXITS FROM THE BIRTHDAY PARTY

**Assess room layout:** identify exit points including doors, windows.

**Entrance supervision:** designate one entrance, position adult to monitor. Childproof door locks out of reach. Safety gates or barriers blocking doorways. Window locks and guards. Visible signage near exits. Assign adults to monitor exits. Engaging activities to captivate attention. Strategic seating arrangements. Appropriate adult-to-child ratio.

**Emergency preparedness:** adults aware of routes, evacuation procedures. Communicate with parents about safety measures. Keep celebrations indoors if weather permits. Regular visual checks. Proactive planning, vigilant supervision creates safe birthday.

---

<u>**Birthdays**</u>
Infant/Non-mobile: (Birth - 6 months)
Infant crawl/roll: (5 months - 1 year)
→ **Toddler/Pre-school: (1 year - 4 years)**
→ **School-age: (5 years - 6+ years)**

# DO NOT USE SHARP OR HEAVY OBJECTS

**Choose soft, lightweight, child-friendly objects.** Thorough preparations: plan games in advance. Inspect all materials. Use artificial props made from soft materials. Soft targets for throwing games. Assign adults to supervise. Clear instructions. Age-appropriate games. Alternative activities. Safe props: child-safe from foam, plastic. Education and awareness. Adaptation and modification: foam balls, pull-string piñatas. Prioritize fun and safety. Creating child-safe environment ensures delightful, accident-free experience.

---

<u>**Birthdays**</u>
→ **Infant/Non-mobile: (Birth - 6 months)**
→ **Infant crawl/roll: (5 months - 1 year)**
→ **Toddler/Pre-school: (1 year - 4 years)**
→ **School-age: (5 years - 6+ years)**

# NO PETS AT BIRTHDAY CELEBRATIONS

**Over 1,200 children yearly suffer injuries from balloons and ties (CPSC).**

**Unpredictable reactions:** overwhelming for pets. Allergies and sensitivities.

**Safety concerns:** unpredictable child behavior. Food hazards. Escape risk. Agitation and stress. Distractions and responsibilities. Preventing accidents.

**Guest comfort:** some have phobias.

**Pet's well-being:** calm, stress-free environment. Opting for no pets creates controlled, secure environment.

---

# Popped/Un-popped Balloons

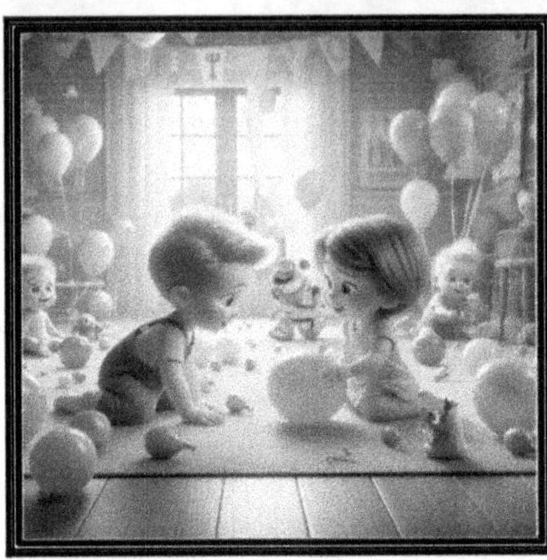

Each year, **over 1,200 children** in the US. suffer injuries from balloons and balloon ties, including choking and strangulation incidents. (Source: US. Consumer Product Safety Commission (CPSC) - Balloon Safety) Balloons are a staple of celebrations, adding a festive touch to birthdays, parties, and special occasions. While they bring joy and color to any event, it's important to be mindful of both popped and un-popped balloons to ensure child safety. Latex balloons leading cause of toy-related choking deaths. Over 110 suffocation deaths since 1973, mostly under 6. From 1990 to 2004: **at least 68 U.S. children died choking on balloons** (CPSC).**Popped:** choking hazard from fragments, loud noise startles. **Unpopped:** choking if put in mouth, swallowing risk. Always supervise. Proper inflation to safe size. Secure, short strings. Adult assistance for inflation. Immediately discard popped balloons. Choose natural latex. Age-appropriate play. Educate guests. Vigilance, proactive measures ensure safe balloon-filled celebrations.

---

🍎 Latex balloons are the leading cause of toy-related choking deaths among children and tragically, over 110 suffocation deaths have occurred since 1973, mostly among kids under six. **From 1990 to 2004 alone, at least 68 U.S. children died from choking on balloons, often in just seconds. Pediatricians describe balloon fragment asphyxia as one of the most terrifying emergencies they encounter.** *-U.S. Consumer Product Safety Commission (CPSC)*

# Long Hair Near Candles

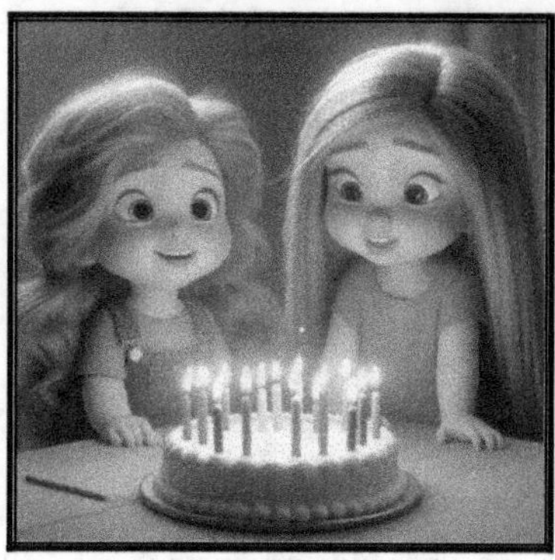

**Fire risk:** hair catches fire easily. Entanglement in burning candle. Secure hair in bun, ponytail, updo. Choose candle placement. Supervise children with long hair. Wear protective hairstyles: braids, tucked under hat. Keep hair elevated when near candles. Blow out candles before leaning over. Use flameless alternatives. Educate children. Stay alert. Adult supervision. Proactive, mindful about hair safety ensures safe, enjoyable candle environment.

---

**<u>Birthdays</u>**
Infant/Non-mobile: (Birth - 6 months)
Infant crawl/roll: (5 months - 1 year)
→ **Toddler/Pre-school: (1 year - 4 years)**
→ **School-age: (5 years - 6+ years)**

# Plastic Birthday Cake Decorations

**Choking hazard:** small pieces. Swallowing risk. Sharp edges. Opt for larger decorations. Age-appropriate. Secure placement on cake. Avoid sharp edges. Remove before serving slices. Supervision.

**Use edible alternatives:** fondant, icing. Prevent access to leftover decorations. If using on cupcakes, ensure secure positioning. Dispose properly after. Read labels for safety. Informed choices ensure safety during celebrations.

---

# Beware of Lawn Chemicals During Egg Hunts

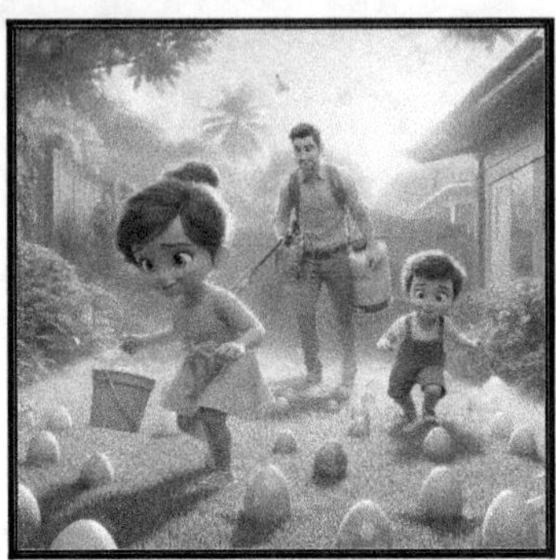

Chemical exposure through skin or ingestion. Skin irritation, rashes, allergic reactions. Inhalation risk. Choose safe location free from recent treatments. Read labels, follow instructions. Schedule hunt well after application. Mark treated areas. Protective clothing: long sleeves, pants, closed-toe shoes. Hand washing after hunt. Supervision. Use alternative areas: community park. Rinse eggs before decorating or consuming. Educate participants. Natural lawn care methods. Create safe, enjoyable egg hunt without compromising well-being.

---



# Small Easter Treats

**Size matters:** small enough to fit in mouth. Texture: hard, round, smooth surface.

**Components: small, detachable parts. Choose age-appropriate treats.**

**Supervision:** sit down while eating. Inspect treats, remove hazards. Cut foods into smaller pieces. Educate older siblings. Offer safe alternatives.

**Teach proper eating:** small bites, chew thoroughly.

**Choking rescue knowledge:** CPR, Heimlich. Stay informed about recalls. Open treats carefully. Clear eating area. Lead by example.

---

**4<sup>th</sup> of July**
→ **Infant/Non-mobile: (Birth - 6 months)**
→ **Infant crawl/roll: (5 months - 1 year)**
→ **Toddler/Pre-school: (1 year - 4 years)**
→ **School-age: (5 years - 6+ years)**

# Firework Concerns

**Annually over 5,000 children injured by fireworks (CPSC).**
Burns vary in severity. Risk of cuts, bruises from debris. Educate about dangers. Maintain safe distance. Choose safe locations. Proper supervision. Protective gear: safety glasses. First aid preparedness. Emergency contacts. Choose public displays with safety measures. Provide ear protection: earmuffs, earplugs. Limit exposure. Explain dangers. Prevent close proximity. Quiet viewing areas. Alternatives: televised displays. Monitor reactions. Education on hearing protection. Professional displays. Healthy hearing habits. Regular hearing checkups.

---

**Thanksgiving**
Infant/Non-mobile: **(Birth - 6 months)**
Infant crawl/roll: **(5 months - 1 year)**
→ **Toddler/Pre-school: (1 year - 4 years)**
→ **School-age: (5 years - 6+ years)**

# Turkey Fryer Concerns

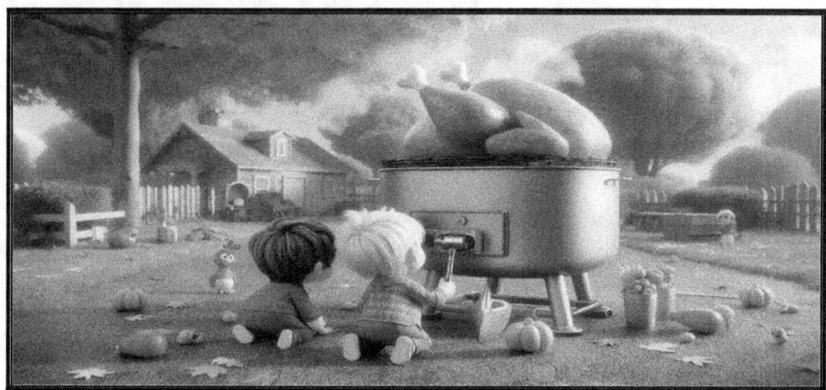

Deep-fryer incidents cause about 60 injuries nationwide yearly. Half of pediatric hot-oil burns linked to these (NFPA, FDNY). Roughly 10 to 11 children yearly, most under 6, suffer serious grease burns.

Establish kid-free zone. Mark and educate. Physical barrier: baby gate, playpen. Stable setup on flat surface. Constant supervision. Secure tools, accessories, hot liquids out of reach. Cooling time after frying.

**Emergency preparedness:** fire extinguisher, first aid kit. Engage children in safe activities away from area. Another adult monitors children.

---

<u>**Thanksgiving**</u>
Infant/Non-mobile: (Birth - 6 months)
Infant crawl/roll: (5 months - 1 year)
→ **Toddler/Pre-school: (1 year - 4 years)**
→ **School-age: (5 years - 6+ years)**

# CHILD-FRIENDLY ZONE

Create zone with festive decorations, crafts, toys. Involve in safe cooking activities. Cozy corner for parade viewing. Organize fun safety games, role-play. Secure heavy furniture. Install stair gates. Manage cords effectively. Fostering festive, secure environment.

---

**Notes:**

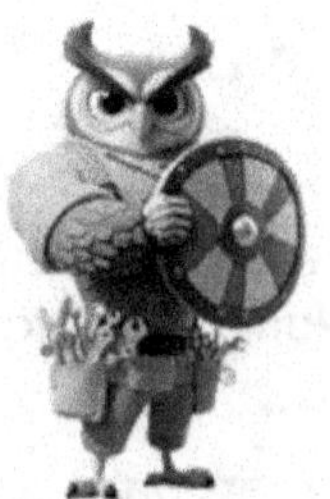

**Caretaker/Grandparents**
→ Infant/Non-mobile: (Birth - 6 months)
→ Infant crawl/roll: (5 months - 1 year)
→ Toddler/Pre-school: (1 year - 4 years)
→ School-age: (5 years - 6+ years)

# GRANDPARENT SAFETY

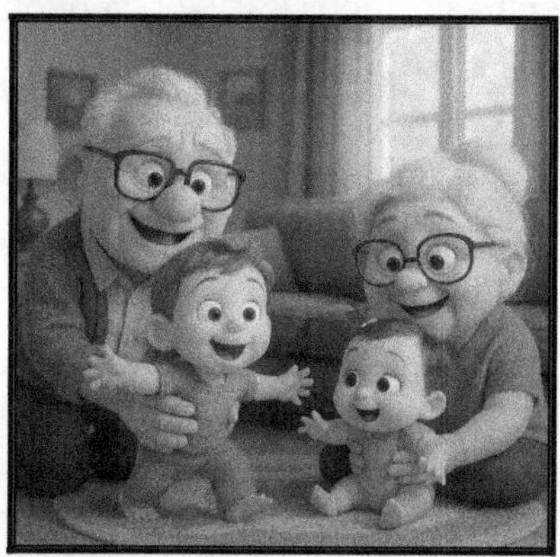

**Medication safety:** locked cabinet out of reach. Remove small-object choking hazards. Cover electrical outlets, secure cords. Window locks or guards. Lock outside doors or childproof.

**Kitchen:** lock sharp knives, utensils, cleaning supplies; hot liquids away from edges.

**Stairway and balcony:** safety gates, childproof locks. Anchor furniture to wall.

**Fireplace, stove:** safety gates or screens; store matches, lighters out of reach.

**Bathroom:** toilet locks, remove cleaning supplies, toiletries.

**Pet safety:** controlled, supervised; teach safe interaction. Emergency contacts, allergy information.

**Safe sleep environment:** cribs meeting standards; back sleeping for infants. Remove toxic plants. Securely store chemicals. Safety gear correctly installed. Supervision, communication. Home security functioning. Store personal items, purses, bags out of reach. Well-stocked first aid kit accessible.

# Caretaker/Babysitter Safety

**Ensure knowledge of emergency procedures:** first aid, emergency contacts.

**Secure hazardous areas:** kitchen, bathroom, heavy furniture, sharp corners; store cleaning agents, medicines. Communicate allergies, know how to respond.

**Educate about choking hazards;** supervise meals, play. Inform about correct sleeping positions (SIDS prevention).

**Familiarize with fire safety:** extinguishers, exit routes.

**Open communication line. Information sheet**: routines, preferences. First visit orientation. Feedback and learning. Thorough preparation, open communication creates safe childcare experience.

---

**Notes:** (Based of your caretaker/babysitter's personality and experience.)

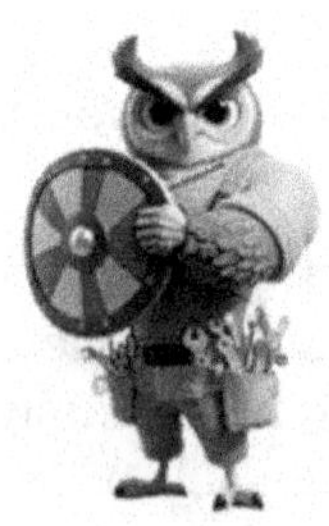

# |Ch. 28| Child Internet Safety



Infant/Non-mobile: (Birth - 6 months)
Infant crawl/roll: (5 months - 1 year)
Toddler/Pre-school: (1 year - 4 years)
→ **School-age: (5 years - 6+ years)**

**Educate about online risks:** cyberbullying, predators, phishing, inappropriate content. Privacy importance, digital footprint.

**Set clear rules:** screen time, activities, appropriate sites/apps. Family media plan. Age-appropriate social media guidelines. Use parental control software, safe search filters.

**Create safe online environment:** devices in common areas, child accounts with restrictions.

**Teach responsible behavior:** kindness, critical thinking.

**Monitor activities:** check browsing history.

**Be involved:** engage together.

**Address cyberbullying:** block, report. Stay informed, updated. Combination of strategies creates safer online environment, promoting responsible digital citizenship.

---

**Notes:**

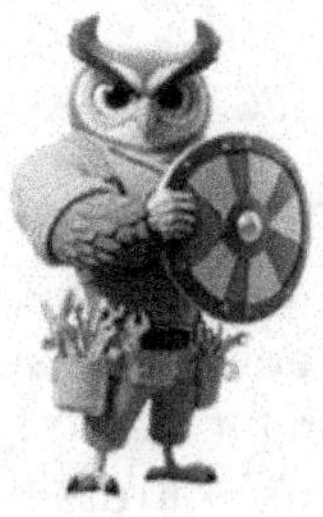

# |Ch. 29| Intruder and Child Abduction Protection

**Intruder and Child Abduction Protection**
→ Infant/Non-mobile: (Birth - 6 months)
→ Infant crawl/roll: (5 months - 1 year)
→ Toddler/Pre-school: (1 year - 4 years)
→ School-age: (5 years - 6+ years)

## INTRUDER AND CHILD ABDUCTION PROTECTION

Ensuring your child's safety from potential intruders and abduction threats requires a comprehensive approach that combines home security measures, education, communication, and vigilance.

**Home security:** secure entry points with locks, deadbolts, bars. Window coverings. Alarm system. Outdoor lighting.

**Stranger awareness:** teach dangers; safe passwords; emergency contacts. Scheduled activities: know child's schedule, whereabouts. Designated meeting points. Home safety zones.

**Open communication:** foster dialogue. School, activity policies. Internet safety: rules, privacy settings.

**Family emergency plan:** escape routes, meeting points, roles; practice drills.

**Community awareness:** registered sex offenders; neighbors network.

**Identification:** child ID kit with photos, fingerprints.

**Travel precautions:** inform neighbors, choose secure accommodations. Trust child's instincts.

## TRACK YOUR CHILD!

Wearable GPS trackers. Sound-activated tags. Temporary tattoos with contact info. Call-and-response games. Clothing with reflective patches or bright colors. Light-up shoes. Safety word system. Motion-activated alarms. Mirrors, cameras in blind spots. Hidden tracking stickers. Balloon or flag system for play areas. Mix of tools, techniques increases chances of quickly finding missing child.

 # Government Agencies



Several U.S. agencies work to protect children by enforcing safety regulations, promoting injury prevention, and providing childproofing guidelines to create safer environments for young children. These agencies focus on different aspects of child safety, from product regulations to poisoning prevention and digital security.

## Key Agencies & Their Responsibilities

### Consumer Product Safety Commission (CPSC)

- Regulates children's products such as cribs, car seats, and safety gates.

- Issues recalls on dangerous toys, furniture, and baby products.

- Provides childproofing guidelines for home safety

### Centers for Disease Control and Prevention (CDC)

- Focuses on injury prevention, including falls, burns, drowning, and poisoning.

- Promotes safe sleep practices to reduce Sudden Infant Death Syndrome (SIDS).

- Provides guidelines for preventing household accidents.

### U.S. Food and Drug Administration (FDA)

- Ensures baby food, formula, and medications are safe for children.

- Regulates packaging and labeling to prevent accidental poisoning.

- Issues warnings on unsafe substances and recalled products.

### National Highway Traffic Safety Administration (NHTSA)

- Enforces child car seat regulations and crash safety standards.

- Provides installation guidance and recalls defective car seats.

- Educates parents on preventing hot car deaths

<u>**Environmental Protection Agency (EPA)**</u>
- Regulates exposure to hazardous materials such as lead, asbestos, and mold.

- Promotes clean air and water for child health.

- Provides resources on household toxin reduction

<u>**U.S. Fire Administration (USFA)**</u>
- Educates families on fire prevention and emergency planning.

- Recommends installing smoke and carbon monoxide detectors.

- Provides guidance on safe use of electrical outlets and heating devices.

<u>**Poison Control Centers (AAPCC)**</u>
- Offers a 24/7 emergency hotline (**1-800-222-1222**) for poisoning incidents.

- Educates families on safe storage of medications and household chemicals.

- Provides immediate treatment advice for accidental ingestion.

<u>**Administration for Children and Families (ACF) – U.S. Department of Health and Human Services (HHS)**</u>
- Oversees child abuse prevention programs and ensures child welfare.

- Provides funding and resources to help families create safe home environments.

- Supports early childhood safety education programs.

<u>**Office of Juvenile Justice and Delinquency Prevention (OJJDP) – U.S. Department of Justice (DOJ)**</u>
- Protects children from abuse, exploitation, and endangerment.

- Funds programs aimed at preventing child trafficking and online threats.

- Works with law enforcement to enhance child safety initiatives

<u>**National Center for Missing & Exploited Children (NCMEC)**</u>
- Assists in locating missing children and preventing abductions.

- Provides digital safety resources for families and children

Operates a tip line for reporting child exploitation and suspicious activity.

# Conclusion

**Congratulations!**

**Pat yourself on the back**, diligent guardian of tiny daredevils! You have successfully navigated the perilous journey of childproofing your home, transforming it into a fortress of safety and fun for your little adventurer. Oh, the countless stubbed toes and bumped heads you've prevented! Your home is now less of a danger zone and more of a secure play paradise.

Not only have you mastered the art of spotting a choking hazard from a mile away, but you've also become fluent in the language of "Baby-ese" and can now differentiate between a cry of hunger and a cry of "I've just found another thing to get into!"

Your new eagle-eyed vigilance means that every sharp corner is cushioned, and every electrical outlet is covered. Your child might think they've got the upper hand, but little do they know, they're up against a childproofing ninja, a safety virtuoso, and a maestro of baby-proof barricades!

But remember, childproofing isn't just about keeping those little rascals safe; it's about fostering a space where their curiosity and imagination can run wild without you having to run behind them with a first-aid kit.

So, here's to you, brave protector of tiny humans! You've climbed the mountains of baby gates, sailed the seas of spill-proof sippy cups, and emerged victorious. Now, go ahead and enjoy a well-earned cup of coffee or perhaps a nap. (We won't tell if you do.) Your home is now a childproofed haven, a place where your child can explore, play, and grow under the loving watch of the world's newest childproofing champion - You!

**Remember, in the grand playground of life, it's always better to be safe than sorry!**

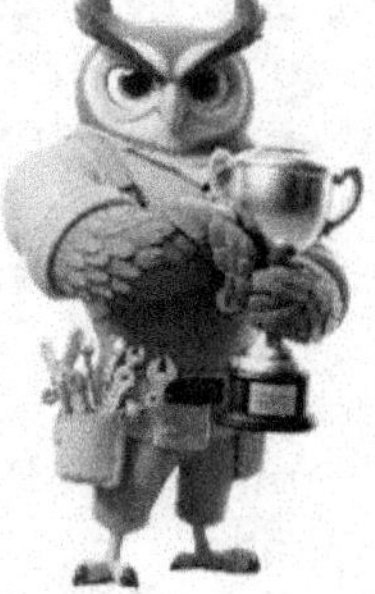

# Ultimate Childproofing Checklist

*(A Quick Reference Guide)*

### Home Entry & Exits

☐ Install **doorknob covers** or lever locks on doors leading outside.

☐ Secure **deadbolts and peepholes** out of children's reach.

☐ Use **door stoppers** to prevent finger pinching.

☐ Set up **video doorbells** or security systems.

☐ Keep **keys and garage openers** out of reach.

☐ Ensure **screens on windows** are secure and childproof.

---

### Living Room & Common Areas

☐ Cover **sharp furniture corners and edges** with padding.

☐ Secure **TVs, bookcases, and heavy furniture** to the wall.

☐ Keep **cords, chargers, and electrical outlets** covered.

☐ Install **cordless window blinds** or secure loose blind cords.

☐ Store **remote controls, small objects, and choking hazards** out of reach.

☐ Use **fireplace screens** and store matches/lighters safely.

☐ Keep **houseplants out of reach** (some can be toxic).

☐ Secure **pet food and water bowls** (choking and drowning hazard).

---

### Nursery & Bedroom

☐ Use a **firm crib mattress** with a fitted sheet (no loose blankets or pillows).

☐ Keep **cribs away from windows, blinds, and heaters.**

☐ Install **drawer and dresser anchors** to prevent tipping.

☐ Secure **diaper creams, lotions, and small items** in locked drawers.

☐ Use **nightlights with cool-to-touch bulbs** and keep lamps out of reach.

☐ Ensure **mobiles and wall decorations** are well secured and out of baby's reach.

☐ Use **cordless baby monitors** or secure monitor cords away from cribs.

☐ Remove **stuffed animals and bumpers** from cribs to prevent suffocation.

---

## Kitchen

☐ Install **stove knob covers** and use back burners for cooking.
☐ Secure **cabinets and drawers** with childproof locks.
☐ Store **knives, sharp objects, and cleaning supplies** in locked drawers.
☐ Keep **hot liquids and foods** away from edges of tables and counters.
☐ Use **appliance locks** on the fridge, oven, and dishwasher.
☐ Set the **water heater to 120°F (49°C)** to prevent burns.
☐ Store **breakable dishes and glassware** out of reach.
☐ Keep **small magnets and fridge decorations** out of reach (choking hazard).
☐ Use **high chairs with secure straps and never leave child unattended**.
☐ Keep **plastic bags and cling wrap** stored safely.

---

## Bathroom & Laundry Room

☐ Use **toilet locks** to prevent drowning hazards.
☐ Secure **medications, toiletries, and cleaning supplies** in locked cabinets.
☐ Install **non-slip mats** inside and outside the bathtub.
☐ Always **unplug hair dryers, curling irons, and electric razors** after use.
☐ Keep the **washer and dryer doors closed and locked** when not in use.
☐ Store **laundry detergent pods** in a locked cabinet.
☐ Use **a thermometer to test bathwater temperature** before placing a child in.
☐ Ensure **razors, scissors, and tweezers** are stored out of reach.

---

## Stairs & Hallways

☐ Install **safety gates** at the top and bottom of stairs.
☐ Secure **loose rugs and carpets** to prevent tripping.
☐ Use **motion-sensor nightlights** in hallways and staircases.
☐ **Banister gaps are too narrow for a child's head to fit through.**
☐ Keep **hallways free of clutter** to avoid tripping hazards.

---

## Playroom & Toy Safety

☐ Choose **age-appropriate toys** without small, detachable parts.
☐ Keep **batteries, especially button batteries, locked away.**
☐ Store toys in **open bins (not heavy-lid toy chests)** to prevent trapped fingers.
☐ Regularly **inspect and clean toys** for damage or choking hazards.
☐ Avoid **balloons or plastic wrappers** that pose a suffocation risk.
☐ Anchor **bookshelves and play furniture** to the wall.

---

**<u>Outdoor & Garage Safety</u>**
☐ Install **fences around pools, ponds, or water features** with self-latching gates.
☐ Keep **garage tools, chemicals, and gas cans** in locked cabinets.
☐ Ensure **playground equipment** is sturdy and placed over soft ground (e.g., mulch, rubber).
☐ Store **bicycles, scooters, and helmets** in an organized area.
☐ Keep **grills, fire pits, and propane tanks** locked or covered.
☐ Secure **garden hoses and electrical outlets**.
☐ Ensure **fences and gates are properly maintained** to prevent escape.

---

**<u>Car Safety</u>**
☐ Use an **age-appropriate car seat** and install it correctly.
☐ **Never leave a child alone in a car, even for a minute.** ☐ Keep **loose items secured** to prevent them from becoming projectiles in a crash.
☐ Use **child safety locks** on doors and windows.
☐ Keep **emergency roadside supplies** (first-aid kit, flashlight, blanket, water).
☐ Store **car cleaning supplies and tools** in a locked trunk or cabinet.

---

**<u>Emergency & First Aid</u>**
☐ Keep a **fully stocked first-aid kit** in an accessible place.
☐ Install **smoke detectors and carbon monoxide detectors** on every floor.
☐ Test **smoke alarms monthly** and replace batteries yearly.
☐ Teach **fire escape plans** and practice them regularly.
☐ Have **emergency contact numbers** posted in a visible area.
☐ Keep **a fire extinguisher in the kitchen and know how to use it**.
☐ Create and review **a choking response plan** for all caregivers

---

**<u>Final Safety Reminders</u>**
☐ Always **supervise young children, especially in high-risk areas**.
☐ Regularly **inspect and update safety measures** as your child grows.
☐ Stay informed about **recalls on child safety products and toys**.
☐ Teach **older siblings and caregivers** about childproofing rules.

---